CHEST PAIN WITH NORMAL CORONARY ANGIOGRAMS:
PATHOGENESIS, DIAGNOSIS AND MANAGEMENT

198. Antoine Lafont, Eric Topol (eds.): *Arterial Remodeling: A Critical Factor in Restenosis.* 1997   ISBN 0-7923-8008-8
199. Michele Mercuri, David D. McPherson, Hisham Bassiouny, Seymour Glagov (eds.):*Non-Invasive Imaging of Atherosclerosis*   ISBN 0-7923-8036-3
200. Walmor C. DeMello, Michiel J. Janse(eds.): *Heart Cell Communication in Health and Disease*   ISBN 0-7923-8052-5
201. P.E. Vardas (ed.): *Cardiac Arrhythmias Pacing and Electrophysiology.* The Expert View. 1998   ISBN 0-7923-4908-3
202. E.E. van der Wall, P.K. Blanksma, M.G. Niemeyer, W. Vaalburg and H.J.G.M. Crijns (eds.) *Advanced Imaging in Coronary Artery Disease, PET, SPECT, MRI, I VUS, EBCT. 1998*   ISBN 0-7923-5083-9
203. R.L. Wilensky (ed.) *Unstable Coronary Artery Syndromes, Pathophysiology, Diagnosis and Treatment. 1998.*   ISBN 0-7923-8201-3
204. J.H.C. Reiber, E.E. van der Wall (eds.): *What's New in Cardiovascular Imaging?* 1998   ISBN 0-7923-5121-5
205. Juan Carlos Kaski, David W. Holt (eds.): *Myocardial Damage Early Detection by Novel Biochemical Markers. 1998.*   ISBN 0-7923-5140-1
207. Gary F. Baxter, Derek M. Yellon, *Delayed Preconditioning and Adaptive Cardioprotection. 1998.*   ISBN 0-7923-5259-9
208. Bernard Swynghedauw, *Molecular Cardiology for the Cardiologist, Second Edition* 1998.   ISBN 0-7923-8323-0
209. Geoffrey Burnstock, James G.Dobson, Jr., Bruce T. Liang, Joel Linden (eds): *Cardiovascular Biology of Purines. 1998.*   ISBN: 0-7923-8334-6
210. Brian D. Hoit, Richard A. Walsh (eds): *Cardiovascular Physiology in the Genetically Engineered Mouse.* 1998.   ISBN: 0-7923-8356-7
211. Peter Whittaker, George S. Abela (eds.): *Direct Myocardial Revascularization: History, Methodology, Technology* 1998.   ISBN: 0-7923-8398-2
212. C.A. Nienaber, R. Fattori (eds.): Diagnosis and Treatment of Aortic Diseases. 1999.   ISBN: 0-7923-5517-2
213. Juan Carlos Kaski (ed.): *Chest Pain with Normal Coronary Angiograms: Pathogenesis, Diagnosis and Management. 1999.*   ISBN: 0-7923-8421-0

Previous volumes are still available

KLUWER ACADEMIC PUBLISHERS - DORDRECHT/BOSTON/LONDON

Chest Pain with Normal Coronary Angiograms: Pathogenesis, Diagnosis and Management

edited by

Juan Carlos Kaski MD, MRCP, FACC, FESC

BHF Sugden Reader in Clinical Cardiology and Consultant Cardiologist, Head of Coronary Artery Disease Research Group, St George's Hospital Medical School, London, UK

KLUWER ACADEMIC PUBLISHERS
Boston/Dordrecth/London

Distributors for North, Central and South America:
Kluwer Academic Publishers
101 Philip Drive
Assinippi Park
Norwell, Massachusetts 02061 USA

Distributors for all other countries:
Kluwer Academic Publishers Group
Distribution Centre
Post Office Box 322
3300 AH Dordrecht, THE NETHERLANDS

Library of Congress Cataloging-in-Publication Data

Printed on acid-free paper.

Printed in the United States of America

Table of Contents

List of Contributors   ix

Foreword   xiii

Preface   xvii

Chapters

1. **Cardiac syndrome X and microvascular angina**   1
   Juan Carlos Kaski

2. **Chest pain with normal coronary arteries: psychological aspects**   13
   Steve G. Potts and Christopher Bass

3. **Esophageal chest pain**   33
   John S. de Caestecker

4. **Esophageal abnormalities and "Linked - Angina" in syndrome X**   49
   Anoop Chauhan

5. **Abnormal pain processing in syndrome X**   61
   Ole Frøbert, Lars Arendt-Nielsen and Jens Peder Bagger

6. **Insights into the pathophysiology of syndrome X obtained using
   positron emission tomography (PET)**   69
   Stuart D. Rosen and Paolo G. Camici

7. **Myocardial metabolism in cardiac syndrome X**   81
   Jens Peder Bagger

8. **Endothelial dysfunction in cardiac syndrome X (microvascular
   angina)**   91
   Kensuke Egashira, Masahiro Mohri and Akira Takeshita

9. **Endothelin: an important mediator in the pathophysiology of
   syndrome X**   101
   Ian D. Cox and Juan Carlos Kaski

10. Estrogen deficiency and syndrome X   115
    Peter Collins

11. Alternative mechanisms for myocardial ischemia in
    syndrome X - New diagnostic markers   123
    Filippo Crea, Antonio Buffon, Achille Gaspardone
    and Gaetano Lanza

12. Increased plasma membrane ion-leakage: A new hypothesis
    for chest pain and normal coronary arteriograms   135
    Anders Waldenström and Gunnar Ronquist

13. A possible cell membrane defect in chronic fatigue syndrome
    and syndrome X   143
    Walter S. Watson, Abhijit Chaudhuri, Georgina T. McCreath
    and Peter O. Behan

14. The changing concept of syndrome X   151
    Attilio Maseri, Gaetano Antonio Lanza and Antonino Buffon

15. Assessment of coronary blood flow reserve -
    Techniques and limitations   159
    Antonio L'Abbate

16. The role of echocardiography in diagnosis and
    management of cardiac syndrome X   171
    Petros Nihoyannopoulos

17. Imaging in microvascular angina – what's new?   181
    Ann Tweddel

18. Assessment of quality of life in patients with syndrome X   187
    Felipe Atienza and José A. de Velasco

19. Treatment of patients with angina and normal coronary
    arteriograms   195
    Giuseppe M.C. Rosano, Gabriele Fragasso and Sergio L. Chierchia

20. Management strategies for chest pain in patients with
    normal coronary angiograms   203
    Richard O. Cannon III

21. Abnormal autonomic nervous control of the cardiovascular
    system   211
    Giuseppe M.C. Rosano, Gabriele Fragasso, Sergio L. Chierchia

22. **The metabolic syndrome**   221
    Francisco Leyva and John C. Stevenson

23. **Two syndromes X**   243
    Andrew Henderson

24. **Hyperlipidemia and endothelial vasodilator dysfunction:**
    The pathogenetic link to myocardial ischemia   251
    Andreas M. Zeiher

25. **Microvascular dysfunction in patients with systemic**
    hypertension without left ventricular hypertrophy:
    The role of nitric oxide   259
    Julio A. Panza

26. **Microvascular angina and hypertensive left ventricular**
    hypertrophy   269
    Wolfgang Motz and Sibylle Scheler

27. **Myocardial ischemia in hypertrophic cardiomyopathy:**
    Clinical assessment and role in natural history   281
    Perry M. Elliott

28. **Microvascular endothelial dysfunction after heart**
    transplantation   293
    Giuseppe Vassalli and Augusto Gallino

Index   305

List of Contributors

Lars Arendt-Nielsen, MsSc
Laboratory for Experimental Pain Research, University of Aalborg, Aalborg, Denmark

Filipe Atienza, MD
Cardiology Department, Hospital General Universitario, Valencia, Spain

Jens Peder Bagger, MD
Division of Cardiology, Imperial College School of Medicine, Hammersmith Hospital, London, UK

Christopher Bass, MA, MD, FRCPsych
Consultant in Liaison Psychiatry, Department of Psychological Medicine, John Radcliffe Hospital, Oxford, UK

Peter O. Behan, MBChB, MD, DSc, FACP, FRCP(Glas, Lond, Ire)
University Department of Neurology, Institute of Neurological Sciences, Southern General Hospital NHS Trust, Glasgow, Scotland, UK

Antonino Buffon, MD
Institute of Cardiology, Universita Cattolica del Sacro Cuore, Rome, Italy

Paolo G. Camici, MD, FRCP FESC, FACC
MRC Clinical Sciences Centre, RPMS, Hammersmith Hospital, London, UK

Richard O. Cannon III, MD
Cardiology Branch, NHLBI, National Institutes of Health, Bethesda, Maryland, USA

Abhijit Chaudhuri, DM, MD, MRCP(UK)
University Department of Neurology, Institute of Neurological Sciences, Southern General Hospital NHS Trust, Glasgow, Scotland, UK

Anoop Chauhan, MD, MRCP
Consultant Cardiologist, Regional Cardiac Unit, Victoria Hospital, Blackpool, UK

Sergio L. Chierchia, MD, FACC, FESC
Professor of Cardiology, Department of Cardiology, Istituto H San Raffaele, Milano and Roma, Italy

Peter Collins, MA, MD(Cantab), FRCP, FESC, FACC
National Heart and Lung Institute, Imperial College School of Medicine, London, UK

Ian D. Cox, MA, MRCP
Coronary Artery Disease Research Group, Department of Cardiological Sciences, St George's Hospital Medical School, London, UK

Filippo Crea, MD, FACC, FESC
Senior Lecturer in Cardiology, Institute of Cardiology, Universita Cattolica del Sacro Cuore, Rome, Italy

John S. de Caestecker, MD, FRCP, FRCP(E)
Consultant Gastroenterologist, The Glenfield Hospital and Honorary Senior Lecturer, Division of Gastroenterology, University of Leicester Medical School, Leicester, UK

Kensuke Egashira, MD, PhD
Research Institute of Angiocardiology and Cardiovascular Clinic, Kyushu University Faculty of Medicine, Fukuoka, Japan

Perry M. Elliott, MRCP
Department of Cardiological Sciences, St George's Hospital Medical School, London, UK

Gabriele Fragasso, MD
Senior Lecturer, Department of Cardiology, Istituto H San Raffaele, Milano and Roma, Italy

Ole Frøbert, MD
Department of Cardiology, Skejby Section, Aarhus University Hospital, Aarhus, Denmark

Augusto Gallino, MD, FACC, FESC
Specialista FMH Medicina Interna, Cardiologia E Angiologia, Primario Ospedale San Giovanni, Bellinzona, Switzerland

Achille Gaspardone, MD, FESC
Cattedra di Cardiochirurgia, Universita Tor Vergata, Rome, Italy

Andrew Henderson, FRCP, FESC
Department of Cardiology, University of Wales College of Medicine, Cardiff, Wales, UK

Juan Carlos Kaski, MD, MRCP, FESC, FACC
Reader in Clinical Cardiology and Consultant Cardiologist, Head of Coronary Artery Disease Research Group, St George's Hospital Medical School, London, UK

Antonio L'Abbate, MD
CNR Clinical Physiology Institute, via Savi 8, Pisa, Italy

Gaetano Antonio Lanza, MD, FESC
Institute of Cardiology, Universita Cattolica del Sacro Cuore, Rome, Italy

Francisco Leyva, MB, ChB, BSc (Hons), MRCP
Department of Cardiac Medicine, Royal Brompton Hospital, London, UK

Georgina T. McCreath, MBChB, DMRD, FRCR, FRCP(Glas)
Department of Radiology, Southern General Hospital NHS Trust, Glasgow, Scotland, UK

Attilio Maseri, MD, FACC, FESC, FRCP
Professor of Cardiology, Director Institute of Cardiology, Universita Cattolica del Sacro Cuore, Rome, Italy

Masahiro Mohri MD, PhD
Research Institute of Angiocardiology and Cardiovascular Clinic, Kyushu University Faculty of Medicine, Fukuoka, Japan

Wolfgang Motz, MD, PhD, Professor of Medicine
Herz- und Diabeteszentrum Mecklenburg-Vorpommern, Klinik für Kardiologie, Karlsburg, Germany

Petros Nihoyannopoulos, MD, FACC, FESC
Senior Lecturer and Consultant Cardiologist, Cardiology Division, Imperial College School of Medicine, National Heart & Lung Institute, Hammersmith Hospital, London, UK

Julio A. Panza, MD
Vascular Physiology Laboratory, Section on Echocardiography, Cardiology Branch, National Heart, Lung & Blood Institute, National Institutes of Health, Bethesda, USA

Stephen Potts, MA, BM, BCh, MRCPsych
Department of Psychological Medicine, Royal Infirmary (Edinburgh), Edinburgh, Scotland, UK

Gunnar Ronquist, MD, PhD
Department of Clinical Chemistry, University Hospital, Uppsala, Sweden

Giuseppe M.C. Rosano, MD, FACC
Senior Lecturer, Department of Cardiology, Istituto H San Raffaele, Milano and Roma, Italy

Stuart D. Rosen, MA, MD, MRCP, FESC, FACC
Honorary Consultant Cardiologist, MRC Cyclotron Unit, Imperial College School of Medicine, Hammersmith Hospital, London, UK

Sibylle Scheler, MD
Herz- und Diabeteszentrum Mecklenburg-Vorpommern, Klinik für Kardiologie, Karlsburg, Germany

John C. Stevenson, MB BS, FRCP, FESC
Reader and Honorary Consultant Physician and Head of Rosen Laboratories of the Wynn Institute, Endocrinology and Metabolic Medicine, Imperial College School of Medicine, London, UK

Akira Takeshita, MD, PhD
Research Institute of Angiocardiology and Cardiovascular Clinic, Kyushu University Faculty of Medicine, Fukuoka, Japan

Ann Tweddel, MB, ChB, Dip Mgmt (Open), MD, MRCP, FESC
Director of Nuclear Cardiology, Department of Cardiology, University of Wales College of Medicine, Cardiff, Wales, UK

Giuseppe Vassalli, MD
Division de Cardiologie, Centre Hospitalier Universitaire Vaudois, Lausanne, and Ospedale San Giovanni, Bellinzona, Switzerland

José A. de Velasco, MD
Cardiology Department, Hospital General Universitario, Valencia, Spain

Anders Waldenstrom, MD, PhD
Associated Professor of Cardiology, Department of Internal Medicine, Umea University, Umea, Sweden

Walter S. Watson, BSc, PhD, CPhys, FIPEMB, FInstP
Principal Physicist, Nuclear Medicine Department, Southern General Hospital NHS Trust, Glasgow, Scotland, UK

Andreas M. Zeiher, MD
Head, Department of Internal Medicine IV, Division of Cardiology, Klinikum der Johann Wolfgang Goethe Universitat, Frankfurt, Germany

Acknowledgement

We are grateful to

Nicola H. Tansey
Medical Education Co-ordinator, Cardiological Sciences, St George's Hospital, London

For all her endeavors in co-ordinating and formatting this book.

Foreword

This book is timely and challenging. Within its pages are commentaries and opinions on the scientific background and explanatory ideas for a complex of symptoms and investigations known as syndrome X.

The commonest cause by far of angina pectoris is coronary artery obstruction due to atheromatous lesions both within the wall of the artery and intruding into the lumen; in such patients it is expected that there maybe ST segment depression on atrial pacing or on an exercise test indicating myocardial ischemia. Syndrome X was a term first used in an editorial written by Kemp in 1973. He was referring to patients in group X in a paper from Arbogast and Bourassa. Patients in group X had three features, namely angina as judged on a clinical history, alterations of the ST segment on the electrocardiogram during atrial pacing and smooth unobstructed coronary arteries (presumed normal) as assessed by the technique of coronary angiography. The changes on the electrocardiogram, conventionally indicative of myocardial ischemia, could not be explained on the basis of any abnormality of the coronary arteries and Kemp named the complex of findings syndrome X because of this seeming paradox and the lack of a single explanation. In the last thirty-one years there has been substantial scientific interest in this syndrome giving rise to a large number of publications.

The name syndrome X has led to considerable confusion. Physicians are familiar with the X chromosome and with X linked congenital disorders. Fragile X syndrome is the most common inherited form of mental retardation. In 1998 Reaven commenting on the role of insulin resistance in human disease referred to the constellation of findings associated with insulin resistance as syndrome X. There, thus emerged two syndromes X, a cardiac syndrome X and a metabolic syndrome X. Worse was to follow when some authors showed an association between the two. This book is primarily concerned with what is often referred to as cardiac syndrome X.

It may seem odd that an entire book should be devoted to such a syndrome. There are two major reasons. The first reason is that syndrome X, although not associated with an increased mortality or an increased risk of coronary events, is a debilitating disorder which can severely disrupt patients lives and leads to considerable costs in terms of medical care, numerous investigations and hospital admissions. Approximately 20% of coronary angiograms undertaken in the western world in patients with the clinical diagnosis of angina, usually attributed to coronary heart disease, turn out to be normal as judged by angiography. A proportion of those will have syndrome X. The disorder is not, therefore, that uncommon and naturally persons with chest pain suggestive of angina are extremely concerned that they may have important heart disease and are not easily satisfied without a full explanation. That is usually not forthcoming. The second reason for interest in syndrome X is because the syndrome requires an explanation. Numerous ideas have been put forward and some challenge the very foundations of our knowledge of abnormalities of the heart and of the coronary vasculature. It is possible and indeed even probable that understanding entities such as syndrome X will greatly increase our knowledge with regard to other disorders of the heart and thereby result in improved treatments for a much larger group of patients.

Syndrome X is a heterogeneous group of disorders. Essential requirements are the presence of a pain, which has many of the features and can be considered as angina pectoris, and normal coronary arteries. Some authors have included patients whose arteries are near normal rather than totally smooth as viewed by coronary angiography. There is always the possibility that there may be disease in the wall of the vessel which is not detected by coronary angiography. In addition there must be some further evidence that the abnormality is in the heart. Kemp used atrial pacing but others have used exercise testing (the most common investigation and criterion), radionucleide investigations, positron emission tomography and measurements of blood flow. In any one patient all these tests rarely give consistent and positive results. Thus several groups of patients can be identified and real differences may exist between them.

Within this book will be found several explanations for syndrome X and there is probably truth in many. The greatest divide is between those physicians and scientists who believe that the pain is the consequence of myocardial ischemia and those who believe that the syndrome has a more complex metabolic or structural cause. The difficulty with asserting that the syndrome is due to ischemia, "microvascular angina", is that in most patients there is a lack of evidence for ischemia in the traditional sense of that word. The temptation to attribute the syndrome to ischemia arises, of course, because in patients who have known fixed obstructions in the coronary arteries, the positive tests usually do indicate ischemia. Other explanations for syndrome X include abnormalities of central perception of pain, psychiatric disturbances, abnormalities of the esophagus and gut and many others. Perhaps the two hypotheses which are being investigated most widely at the moment are that syndrome X is attributable to subtle changes in the distribution of blood flow in the microvasculature between the endocardium and epicardium. This might be linked to alterations of adenosine release, abnormal presence or function of adenosine receptors or modified nitric oxide production. Alternatively the abnormality could be one of structure and function of the myocardial cell releasing metabolites such as potassium or adenosine in such a way as to give rise to pain and possibly but not crucially modify blood flow in the myocardium. The hypothesis that the abnormality is myocardial would be supported by the observation that ischemia is observed or proven in syndrome X in only about 25% of patients. Hypotheses relating to the maldistribution of flow in the microvasculature need to explain (and often can) how it is that gross investigations have failed to detect what may be ischemia localized to the microvascular circulation.

The treatment of syndrome X remains elusive. Several therapies have been shown to give rise to marginal benefits but are far from providing a cure. Syndrome X remains a difficult and even tiresome entity which often irritates cardiovascular physicians probably because of their inability to resolve what is often a non and chronic disability. Lack of understanding of a syndrome should not result in disregard for the clinical problem.

This book is a fair summary of the opinions of leading research workers with regard to syndrome X and brings together a literature which is disparate and difficult to find. The book presents the clinical and scientific problems, describes our current knowledge and must therefore be a major platform for future endeavor.

Philip A Poole-Wilson, MD, FRCP, FACC, FESC
Head, National Heart & Lung Institute
Imperial College School of Medicine
Dovehouse Street
London

Preface

The problem of chest pain with normal coronary arteriograms ("syndrome X") continues to represent a major challenge to contemporary cardiology. Progress has been made in recent years regarding the pathophysiology and management of this condition. However, information contained in the medical journals continues to be conflicting and controversial. Physicians still face the difficult problem of the overall meaningful synthesis of this ever-growing flow of information. This is particularly problematic as new concepts have emerged as a result of recent clinical observations and scientific discoveries.

Chest pain with normal coronary arteriograms is a relatively common syndrome. It affects 10-30% of patients undergoing cardiac catheterization for the assessment of chest pain suggestive of myocardial ischemia. The syndrome of angina and normal coronary arteriograms is obviously heterogeneous. Cardiac and extra-cardiac causes have been identified and it has become apparent that the underlying pathophysiological mechanisms may be different in different patients. In managing these patients it is therefore imperative that these mechanisms are identified.

This monographic work brings together leading authorities in the fields of chest pain and microvascular dysfunction. This book addresses specifically the cardiac causes of chest pain with normal coronary arteriograms and also the various extra-cardiac mechanisms known to play a role, including esophageal abnormalities, psychological conditions and the recently described "metabolic syndrome X".

Although patients with cardiac syndrome X have good prognosis regarding survival, morbidity is highly prevalent. The prognosis and management of patients with chest pain and normal coronary arteriograms, as well as the assessment of quality of life in these patients is specifically addressed.

The problem of microvascular angina as one of the important pathogenic mechanisms of cardiac syndrome X is thoroughly discussed. Microvascular angina is also discussed in the context of other conditions, such as, dilated and hypertrophic cardiomyopathy, hypertension and hyperlipidemia. There is a high prevalence of women in syndrome X and therefore estrogen deficiency has been suggested to play a pathogenic role. This book specifically discusses the important and clinically relevant issue of estrogen deficiency and endothelial dysfunction in cardiac syndrome X.

The diagnosis of chest pain with normal coronary arteriograms is costly and patients usually undergo a large series of invasive and non-invasive investigations. This obviously represents a major financial burden and is a matter of great concern. Cost-effective diagnostic strategies are proposed in the book. The role of different diagnostic tools, including nuclear imaging, echocardiography, positron emission tomography and the electrocardiogram is discussed in different chapters.

This book thus provides a comprehensive clinical and pathophysiological review of syndrome X. The whole spectrum of the syndrome is scrutinized, including clinical features, mechanisms, diagnosis, treatment and prognosis.

Juan Carlos Kaski

Chapter 1

CARDIAC SYNDROME X AND MICROVASCULAR ANGINA

Juan Carlos Kaski

Chest pain suggestive of myocardial ischemia occurs in approximately 20-30 % of patients in the absence of angiographically obvious coronary artery disease, as suggested by findings in large studies [1-3]. The presence of angina-like chest pain in subjects with normal coronary arteriograms is often referred to as "syndrome X". The term "syndrome X" was used for the first time by Kemp [4] in 1973 in an editorial comment of a paper by Arbogast and Bourassa [5] who compared the effects of atrial pacing on the left ventricular function of patients with coronary artery disease and patients with normal coronary arteriograms (termed "group X"). Arbogast and Bourassa were puzzled by the observation that patients of "group X" had normal ventricular performance despite the occurrence of typical ischemic electrocardiographic changes and metabolic evidence of ischemia, such as myocardial lactate production. In his editorial article, over 25 years ago, Kemp [4] highlighted several important aspects of the syndrome. In particular, the heterogenous nature of syndrome X, the possibility of more than one etiologic cause and the fact that a different form of myocardial ischemia could play a pathogenic role in this condition.

The clinical problem posed by the occurrence of angina pectoris in the absence of "arterio-sclerosis" was identified many years before the advent of coronary arteriography. Indeed, in 1901, William Osler [6] refers to "hysterical or pseudo-angina" as a form of angina that represents "the chief difficulty" in the diagnosis of "true" angina pectoris (the one associated with coronary artery disease). Prior to the article of Arbogast and Bourassa in 1973 [5] and soon after the advent of coronary arteriography, it became apparent that a significant proportion of patients with symptoms suggestive of obstructive coronary artery disease had only minimal coronary artery stenosis or even completely normal coronary arteriograms. In non-diabetic women, Likoff *et al* [7] observed the occurrence of exertional chest pain and ischemia-like electrocardiographic changes in the absence of obstructive coronary artery disease. Women in this study [7] were normotensive but had "non-specific" abnormalities of the resting electrocardiogram (ECG). During exercise stress testing they had a normal hemodynamic response despite the occurrence of angina and ST segment shifts. Later studies [8] confirmed Likoff *et al's* [7] initial findings and showed that patients with "angina pectoris and normal coronary arteries" often have severe chest pain which is refractory to conventional forms of therapy. Some of these patients were found to have not only ischemic ECG changes but also, more objective, metabolic evidence of myocardial ischemia [8]. In the past 30 years numerous investigations have been carried out in patients with chest pain and normal coronary arteriograms in an attempt to define the pathogenic mechanisms and devise rational therapies. Despite these efforts, uncertainties exist as to the nature of the condition that we continue to call syndrome X. One of the major reasons for our uncertainties is the lack of an accepted definition for syndrome X and its heterogeneous nature.

Problems associated with the definition of syndrome X

Although the term syndrome X is widely used, particularly in Europe, to label patients with typical exercise-induced angina and normal coronary arteriograms, no agreed definition exists for syndrome X. The reasons for this are probably severalfold and include the fact that the syndrome of chest pain with normal coronary arteriograms is heterogeneous and encompasses a multitude of pathogenic mechanisms. Adopting a broad definition for syndrome X (e.g. chest pain without coronary artery disease) is problematic as both patients with cardiac and non-cardiac causes would be included, further clouding the issue. The exclusion of extra-cardiac causes of chest pain is vital from a clinical point of view, e.g. patient management, prognosis, the psychological implications of the diagnosis of 'angina pectoris', etc.

Extracardiac causes

Chest pain in the absence of obstructive coronary artery disease is frequently non-cardiac in origin. Thoracic pain, esophageal abnormalities and psychosomatic symptoms referred to the heart often mimic angina pectoris. Pain of extracardiac origin and cardiac ischemic pain may be indistinguishable in character and circumstances of occurrence and relief. These mechanisms and their role in syndrome X are discussed in other chapters of this book.

Cardiac chest pain

In defining syndrome X, attempts should be also made to rule out well known causes of cardiac chest pain which may develop despite the presence of normal coronary arteriograms, such as left ventricular hypertrophy (LVH) and coronary artery spasm. The mechanisms whereby these conditions cause chest pain are well established and specific therapies exist to improve symptoms in patients who are affected by them, as described in other chapters of this book.

In my view, the definition of syndrome X should, in first place, serve a clinical purpose. That is to provide the managing physician with a tool for the identification of the different patients subgroups who may benefit from different therapeutic modalities (specific, if available). We should not forget that syndrome X is a syndrome and not a disease with a unique etiology. What patients with syndrome X have in common is simply the clinical presentation with ischemia like chest pain and the absence of angiographic coronary disease. The mechanism responsible for these symptoms, however, differ in different patients. Our attempts should therefore be directed to the understanding of the mechanism, or mechanisms, responsible for the syndrome in the individual patient. The term syndrome X just indicates a series of symptoms and ECG findings; if and when an etiologic cause is identified in a given patient or groups or patients, syndrome X ceases to exist as such. This phenomenon is analogous to the evolution of the concept of "dropsy" in the history of Medicine.

At present it is accepted that patients with syndrome X have typical chest pain, ECG shifts suggestive of transient myocardial ischemia and completely normal coronary arteriograms.

ST segment depression as a diagnostic criterion for syndrome X

Attempts to focus on cardiac mechanisms led some investigators to incorporate the presence of a positive electrocardiographic response during stress testing as a criterion for the definition of syndrome X [9, 10]. However, there is no guarantee that only "cardiac" patients will be identified when using this diagnostic criterion. Undoubtedly, a proportion of patients with typical chest pains but "negative" exercise tests are likely to have a cardiac origin of their chest discomfort and, *viceversa*, a proportion of patients with "positive" stress tests will have a non cardiac cause. There is also the problem of those patients who have baseline electrocardiographic abnormalities such as LBBB and in whom the interpretation of the response to conventional stress testing is precluded. Thus, although useful as a broad selecting tool, the ST segment criterion has important limitations. Indeed, both symptoms and response to treatment of patients selected on the basis of an ischemic-appearing ECG response to stress testing, are similar to those of patients without ischemic electrocardiograms. The proportion of patients with typical chest pain in Kaski *et al's* [11] patients with "syndrome X" selected on the basis of an ischemic ECG during exercise is similar to that of Cannon *et al's* [12] and the Duke Data Bank [13] patients, who were not selected on the basis of abnormal ECG responses to exercise.

Myocardial ischemia as a diagnostic criterion

Some clinicians and investigators consider that the presence of "documented" myocardial ischemia should be a *sine qua non* for the diagnosis of syndrome X. There are, however, several problems with this notion; in particular, 1) the problem that the "objective" diagnosis of myocardial ischemia is difficult in the clinical setting and 2) the fact that myocardial ischemia is probably one of the many causes of syndrome X. Regarding the first point, I find it hard to accept that ECG abnormalities or myocardial perfusion defects can be considered objective evidence of myocardial ischemia in patients without obstructive coronary artery disease. Metabolic markers, such as lactate production, abnormal ATP fluxes and pH changes in the coronary sinus blood may provide more objective information, but these tests are usually performed in the experimental setting.

Is there an accepted definition?

In general, it is accepted that the presence of typical, ischemia like, chest pain and ECG changes during pain in patients with normal coronary arteriograms defines syndrome X. The absence of extracardiac causes, coronary artery spasm, systemic hypertension and left ventricular hypertrophy is also required.

It has recently been suggested that the term syndrome X has outlived its usefulness. However, this name continues to be widely used and syndrome X continues to capture the imagination of clinicians and researchers alike.

The relatively recent description of a "new" syndrome X by Reaven [14] (who was unaware of the existence of the cardiac syndrome X) has introduced yet another confounding variable to the already complex picture. This new metabolic entity is characterized by the presence of hyperlipidemia, insulin resistance, hypertension and coronary artery disease. A possible link between the two syndromes "X" has been suggested and this subject will be addressed by other authors in the book.

Microvascular angina

The concept of microvascular angina

Several reports of limitation in coronary flow reserve have supported the possibility of an ischemic mechanism in at least some patients with chest pain and normal coronary arteries. Observations by Opherk *et al* [15] that coronary blood flow reserve was reduced in patients with syndrome X, and that patients with this abnormality also had metabolic evidence of myocardial ischemia, stimulated the notion of syndrome X as an ischemic syndrome. Expanding on Opherk *et al's* [15] findings, Cannon and Epstein [16] suggested that patients with chest pain and normal coronary arteries had abnormal coronary microvessel dilator responses (located at the pre-arteriolar level) and coined the term "microvascular angina" to define this condition. Their suggestion was based on observations carried out in the early 1980's. They reported a limitation in great cardiac vein flow responses to atrial pacing in patients who had typical chest pain during that stress [17]. Patients in the NIH study [17] were not selected on the basis of characteristics of the pain or the results of non-invasive testing. To assess whether a dynamic component to this flow limitation was present, 0.15 mg ergonovine was administered intravenously after the initial pacing stress, with repeat flow measurement during pacing stress at the same paced heart rate (150 beats/minute). Great cardiac vein flow increased less in patients who experienced their typical pain during pacing and ergonovine administration than in those who remained symptom-free during testing. In subsequent studies, patients with "microvascular dysfunction" were found to extract more oxygen during pacing stress than those who did not show a microvascular constrictor response [18]. In Cannon's study, lactate consumption during pacing was significantly lower in patients with a microvascular constrictor response to ergonovine. However, actual myocardial lactate production was demonstrable in only 10% of patient during pacing stress. The finding of a microcirculatory vasodilator derangement is the hallmark of the syndrome of microvascular angina. Coronary microvascular dysfunction, usually associated with endothelial dysfunction, has been reported in different conditions, including systemic hypertension, LV hypertrophy, dyslipidemia, estrogen deficiency, aging, etc. The demonstration of coexisting abnormal forearm responses to ischemia [19], esophageal motility abnormalities [20], and bronchoconstrictor responses [21] led the NIH investigators to postulate that some patients with coronary microvascular dysfunction may have a generalized disorder of vascular and non-vascular smooth muscle function.

One of the major problems with the definition of microvascular angina is that the diagnosis of this condition largely depends on the accuracy of current techniques to identify the presence of a reduced flow reserve. It is established that invasive studies of coronary flow suffer from methodological limitations. Moreover, few angiographic studies to date have provided data on normal controls. Non-invasive studies, however, have reported coronary flow responses to pharmacologic vasodilators in both patients with chest pain and normal coronary angiograms and normal volunteers. Geltman *et al* [22] studied 17 patients using positron emission tomography (PET) with ^{15}0-labelled water. There were no differences in myocardial perfusion after the administration of dipyridamole between patients and control subjects. However, more patients than controls had flow increases < 2.5 times over baseline, and differences in the homogeneity of myocardial perfusion were also detected between patients and controls. Camici *et al*

[23] studied 45 normotensive patients with chest pain (29 with ischemic ECG responses to exercise). Myocardial perfusion increased significantly more in response to dipyridamole in the 16 patients without ECG changes compared to the 29 patients with ischemic ECG responses. In another PET study, Galassi *et al* [24] observed that patients who had chest pain and ST segment depression after dipyridamole infusion had significantly higher resting blood flows than patients without chest pain and ST segment changes, or normal controls.

Syndrome X: clinical features

The clinical characteristics of syndrome X are summarized in Table 1.

Table 1. Main clinical features of syndrome X

Ill defined condition
Typical exercise induced chest pain
Positive responses to exercise stress testing
Completely normal coronary arteriograms
More common in women with estrogen deficiency
Atypical features of chest pain e.g. prolonged duration of episodes and poor response to sublingual nitrates in 50 % of cases
Good prognosis regarding survival
Poor quality of life in a proportion of patients
Multiple pathogenic mechanisms
Abnormal pain perception in a large number of cases
Microvascular angina associated in a proportion of patients
Antianginals ineffective in approximately 50 % of patients

Chest pain and electrocardiographic changes

Chest pain in patients with syndrome X is typically exertional and similar in character and radiation to that observed in patients with obstructive coronary artery disease. Despite its typical features, chest pain in patients with syndrome X (and those with microvascular angina) has several atypical features. It occurs at rest in a large proportion of syndrome X patients (41%) [11] and tends to be long lasting. The response of chest pain to sublingual nitrates is, in our experience [11] excellent in less than 50% of patients. Lanza *et al* [25] have recently reported that nitrate administration is associated with an impaired exercise capacity in syndrome X patients. Although a smaller proportion of patients with syndrome X than coronary artery disease patients respond to the administration of sublingual nitrates, there is no clinical evidence that nitrate administration is detrimental in syndrome X patients.

Chest pain in syndrome X patients may be severe and often frightening but, interestingly, it is not associated with LV dysfunction as assessed by nuclear techniques, hemodynamic measurements [5] and echocardiography [26, 27]. This clearly differs from findings in patients with obstructive coronary artery disease in whom ischemic chest pain is most often associated with regional wall motion abnormalities.

The exercise response of patients with syndrome X is frequently indistinguishable from that of patients with coronary artery disease. Although, on average, syndrome X patients tend to develop ischemia-like ST-segment changes at a higher rate-pressure product than patients with coronary artery disease [28], patterns of onset and offset of ST-segment depression are similar in syndrome X and patients with coronary artery disease, as described by Pupita *et al* [28]. Heart rate-recovery loops are also similar in coronary artery disease and syndrome X patients [29].

Continuous ambulatory ECG monitoring in patients with syndrome X has revealed the presence of ST-segment changes during their daily activities, indistinguishable from episodes observed in patients with coronary disease. The circadian distribution of these episodes is also similar to that observed in coronary artery disease patients and clearly opposite to that in Prinzmetal's variant angina. Indeed, patients with syndrome X develop ST segment shifts predominantly during waking hours. Episodes are similar in character to those of coronary artery disease patients. However, prolonged ST-segment depression associated with anginal symptoms is not infrequent in syndrome X. Silent ST-segment depression and angina without ST-segment shifts are also frequently found in patients with syndrome X [9]. The large majority of ischemic episodes are heart rate related but a significant proportion are not preceded by increases of heart rate [9]. This suggests the possibility of a reduced flow supply to the myocardium due to microvascular coronary constriction.

Female prevalence and coronary risk factors

Syndrome X commonly occurs in peri- or post-menopausal women. The high prevalence of menopausal women in the majority of the studies suggests that estrogen deficiency could play a pathogenetic role in syndrome X. Indeed, estrogen deficiency associated with hysterectomy or natural menopause is common in women with syndrome X [30]. The role of estrogen deficiency in syndrome X is discussed by P. Collins in another chapter of this book.

Risk factors for coronary artery disease, including hyperlipidemia, smoking, obesity and family history are similar in syndrome X and the general population. Usually, hypertension and diabetes mellitus are excluded from syndrome X series.

Left ventricular function in syndrome X

A proportion of patients with microvascular angina exhibit an abnormal ejection fraction response during exercise [31]. Cannon *et al* [32] have looked at the relationship between LV function and ST-segment shifts during exercise stress and found that 35% of patients who do not show exercise-induced ECG changes have an abnormal wall motion response, whereas 53% of those with ischemia-like ST-segment changes and 64% of those with LBBB have a reduced ejection fraction during exercise. Thus a substantial proportion of patients with angina and normal coronary arteriograms have a reduced vasodilatory capacity of the microcirculation, which is also associated with an abnormal LV function during stress. Contrary to findings in patients with microvascular angina, in patients with syndrome X, Nihoyannopoulos *et al* [26] and, more recently Panza *et al* [27] were unable to demonstrate an abnormal LV function in response to stress, as assessed by 2-D echocardiography.

Long-term left ventricular function

Deterioration of LV function is a rare event in patients with angina and normal coronary arteriograms [11]. Recently Kaski *et al* [11] reported preserved resting LV function in 98 of 99 patients followed for an average of 6.7 years, selected on the basis of an ischemic ECG response to exercise. Other studies [33], however, suggest that certain patient subgroups may experience deterioration in LV function over time. Opherk *et al* [33] reported that of 40 patients with syndrome X, patients with LBBB present on resting or exercise ECGs, commonly demonstrated deterioration in rest and exercise LV ejection fraction over an average follow-up of four years. Cannon *et al* [34] studied the 4.5 year follow-up of 61 patients with microvascular angina; 25% showed significant deterioration in resting LV ejection fraction or new wall motion abnormalities. In contrast to findings by Opherk [33] in this preliminary report, Cannon *et al* [34] observed that decline in LV function was not restricted to patients with LBBB. Furthermore, a decline in function was actually seen more commonly in patients without ischemic appearing ECG responses to exercise stress. None of the patients in Cannon's study [34] showed evidence of inflammation or amyloid deposition. Whether this progressive dysfunction was a consequence of limited coronary flow reserve, potentially reflecting microvascular dysfunction, or some cardiomyopathic or metabolic process with associated limitation in flow reserve, is not known. In Cannon's study, patients with abnormal left ventricular ejection fraction responses to exercise did not convert their ECG to LBBB during exercise prior to developing deterioration in LV function. Left ventricular endocardial biopsies performed in 5 patients with LBBB, and 5 patients with normal ECGs but similar depression in LV function, revealed no histological differences.

Syndrome X: pathogenic hypotheses

The pathophysiological mechanisms of chest pain in patients with normal coronary angiograms are controversial, as evidenced by the conflicting results of studies performed over the past 30 years and various opinions expressed in editorials [35, 36]. Several pathogenetic mechanisms have been proposed and they are listed in Table 2.

Myocardial ischemia

The search for an ischemic mechanism for syndrome X is justifiable in view of the clinical, electrocardiographic and metabolic findings. Chest pain and exercise-induced ST-segment changes in patients with syndrome X are suggestive of myocardial ischemia and these patients are frequently referred for coronary arteriography to rule out obstructive coronary lesions. However, for the accurate definition of an ischemic syndrome, it is required that objective evidence of ischemia is obtained and, if possible, the mechanisms responsible for this are identified. The concept of microvascular angina is based on the demonstration of a reduced coronary blood flow reserve. Obviously, ECG shifts are inadequate and conventional nuclear studies also have limitations. The techniques routinely used for the measurement of coronary flow reserve also are far from ideal, as discussed by L'Abbate in another chapter of this book.

Table 2. Pathogenic mechanisms in cardiac syndrome X

Myocardial ischemia
Microvascular dysfunction
    Estrogen deficiency
    Endothelial dysfunction
    Coronary artery hyperreactivity (microvascular spasm)
    Increased sympathetic tone
    Release of endogenous peptides (NPY, endothelin-1)
    Structural abnormalities of the coronary microvessels
    Prearteriolar constriction and "patchy" release of adenosine

Diffuse epicardial and microvascular coronary constriction

Non ischemic mechanisms
    Increased pain perception
    Abnormal interstitial release of potassium
    Myocardial metabolic abnormality
    Insulin resistance
    Early cardiomyopathy

The initial observations of Opherk *et al* [15] and Cannon *et al* [16, 37] gave support to the ischemic hypothesis. Opherk *et al* [15] reported that a reduced vasodilator capacity of the coronary microcirculation was apparent in patients with syndrome X, as assessed by the argon washout method, after the infusion of dipyridamole. Three of their patients also showed lactate production in association with the reduced flow reserve, during rapid atrial pacing. In 1983 Cannon *et al* [37] reported limitation in great cardiac vein flow response to atrial pacing (coronary sinus thermodilution method) in patients with typical angina and normal coronary arteriograms. Repeat flow measurements during pacing stress, but after the administration of ergonovine, showed further limitation of flow reserve with increase of coronary resistance in patients with chest pain but not in those who remained symptom free. As angiography during ergonovine demonstrated no change in epicardial coronary dimensions, Cannon *et al* [37] concluded that the increase of coronary resistance was caused by constriction of the microcirculation. Lactate production was found in 10% of their patients with pacing-induced chest pain. Cannon and Epstein [16] used the term "microvascular angina" to indicate what appeared to be an increased sensitivity of the coronary microcirculation to vasoconstrictor stimuli. The authors proposed that an abnormal vasodilator capacity of the pre-arteriolar vessels was the cause of ischemia in syndrome X.

Cannon *et al* [32] performed studies of coronary flow velocity in 47 consecutive normotensive patients (33 women and 14 men; age 49 years, range 28 to 70 years). All had angina-like chest pain and completely normal coronary angiograms, normal M-mode and 2D echocardiograms, and had no conduction abnormalities. Of the 33 women, 73% were postmenopausal; of these 24 women, 13 (54%) were on estrogen replacement therapy at the time of their study. Of the 47 patients, 36 had normal radionuclide angiographic studies whilst 11 had abnormal findings, including a fall in ejection fraction and/or the development of wall motion abnormalities. Of the 36 patients with normal radionuclide studies, 24 also underwent exercise thallium study; only 1 patient had reversible perfusion abnormalities. In contrast, of the 11 patients with abnormal radionuclide angiographic studies, 5 of 8 who also underwent exercise thallium scintigraphy had reversible perfusion abnormalities.

Evidence of myocardial ischemia in patients with syndrome X and microvascular angina

Myocardial ischemia has been documented objectively in a variable proportion of syndrome X patients. Myocardial lactate production, an accepted index of myocardial ischemia, has been found in 13% - 100% of patients with angina and normal coronary arteriograms in different series [10], and it has been suggested that "lactate producers" have marked ST-segment changes during atrial pacing [38]. Chest pain alone does not seem to correlate with lactate production [39]. In patients with microvascular angina, evidence of lactate production has also been obtained [40, 41].

As mentioned above, studies of myocardial perfusion and LV function using radionuclides have convincingly shown changes compatible with transient myocardial ischemia in approximately 20%- 30% of syndrome X and microvascular angina patients[3, 11]. However, ischemia cannot be documented in the large majority of patients with syndrome X. This may have different explanations. Among these: 1) No ischemia is present; syndrome X is heterogeneous and mechanisms other than myocardial ischemia may be responsible for the condition 2) ischemia is of mild intensity and below the threshold of our diagnostic techniques, 3) ischemia is patchy or limited to the subendocardium.

Specific chapters in this book will address the different pathogenic mechanisms of syndrome X, both ischemic and non ischemic. These will include:

1) the problem of pre-arteriolar constriction and adenosine release, as recently suggested by Maseri et al [42]. These authors proposed that as a result of increased resistance at a pre-arteriolar level, local release of adenosine may occur. Distal to the most constricted arterioles, a compensatory increase of adenosine may take place, which could cause angina even in the absence of myocardial ischemia.

2) Increased pain perception. Patients with chest pain and normal coronary arteries have atypical pain features (e.g. chest pain is severe, long lasting and not associated with objective signs of myocardial ischemia in the majority of cases) and there is evidence that many patients have an exaggerated or abnormal cardiac sensitivity [43-46]. These observations have led investigators to consider abnormal pain perception as the underlying mechanism of the syndrome in some patients. Turiel et al [43] showed that women with syndrome X had a reduced pain threshold for forearm ischemia and electrical skin stimulation. Shapiro et al [44] and Cannon et al [45] observed that catheter manipulation within the heart chambers of patients with chest pain and normal coronary arteriograms (syndrome X and microvascular angina patients, respectively) resulted in typical chest pain. These findings are also consistent with recent observations by Cannon et al. [47] who reported a beneficial effect of imipramine, a tricyclic antidepressant used in the management of chronic pain syndromes, in patients with chest pain and normal coronary arteriograms undergoing a randomized, double-blind, placebo-controlled trial.

3) Cardiomyopathy: coronary microvascular dysfunction has been observed in patients with dilated [48, 49] and hypertrophic [50] cardiomyopathy. Moreover, some patients with syndrome X may evolve towards dilated cardiomyopathy. Opherk et al [33] and Cannon et al [34] have suggested that a subgroup of patients with microvascular angina

may experience deterioration of left ventricular function over time. A pathogenic link between microvascular dysfunction and certain forms of cardiomyopathy has therefore been suggested.

4) Endothelial dysfunction, estrogen deficiency and insulin resistance, are also important mechanisms which will be discussed in other chapters.

Summary and conclusions

Syndrome X defines patients with typical ischemia-like chest pain, positive responses to stress testing and completely normal coronary arteriograms. This syndrome is heterogeneous and encompasses a number of different pathogenic mechanisms. Syndrome X is more common amongst peri- or post-menopausal women, which suggests a role for estrogen deficiency. Prognosis is good regarding survival but quality of life is poor in a proportion of patients due to chest pain. Antianginals are effective in less than 50% of patients and pain perception abnormalities appear to play a major pathogenic role. Anti-nociceptive therapy offers promise, but a larger experience will be required to define the role of drugs useful in chronic pain syndromes in managing syndrome X patients.

Despite suggestions that the term "syndrome X" has outlived its usefulness and is confusing to physicians, it continues to be used perhaps as a reminder of our ignorance. The mysterious "X" appears to also represent a challenge to continue the search for the mechanisms responsible for the syndrome and for rational therapies to serve our patients better.

References

1. Proudfit WL, Shirley EK, Sones FM. Selective cine coronary arteriography: Correlation with clinical findings in 1,000 patients. Circulation 1966; 33: 901 – 910.
2. Kemp HG, Kronmal RA, Vlietstra RE, Frye RL and the Coronary Artery Surgery Study (CASS) participants. Seven year survival of patients with normal or near normal coronary arteriograms: A CASS registry study. J Am Coll Cardiol 1986; 7: 479 – 483.
3. Cannon R, Camici P, Epstein SE. Pathophysiological dilemma of syndrome X. Circulation 85; 1992: 883 – 892.
4. Kemp HG. Left Ventricular Function in patients with the anginal syndrome and normal coronary arteriograms. Am J Cardiol 1973; 32: 375 – 376.
5. Arbogast R, Bourassa MG. Myocardial function during atrial pacing in patients with angina pectoris and normal coronary arteriograms: Comparison with patients having significant coronary artery disease. Am J Cardiol 1973; 32: 257 – 263.
6. Osler W. Lectures on angina pectoris and allied states. Appleton, New York 1901.
7. Likoff W, Segal BL, Kasparian H. Paradox of normal selective coronary arteriograms in patients considered to have unmistakable coronary heart disease. N Engl J Med 1967; 276: 1063 – 1066.
8. Kemp HG, Vokonas PS, Cohn PF, Gorlin R. The anginal syndrome associated with normal coronary arteriograms: Report of a six year experience. Am J Med 1973; 54: 735 – 742.
9. Kaski JC, Crea F, Nihoyannopoulos P, Hackett D, Maseri A. Transient myocardial ischemia during daily life in patients with syndrome X. Am J Cardiol 1986; 58: 1242 – 1247.
10. Hutchison SJ, Poole-Wilson PA, Henderson AH. Angina with normal coronary arteries: A review. Quart J Med 1989; 72: 677 – 688.
11. Kaski JC, Rosano GMC, Nihoyannopoulos P, Collins P, Maseri A, Poole-Wilson P. Syndrome X - Clinical characteristics and left ventricular function - A long term follow-up study. (In Press).
12. Cannon RO. Microvascular angina: Cardiovascular investigations regarding pathophysiology and management. In Richter JE, Cannon RO, Beitman B (eds.): Unexplained chest pain. Medical Clinics of North America. Philadelphia. WB Saunders, 1991; 75: 1097 – 1118.
13. Papanicolaou MN, Califf RM, Hlatky MA et al. Prognostic implications of angiographically normal and insignificantly narrowed coronary arteries. Am J Cardiol 1986; 58: 1181 – 1187.

14. Reaven G. Banting Lecture 1988: Role of insulin resistance in human diabetes. Diabetes 1988; 37: 1595 – 1607.

15. Opherk D, Zebe H, Wiehe E *et al*. Reduced coronary dilatory capacity and ultrastructural changes of the myocardium in patients with angina pectoris but normal coronary arteriograms. Circulation 1981; 63: 817 – 825.

16. Cannon RO, Epstein SE. "Microvascular Angina" as a cause of chest pain with angiographically normal coronary arteries. Am J Cardiol 1988; 61: 1338 – 1343.

17. Cannon RO, Watson RM, Rosing DR, Epstein SE. Angina caused by reduced vasodilator reserve of the small coronary arteries. J Am Coll Cardiol 1983; 1: 1359 – 1373.

18. Cannon RO, Schenke WH, Leon MB, Rosing DR, Urquhart J, Epstein SE. Limited coronary flow reserve after dipyridamole in patients with ergonovine-induced coronary vasoconstriction. Circulation 1987; 75: 163 – 174.

19. Sax FL, Cannon RO, Hanson C, Epstein SE. Impaired forearm vasodilator reserve in patients with microvascular angina: Evidence of a generalized disorder of vascular function? N Engl J Med 1987; 317: 1366 – 1370.

20. Cannon RO, Cattau EL, Yakshe PN *et al*. Coronary flow reserve, esophageal motility and chest pain in patients with angiographically normal coronary arteries. Am J Med 1990; 88: 217 – 222.

21. Cannon RO, Peden DB, Berkebile C, Schenke WH, Kaliner MA, Epstein SE. Airway hyperresponsiveness in patients with microvascular angina: Evidence for a diffuse disorder of smooth muscle responsiveness. Circulation 1990; 82: 2011 – 2017.

22. Geltman EM, Henes CG, Senneff MJ, Sobel BE, Bergmann SR. Increased myocardial perfusion at rest and diminished perfusion reserve in patients with angina and angiographically normal coronary arteries. J Am Coll Cardiol 1990; 16: 586 – 595.

23. Camici PG, Gistri R, Lorenzoni R *et al*. Coronary reserve and exercise ECG in patients with chest pain and normal coronary angiograms. Circulation 1992; 86: 79 – 186.

24. Galassi AR, Araujo LI, Crea F *et al*. Myocardial blood flow is altered at rest and after dipyridamole in patients with syndrome X. J Am Coll Cardiol 1991; 17: 227A (Abstract).

25. Lanza GA, Manzoli A, Bia E, Crea F, Maseri A. Acute effects of nitrates on exercise testing in patients with syndrome X. Clinical and pathophysiological implications. Circulation 1994; 90:2695 – 2700.

26. Nihoyannopoulos P, Kaski JC, Crake T, Maseri A. Absence of myocardial dysfunction during stress in patients with syndrome X. J Am Coll Cardiol 1991; 18: 1463 – 1470.

27. Panza JA, Laurienzo JM, Curiel RV, Unger EF, Quyyumi AA, Dilsizian V, Cannon RO. Investigation of the mechanism of chest pain in patients with angiographically normal coronary arteries using transesophageal dobutamine stress echocardiography. J Am Coll Cardiol 1997; 29: 293 – 301.

28. Pupita G, Kaski JC, Galassi AR, Gavrielides S, Crea F, Maseri A. Similar time course of ST depression during and after exercise in patients with coronary artery disease and syndrome X. Am Heart J 1990; 120: 848 – 854.

29. Gavrielides S, Kaski JC, Galassi AR *et al*. Recovery-phase patterns of ST-segment depression in the heart rate domain cannot distinguish between anginal patients with coronary artery disease and patients with syndrome X. Am Heart J 1991; 122: 1593 – 1598.

30. Rosano G, Lindsay D, Kaski JC, Sarrel P, Poole-Wilson P. Syndrome X in women: The importance of ovarian hormones. J Am Coll Cardiol 1992; 19: 255A.

31. Cannon RO, Bonow RO, Bacharach SL *et al*. Left ventricular dysfunction in patients with angina pectoris, normal coronary arteries, and abnormal vasodilator reserve. Circulation 1985; 71: 218 – 226.

32. Cannon RO, Quyyumi AA, Dilsizian V. Association of abnormal left ventricular responses to exercise with dynamic limitation in coronary flow reserve in patients with chest pain, angiographically normal coronary arteries. Circulation 1992; 86: I - 588 (Abstract).

33. Opherk D, Schuler G, Wetterauer K, Manthey J, Schwarz F, Kübler W. Four-year follow-up in patients with angina pectoris and normal coronary arteriograms ("syndrome X"). Circulation 1989; 80: 1610 – 1616.

34. Cannon RO, Dilsizian V, Correa R, Epstein SE, Bonow RO. Chronic deterioration in left ventricular function in patients with microvascular angina. J Am Coll Cardiol 1991;17:28A (abstract).

35. Conti CR. What is syndrome X? Clin Cardiol 1993; 16: 1 – 3.

36. Maseri A. Syndrome X: Still an appropriate name. J Am Coll Cardiol 1991; 17: 1471 – 1472.

37. Cannon RO, Watson RM, Rosing DR, Epstein SE. Angina caused by reduced vasodilator reserve of the small coronary arteries. J Am Coll Cardiol 1983; 1: 1359 – 1373.

38. Boudoulas H, Cobb TC, Leighton RF, Wilt SM. Myocardial lactate production in patients with angina-like chest pain and angiographically normal coronary arteries and left ventricle. Am J Cardiol 1974; 84: 501 – 505.

39. Mammohansingh P, Parker JO. Angina pectoris with normal coronary arteriograms: Hemodynamic and metabolic response to atrial pacing. Am Heart J 1975; 90: 555 – 561.

40. Greenberg MA, Grose RM, Neuburger N, Silverman R, Strain JE, Cohen MV. Impaired coronary vasodilator responsiveness as a cause of lactate production during pacing-induced ischemia in patients with angina pectoris and normal coronary arteries. J Am Coll Cardiol 1987; 9: 743 – 751.

41. Cannon RO, Bonow RO, Bacharach SL et al. Left ventricular dysfunction in patients with angina pectoris, normal epicardial coronary arteries, and abnormal vasodilator reserve. Circulation 1985; 71: 218 – 226.

42. Maseri A, Crea F, Kaski JC, Crake T. Mechanisms of angina pectoris in syndrome X. J Am Coll Cardiol 1991; 17: 499 – 506.

43. Turiel M, Galassi AR, Glazier JJ, Kaski JC, Maseri A. Pain threshold and tolerance in women with syndrome X and women with stable angina pectoris. Am J Cardiol 1987; 60: 503 – 507.

44. Shapiro LM, Crake T, Poole-Wilson PA. Is altered cardiac sensation responsible for chest pain in patients with normal coronary arteries? Clinical observation during catheterization. Br Med J 1988; 296: 170 – 171.

45. Cannon RO, Quyyumi AA, Schenke WH et al. Abnormal cardiac sensitivity in patients with chest pain and normal coronary arteries. J Am Coll Cardiol 1990; 16: 1359 – 1366.

46. Cox ID, Salomone O, Brown SJ, Hann CM, Kaski JC. Serum endothelin levels and pain perception in patients with cardiac syndrome X and healthy controls. Am J Cardiol 1997; 80: 637 – 639.

47. Cannon RO, Quyyumi AA, Mincemoyer R et al. Imipramine in patients with chest pain despite normal coronary arteriograms. N Engl J Med 1994; 330: 1411 – 1417.

48. Cannon RO, Cunnion RE, Parrillo JE et al. Dynamic limitation of coronary vasodilator reserve in patients with dilated cardiomyopathy and chest pain. J Am Coll Cardiol 1987; 10: 1190 – 1200.

49. Treasure CB, Vita JA, Cox DA et al. Endothelium-dependent dilation of the coronary microvasculature is impaired in dilated cardiomyopathy. Circulation 1990; 81: 772 – 779.

50. Cannon RO, Rosing DR, Maron BJ et al. Myocardial ischemia in patients with hypertrophic cardiomyopathy: Contribution of inadequate vasodilator reserve and elevated left ventricular filling pressures. Circulation 1985; 71: 234 – 243.

Chapter 2

CHEST PAIN WITH NORMAL CORONARY ARTERIES: PSYCHOLOGICAL ASPECTS

Steve G Potts and Christopher Bass

Although it is only since the development of coronary angiography in the 1960's that the label "chest pain and normal coronary arteries" has been used, accounts of similar patients can be found in the literature up to a century earlier. Most early descriptions emphasize organic abnormalities in explaining the symptoms: but there has been an increasing recognition that psychological abnormalities are also common. Several recent studies, reviewed below, have clearly demonstrated high levels of psychological morbidity, both at the time of angiography, and on follow-up. This observed association could be explained in several ways. The psychological abnormalities observed could simply be *reactions* to the physical symptoms; or they might *cause* those symptoms directly, via a range of possible pathophysiological mechanisms. A third model is suggested below, in which psychological and physical factors *interact* in a variety of ways to precipitate, and especially to maintain, physical symptoms. Such a model indicates a place for psychological approaches in the management of patients with chest pain and normal coronary arteries. The essential elements of a suggested form of psychological treatment are set out below, together with evidence of its efficacy.

Historical background

Since the middle of the 19th century, there have been many descriptions, using a wide variety of terms, of patients who present with cardiorespiratory symptoms (typically chest pain, palpitations, and shortness of breath) unexplained by ischemic or rheumatic heart disease. Hartshorne coined the term "muscular exhaustion of the heart" in describing such symptoms among soldiers at the height of the American civil war [1], and soon afterwards Da Costa gave his classic account of "irritable heart" in men who had served in the same conflict [2]. A pattern was thereby established which persisted for many years: firstly, interest in the condition was greatest among military doctors, and peaked at times of war; and secondly the symptoms were attributed to an organic cause. Hartshorne [1] ascribed the symptoms to over-exhaustion and poor nourishment, whereas Da Costa [2] blamed faulty cardiac innervation. British physicians, on the other hand, saw the cause as over-drilling and tight military garments [3].

In the First World War there was an epidemic of what came to be known as "soldier's heart" or "effort syndrome" in the British Army [4]. Although twenty years earlier, Freud had emphasized the occurrence of cardiovascular symptoms in his description of anxiety neurosis [5], organic explanations of soldier's heart were much preferred, so that even when psychological symptoms were acknowledged they were dismissed as ancillary. Sir Thomas Lewis, in an influential monograph [6], remarked that although his patients were psychologically different from the average soldier, their "nervous manifestations" were "additions", and not essential parts of effort syndrome, which he attributed to the after-effects of various infections. Between the wars other authors paid more attention to psychological factors [7], but it was not until interest in the subject increased again during World War II that their importance was clearly established. In 1941 Paul Wood, a cardiologist based in London, concluded that in cases of what he called Da Costa's syndrome, a primary psychiatric diagnosis could nearly always be made [8]. He pointed out that while the syndrome is common among male soldiers at war, in times of peace it is mainly a complaint of women, suggesting a relationship with environmental stress. His psychiatric colleagues, Aubrey Lewis and Maxwell Jones, argued that while anxiety was the most prevalent psychopathology, depression, hypochondriasis and hysteria were common too [9]. American authors of the period preferred the term "neurocirculatory asthenia" [10]. Although they agreed that psychopathology, mainly in the form of anxiety, was very common, there was dispute about the extent of the overlap between neurocirculatory asthenia and anxiety neurosis. On both sides of the Atlantic the nature of the causal links between these psychiatric states and the presenting somatic symptoms remained obscure. Despite the volume of research in the area since then, and the introduction of new psychiatric categories such as panic disorder, the current position has changed little, and can be summarized thus:

Psychological abnormalities are common, with anxiety disorders predominating, but how they relate to the presenting cardiorespiratory symptoms remains uncertain.

Prevalence and type of psychological abnormality

The development of coronary angiography in the 1960s permitted greater confidence in excluding gross cardiac pathology, particularly coronary artery disease, and contributed to the drive to find a less obvious organic basis for the symptoms, such as mitral valve prolapse or microvascular angina. It also permitted description of the nature and frequency of psychological abnormalities in a more tightly defined group of patients (namely those with chest pain sufficiently suggestive of coronary artery disease to warrant angiography, but who are found to have normal coronary arteries), as well as allowing direct comparison with patients who *do* have coronary artery disease.

The findings of a number of such studies are listed in Table 1. In an early study, Waxler *et al* [11] examined 86 patients with chest pain and normal coronary arteries and found psychological abnormalities in 40% of these patients. These were variously described as "anxiety neurosis", "neurotic personality" and "neurotic or hypochondriacal behavior", although the authors do not make clear the criteria by which the diagnoses were made. Bass and Wade [12] conducted standardized interviews on 99 British patients (53 with significant coronary artery disease, and 46 without) at the time of coronary angiography, with both patient and interviewer blind to the angiogram findings. There was a clear excess of psychiatric abnormality in those without significant coronary artery disease, 40% of whom had anxiety neurosis. Katon *et al* [13] employed similar methods in 74 American patients, but used a different psychiatric classification in which panic disorder replaced anxiety neurosis. They found panic disorder to be significantly more common among those without significant coronary artery disease (43% compared with 7%), as were phobic disorders and both current and lifetime major depression. Beitman *et al* [14], in a study restricted to patients with normal coronary arteries, found similar rates of panic disorder, but lower rates of phobias and major depression. Carney [15] again demonstrated high rates of psychiatric abnormality in patients with chest pain and absent or insignificant coronary artery disease, but found that the commonest psychopathology was current major depression rather than panic disorder.

Table 1. Psychiatric diagnoses in chest pain patients by angiographic findings

	Normal (or near-normal) coronary arteries		Coronary artery disease		p value
Waxler [11]					
Neurotic personality	34/86	40%			
Bass [12]					
Anxiety neurosis	17/46	40%	1/53	2%	0.001
Depression	3/46	7%	4/53	8%	NS
Other psychiatric diagnoses	8/46	17%	7/53	15%	NS
No psychiatric diagnosis	18/46	39%	41/53	77%	0.001
Katon [13]					
Panic disorder	12/28	43%	3/46	7%	0.01
Simple phobia	10/28	36%	7/46	15%	0.05
Major depression (current)	10/28	36%	2/46	4%	0.01
Major depression (lifetime)	18/28	64%	11/46	24%	0.001
No psychiatric diagnosis	6/28	21%	34/46	74%	0.01
Beitman [14]					
Panic disorder	32/94	34%			
Simple phobia	10/94	11%			
Major depression (current)	11/94	12%			
Carney [15]					
Panic disorder	5/48	10%	10/52	19%	NS
Major depression (current)	18/48	38%	0/52	0%	0.001
No psychiatric diagnosis	28/48	58%	42/52	81%	0.05

In a study of what they called "healthy heart-anxious patients", Eifert *et al* [16], once more, found higher levels of anxiety, depression, physical symptoms, obsessive-compulsive features and hypochondriacal beliefs than in cardiac or surgical inpatients or normal controls. The index group also reported more psychological and physical symptoms on hyperventilation. Comparable findings were reported in a Dutch study which compared 67 patients with non-cardiac and 47 with cardiac chest pain [17], and concluded that age, gender, anxiety and hyperventilation were the variables which most clearly discriminated between the two groups. It is not clear however what criteria were used to distinguish the two groups. The paper refers to "extensive cardiological investigation" but does not specify whether this included angiography (even though the groups were labeled NCA and CAD, suggesting that it did).

Alexander et al [18] recently showed similar results in a non-Western population in India. They divided 54 male inpatients with chest pain into ischemic and non-cardiac groups, on the basis of treadmill ECG tests, and undertook blinded psychiatric interviews. DSM-III-R psychiatric diagnoses (mainly panic disorder and major depression) were made in 68% of the non-cardiac and 27% of the ischemic group. In contrast, a large Australian study [19] comparing psychological variables in three groups (defined on the basis of thallium perfusion and history of infarction) found no differences in anxiety, depression, or hypochondriasis.

Relationship between psychological and physical factors

The high prevalence of psychiatric disorder in patients with chest pain and normal coronary arteries could be explained in various ways, several of which have implications for treatment.

Psychological morbidity as reactive

It is possible that the anxiety these patients display is simply a reaction to their physical symptoms, the stress of investigation, and the fear of myocardial infarction or sudden death. While these factors may play a part, they cannot account for the excess of morbidity compared with patients with definite coronary artery disease. As well as the different rates of psychiatric diagnoses described above, there are differences in psychiatric morbidity scores even when these fall short of definite diagnoses. Bass and Wade [12] used an instrument known as the Clinical Interview Schedule (CIS) which yields a total score for psychiatric morbidity, the level above which a subject is designated a psychiatric "case" being 12. The mean score among patients with coronary artery disease was 8.6, while in those with normal or insignificantly narrowed coronary arteries it was 69% higher at 14.5 (p<0.001). Furthermore, the follow-up findings described below indicate that psychological abnormalities are persistent, and not simply transient responses to the stress of angiography.

Psychological morbidity as causative

In the DSM-IV definition of panic disorder [20], chest pain is listed as one of 13 qualifying symptoms, four or more of which are required for a diagnosis of panic attacks. In this context, chest pain is neither a cause nor a result of psychiatric morbidity: it is instead a defining characteristic of that morbidity. Although there is concern that unrecognized organic abnormalities such as paroxysmal SVT may be mis-diagnosed as panic disorder [21], Fleet et al [22,23] recently showed that in patients presenting acutely with chest pain, 75% of whom were discharged with a diagnosis of non-cardiac pain, panic disorder went unrecognized in 98% of cases. Yingling et al [24] found panic disorder or major depression in one third of 334 patients presenting with acute chest pain, but the prevalence of panic disorder in those with and without myocardial ischemia was similar (20% v 17%, NS). In both groups these psychiatric diagnoses predicted higher rates of repeat acute chest pain presentations in the subsequent year. Katon [25] has recently reviewed the evidence about the association between panic disorder, unexplained physical symptoms (including chest pain) and heavy consumption of medical services.

Panic disorder is classified with the anxiety disorders, and there are several plausible mechanisms whereby psychiatric abnormalities, especially anxiety, may cause chest pain, including autonomic overarousal, hyperventilation, skeletal muscle tension, and esophageal dysmotility (see Figure 1).

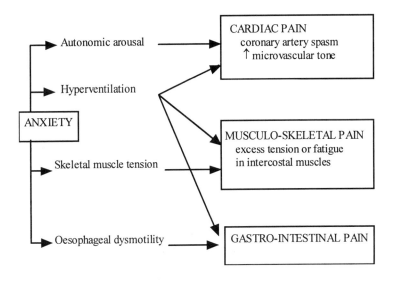

Figure 1. Mechanisms by which anxiety can cause chest pain.

Anxiety may lead to autonomic over-arousal, either by raised levels of circulating catecholamines, increased sympathetic activity, or both. Indeed, observed associations between atypical chest pain and mitral valve prolapse have been explained on the basis that the latter is a marker of a hyper-adrenergic state, which is responsible for both the chest pain and, incidentally, anxiety and panic. Autonomic overarousal could act via either through spasm of the epicardial coronary arteries [26], or increased microvascular tone [27].

Hyperventilation is known to be common among patients with chest pain and normal coronary arteries. Bass *et al* [28] found symptoms suggestive of hyperventilation in 65% of patients with chest pain and normal coronary arteries, as compared with 13% of patients with definite coronary artery disease. Hyperventilation is also known to underlie a proportion of cases presenting acutely with chest pain mistakenly attributed to a heart attack [29].

Hyperventilation provides a plausible link between anxiety and chest pain, as well as to other physical symptoms. Anxiety could lead to overbreathing [30], and thence to alkalosis, which may in turn bring about coronary artery spasm [31] or perhaps increased microvascular tone. Chauhan *et al* [32] recently showed in 10 of 29 patients with syndrome X (defined as typical pain, NCA, and a positive exercise tolerance test) that either hyperventilation or mental stress could reliably induce typical chest pain, and that this was associated with a reduced coronary blood flow suggestive of increased microvascular resistance. Exercise-induced hyperventilation is known to be more common in patients with chest pain and normal coronary arteries than in those with coronary artery disease [33], and may be responsible for some of the observed association between chest pain and exercise in these patients. Furthermore, hyperventilation can cause ECG changes resembling ischemia [34], so exercise-induced hyperventilation could be responsible for some of the positive exercise ECGs encountered in patients with normal coronary arteries. Hyperventilation may exert its effects by altogether different mechanisms, which do not involve the heart. It is known to be capable of inducing esophageal spasm [31], and it may bring about chest pain via fatigue or cramp in overworked intercostal muscles [35], or by aggravating pre-existent chest wall disorders such as fibrositis [36]. The precipitation of chest pain by breath-holding or breathing with a deliberately over-inflated chest [37] supports such a possibility.

Despite this multiplicity of possible linking mechanisms, hyperventilation is unlikely to be a complete explanation, however, since hyperventilation provocation tests reproduce pain in fewer than half of cases [12,38,39] and the test re-test reliability is low [40]. Furthermore, there are other ways in which psychiatric morbidity could be causally linked to chest pain. Anxiety may increase skeletal muscle tone, for example, and lead to spasm or fatigue in the musculature of the thorax. It is also known to cause esophageal dysmotility in healthy normals [41], and may therefore cause or exacerbate dysmotility-induced chest pain in patients with normal coronary arteries. Richter and Bradley [42] have recently reviewed the growing literature on the biopsychosocial dimensions of esophageal diseases, including those with otherwise unexplained chest pain. Carter *et al* [43] present the intriguing possibility that the mechanism involved may not be peripheral at all, but central, the abnormality lying in neural circuits in the anterior limbic system. This suggests potentially fruitful new avenues for research using positron emission tomography.

Plausible mechanisms and observed associations do not prove a causal relationship, however. It is quite possible that in many cases the co-occurrence of pathophysiological abnormalities is epiphenomenal rather than causal. Evidence in favor of this is found in studies showing that esophageal abnormalities, even when present, do not always coincide with episodes of chest pain [44], that effective treatment of esophageal abnormalities does not always relieve chest pain [45], and that treatment with antidepressants can relieve pain in patients with esophageal abnormalities even though these persist [46]. These observations, together with the variety of possible mechanisms discussed above, make it unlikely that any single causal explanation can relate psychiatric morbidity to chest pain.

Psychological morbidity as interactive

As well as the many possible mechanisms linking anxiety and chest pain, a wide variety of *physical* causal mechanisms have been proposed to explain symptom production in patients with chest pain and normal coronary arteries, including microvascular ischemia [47] and esophageal dysmotility and reflux [48]. In all probability, studies on the etiology of chest pain tend to show abnormalities in the organ system that is the special interest of the researchers [49]. This variety strongly suggests that the group as a whole is heterogeneous. Indeed it would be surprising if it were not, since it is defined solely by the occurrence of a common symptom, and the absence of a particular abnormality on investigation.

As well as heterogeneity, there is evidence of substantial overlap, so that several possible causes occur together. This was demonstrated by Cooke *et al* [50], who performed esophageal manometry and pH monitoring, exercise tests with end–tidal pCO2 measurement, and ratings of psychiatric morbidity. One–third of the patients had ST depression on exercise and two–thirds had hypocapnia either on exercise or during the recovery phase. Abnormal psychiatric scores were detected in 50% of the patients and nearly two–thirds had either esophageal reflux or dysmotility. 58% had two or more abnormalities, and esophageal abnormalities co–existed with hypocapnia in one–third and with psychiatric morbidity in one–quarter. Abnormal physiological and psychiatric findings were not associated with descriptions of pain as "typical" or "atypical".

These two features, heterogeneity and overlap, suggest that any attempt to link psychiatric abnormalities and presenting physical symptoms via unitary causal explanations will prove fruitless. It may be better, both in terms of theory and as a guide to management, to adopt instead an interactive model (see Figure 2). According to this view, psychological factors interact with organic factors in a variety of ways, leading to symptom production, consultation, and failure to respond to reassurance after negative investigation.

Community-based studies [51,52] show that chest pain is common in the ostensibly healthy general population, most of whom do not consult doctors for their symptoms: for example, 16% of 2717 healthy relatives of the Framingham cohort reported atypical chest pain [53]. The factors which determine who does and who does not consult are not well understood, but are likely to include personality differences [54], illness fears based on previous experience of illness in oneself or others, or concurrent psychological morbidity. Such psychological factors may act by heightening awareness of bodily sensations which would otherwise be ignored [55]. The sensations in question might be entirely normal (e.g. occasional ectopic beats) or based upon some minor organic abnormalities (e.g. mild esophageal reflux). As well as heightening awareness, psychological factors could act principally as selecting agents, so that those with anxiety disorders or particular personalities are more likely to respond to a given level of symptomatology by consulting doctors.

20

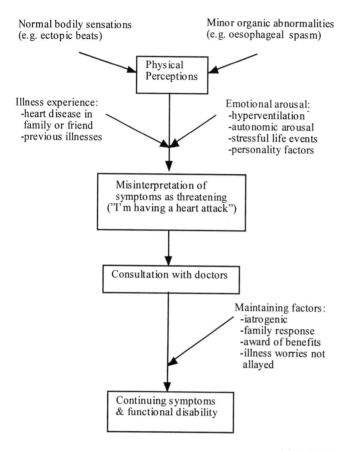

Adapted with permission from Mayou [56].

Figure 2. Proposed interactive model

Cognitive factors, particularly the tendency to "catastrophise", or misattribute innocuous bodily sensations to an imminently life-threatening organic cause such as a myocardial infarction or stroke, are claimed to be important in panic disorder [57], and there is evidence that they operate too in patients with chest pain and normal coronary arteries. Even after explicit reassurance to the contrary following angiography, many such patients continue to believe they have heart disease, especially during episodes of chest pain. Lantinga *et al* [58] found that one year after a negative angiogram, 25% of their chest pain patients believed themselves to have heart disease, while a further 42% remained unsure. Potts and Bass [59,60] found that as long as 11 years after angiography 44% of patients believed they had heart disease, while 17% remained uncertain. This tendency to misattribution has a number of effects. It is likely to heighten any pre-existing health anxiety, which may, in turn, magnify the original symptoms through the various mechanisms described above. It will also select patients for presentation to clinics, and therefore for further investigation.

The power of iatrogenic factors in maintaining symptoms should not be under-estimated. The very process of consultation and investigation may serve to confirm the patient's illness worries, and thereby magnify anxiety, which in turn perpetuates the symptoms. This will be particularly true if patients receive mixed messages. They will often attend cardiac clinics having already been given a diagnosis of "angina" on clinical grounds. If, after angiography, this label is abruptly removed without careful explanation, many patients will fail to be reassured: their worries about the cause of the pain will continue or may even grow worse, which again serves to perpetuate their symptoms. Alternative explanations or reattributions of pain are discussed further below. Any such explanation is likely to be undermined by the continued prescription of cardiac medication or attendance at cardiac clinics, both of which occur commonly in this group [58,59]. As well as the actions of doctors, social and psychological factors relating to the sick role, such as the payment of disability pensions, or family adjustments to the patient's limitations can act as potent factors to maintain symptoms [60].

The range and variety of the possible factors, both physical and psychological, which might be at work in any given case of chest pain and normal coronary arteries, is clearly very wide. Only an interactive model of the type put forward can accommodate them all: unicausal models are unduly restrictive.

Psychological consequences

There have been many follow–up studies of patients with normal coronary arteries (NCA) [See 35 pp.302-306 for review]. Most of these have characterized the extent of functional disability, and described the proportion of patients who continue to report chest pain and other physical symptoms. Relatively few have outlined the psychological and social consequences of a diagnosis of NCA.

About 75% of patients continue seeing a physician, 50% remain, or become, unemployed, and 50% regard their lives as significantly disabled. Only about 30% to 50% of the patients appear reassured that they do not have serious heart disease. About 75% (range 64–100%) report residual chest pain at follow–up. The proportion of patients in whom pain is unchanged or worse is more variable and ranges from 20–70% [35].

There have been very few studies of the psychological and social fate of these patients following coronary angiography. In a prospective study of 46 patients with normal (n=31) and near–normal (n=15) coronary arteries, 21 patients (46%) reported phobic symptoms and 13 (28%) were found by a standardized clinical interview to have psychiatric morbidity 12 months after angiography [61]. This had been evident at the time of catheterization in 28 (61%). The risk of having psychiatric problems at one year was proportional to the severity of the psychiatric disorder at the time of angiography. Furthermore, those patients initially considered to have high levels of psychiatric morbidity and raised neuroticism scores (a measure of "anxiousness"), were more likely to complain of chest pain one year after angiography. The 19 patients (41%) with persistent pain also had significantly higher levels of psychiatric and social morbidity at one year than the 27 patients (59%) whose chest pain had lessened during the follow–up period.

These associations between persistent chest pain and psychiatric morbidity have been confirmed by others [58], and there is a close relationship between residual pain and hypochondriasis (i.e. a patient's continuing belief that he/she has heart disease despite evidence to the contrary [62]). However, in studies of this nature it is not clear whether the psychiatric problems are secondary to the experience of pain or play a causal role.

Panic disorder occurs in 33–46% of patients with NCA [13,14,61]; and may account for some of the long–term problems seen in these patients. In a follow–up study of 72 patients carried out an average of 38 months after angiography, those patients with panic disorder (n=36) had significantly more disability at follow–up than did the other study patients [63]. In particular, they reported more continuing chest pain, worsening of health, greater reduction in exertional capacity, poorer social adjustment, more anxiety symptoms, and more psychological distress than those without panic disorder. A limitation of this study was that several other potentially relevant psychiatric disorders were not systematically examined.

In a cohort study of patients interviewed a mean of 11.4 years after coronary angiography, Potts and Bass [59,60] used standardized interviews and questionnaire ratings of psychiatric morbidity. Eleven year survival in the 46 patients was 91%, and continuing chest pain was reported by 74%. Chest pain outcome was defined by reported intensity and frequency as: good (no pain, n=11), poor (pain described as "severe" and/or occurring at least twice per week, n=16) or intermediate (pain not meeting criteria for poor outcome, n=15). The SCL-90R [64] was used to assess psychological morbidity. This is a widely-used self-report questionnaire, with several subscales, one of which is labeled *Somatization*, and includes 12 items referring to the experience of various physical symptoms within the previous week. Scores for these 12 items, plus another ("heart racing or pounding") from the *Anxiety* subscale for each of the chest pain outcome groups are shown in Figure 3. A poor outcome for chest pain was associated with reporting of other physical symptoms and with increased psychiatric morbidity, which for the entire cohort was higher than at one year after angiography.

Of the 40 patients who were interviewed after 11 years, 22 (55%) had at least one current psychiatric diagnosis. The SCID [65] was used to establish psychiatric diagnoses, and these are shown in Table 2. The most common diagnoses were again anxiety and depressive disorders (n=20), but it is important to note that 7 patients (18%) had a somatoform disorder, i.e. a more chronic, enduring disorder characterized by multiple somatic complaints and high utilization of medical care.

More recently, a five-year follow-up study of 90 consecutive patients previously admitted with acute chest pain found that levels of smoking, alcohol consumption and anxiety were all higher in those with non-specific as apposed to ischemic pain [66]. Levels of continuing chest pain and psychiatric morbidity were high in both groups, even though, in contrast to studies following up patients after angiography, the preponderance were male. Mayou *et al* also found, at 3 years, high levels of continuing physical and psychological symptoms, and associated disability, in an outpatient cohort with either non-cardiac chest pain or benign palpitations [67].

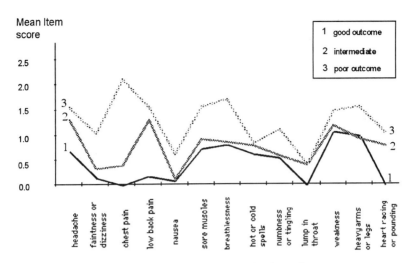

Figure 3. Mean scores on SCL-90R somatisation subscale items by chest pain outcome group

Table 2. DSM-IIIR diagnoses in 40 NCA patients at 11 year follow-up

ANXIETY GROUP:	n=14
Generalized anxiety disorder	3
Panic disorder without agoraphobia	2
Panic disorder with agoraphobia	2
Agoraphobia	2
Simple phobia	5
AFFECTIVE GROUP:	n=6
Bipolar II disorder	1
Major depression	3
Dysthymia	2
SOMATOFORM GROUP	n=7
Somatization disorder	3
Undifferentiated somatoform disorder	2
Hypochondriasis	2

22 of 40 patients had at least one current diagnosis: 27 diagnoses in total

Summary

These findings suggest that a substantial subgroup of patients with chest pain and normal coronary arteries will experience continued pain and incapacity associated with a number of other physical symptoms and psychological distress; that much of this is detectable one year after angiography [61]; and that it persists as long as 11 years later in spite of further medical attention [59,60]. The results of these and other follow-up studies [58,63] suggest that in many of these patients psychological distress makes an important contribution to the chronic pain and disability. If this is the case, then efforts should be directed towards the development of effective psychological treatments (see below), while not disregarding the search for alternative pathophysiological mechanisms for the pain.

Patient management

The interactive model set out above suggests that psychological interventions may be beneficial, whatever organic factors may be involved. Research attention is now moving from the simple demonstration of psychological abnormalities at angiography and subsequently, to trials of psychiatric interventions, both pharmacological and psychological.

Psychological treatment

There is accumulating evidence that psychological treatment is effective in the treatment of non-cardiac chest pain, much of it deriving from a group based in Oxford. Klimes et al [68] treated 31 such patients with persistent non-cardiac pain in a controlled trial of cognitive behavioral treatment (CBT). The average duration of pain was 4.7 years. Patients were randomized either to immediate treatment or to an assessment-only control group. Treatment involved teaching patients how to anticipate and control symptoms, and a modification of inappropriate health beliefs. The average number of sessions given was 7.2. There were significant reductions in chest pain, limitations and disruption of daily life, autonomic symptoms, distress and psychological morbidity in the treated group as compared with the control group who were unchanged. The assessment–only group were treated subsequently and showed comparable changes. Improvements were fully maintained by both treated groups at 4–6 months follow–up.

The treatment was acceptable to all patients, even those who were skeptical about the significance of psychological factors and approach to their complaint. The patients were assured that the physical state could, if necessary, be reassessed at the completion of treatment. Two patients referred with diagnosis of non-cardiac chest pain were diagnosed as suffering from ischemic heart disease during the follow–up stage of the study. One man was reassessed by the cardiac clinic and the diagnosis changed to angina; the other suffered a myocardial infarct during follow–up, having reported improvement during treatment. Both reported that they had found treatment helpful, and it is evident that psychological treatment of anxiety and atypical symptoms can be acceptable to those in whom there is diagnostic uncertainty.

Details of the treatment have been provided elsewhere [69], and are summarized in Table 3. Hyperventilation is a particularly powerful mechanism for the production of chest–localised bodily sensations that become subsequently misinterpreted by the patient as "evidence of heart disease or an imminent heart attack". There is no doubt that breathing retraining can play an important part in the treatment of some patients [70].

Table 3. Key elements in psychological treatment

1.	Explain the possible causal mechanism(s) e.g. stretching of chest muscles caused by hyperventilation (HV)
2.	Encourage patient to reattribute symptoms to non-threatening cause (e.g. muscle pain) by using HV provocation test, etc.
3.	Use breathing control and relaxation exercises to reduce anxiety and control symptoms. (Breathing control especially useful if patient has short breath–holding time, and when HV induces usual chest pain)
4.	Discourage reassurance seeking behavior and checking of body for signs of cardiac disease
5.	Counter negative thoughts and worries about heart disease by encouraging positive "self–statements"
6.	A graded, step-wise return to activity and exercise, where these are avoided because of chest pain, or the fear of it.

A recent Dutch pilot study [71] has also demonstrated the efficacy of CBT. A study carried out in Edinburgh has shown similar results with group treatment [72] and the Oxford group has recently built on their earlier findings. Mayou *et al* [73] conducted a randomized controlled trial comparing this CBT approach to routine cardiac care in a population of 37 patients assessed as having non-cardiac chest pain in a cardiac clinic (though 30 % did not undergo angiography). They demonstrated substantial improvements in frequency and severity of chest pain, mental state, and activity levels, associated with changes in the patients' beliefs about the cause of their symptoms. Most of these gains persisted, although less markedly, at 3 and 6 months follow up.

The authors noted problems with recruitment and retention in the study, with many patients declining to participate, and some dropping out, apparently because they found the approach "too psychological". Similar problems afflicted another study from the same group [74], which examined a brief intervention delivered by a trained cardiac nurse at, or shortly after, angiography in NCA patients, and found a disappointing lack of acceptability or efficacy, as compared with routine cardiac care. In reviewing this and other evidence [75], the authors argue for a stepped approach to intervention (see below).

Pharmacological treatment

Until recently, psychotropic drug treatment for non-ischemic chest pain was entirely grounded in clinical experience, with no evidence base to support it, and extended to the use of antidepressants (tricyclics and mono-amine oxidase inhibitors), anxiolytics (benzodiazapines), and beta-blockers. It was generally held that antidepressants were effective only when chest pain presented as part of a depressive illness or panic disorder, but in 1994 Cannon *et al* [76] showed that low dose imipramine (50mg daily) reduced chest pain by 52%in NCA patients, and that this effect was independent of baseline psychiatric morbidity. They speculated that at these doses, which are well below standard anti-depressant levels, imipramine exerted its effects by a visceral analgesic action. It is also possible that imipramine may act on *central* pain perception pathways, which preliminary Positron Emission Tomography evidence suggests may be overactive in syndrome X [77].

Imipramine and other tricyclic antidepressants have long been a mainstay in the treatment of chronic pain syndromes of all kinds. However they are poorly tolerated, with many patients reporting side effects, sometimes to unacceptable levels. Cox *et al* showed that while imipramine may improve chest pain it does not improve quality of life [78], and they speculate that is because of side effects. It is possible, however, that disability persists because the necessary cognitive and behavioral changes are not brought about by a drug treatment. There is a widespread clinical impression that NCA and other pain patients are more sensitive to side effects than other groups, but little firm evidence on which to base this view. Monoamine oxidase inhibitors have been used in a similar way in the past, but again evidence of efficacy is lacking. Attention is now shifting, as in other pain syndromes, to the use of the SSRI antidepressants. Trials currently being set up in Holland and the United States will compare the effects of SSRI antidepressants with those of a cognitive behavioral approach. Previous work in patients with depression suggests that the best approach may be a combination of drug and psychological treatment, especially given the high relapse rate on discontinuing imipramine [79].

Benzodiazepines appear to be more widely used in these patients in the United States than elsewhere, and in a trial of alprazolam, seven of eight chest pain patients without ischemic heart disease and with panic disorder experienced a fifty per cent reduction in panic frequency as well as decreases in anxiety and depression [80]. However, the trial lasted only 8 weeks and did not include a taper phase, and the drug carries the risk of dependence and withdrawal symptoms.

Although there have been no trials, beta-blockers may be useful in patients who have sympathetically mediated symptoms such as palpitations, trembling, and sweating in addition to the chest pain.

"Stepped" care

The growing awareness of the physiological heterogeneity within this population is now paralleled by recognition of the variety of psychological factors at play, in different sub-groups and at different stages, and the need for psychological approaches to investigation and treatment to be adapted accordingly. Chambers [81] argues that a general practitioner who assesses newly presenting chest pain patients under four headings (cardiac risk factors, quality of the pain, psychiatric risk factors, reason for consultation) can minimize unnecessary cardiology referral and subsequent investigation, with all that implies for iatrogenic aggravation of the presenting problem. Cooke *et al* [82] have shown that three simple clinical questions can discriminate effectively between NCA and CAD patients. Responses to the questions are classified into "typical" and "atypical" as follows:

	Typical	Atypical
If you go up a hill on 10 separate occasions, on how many do you get the pain?	10/10	<10/10
If you have 10 pains in a row, how many occur at rest?	<2/10	>1/10
How many minutes does the pain last	<5	>5

"Atypical" answers to all three questions are associated with a 2% chance of CAD in patients younger than 55, and 12% in those older.

There is continuing debate about the best approach to investigation and treatment once patients have been referred. Many centers operate, in a pragmatic way, a sequence of cardiology investigation, followed by esophageal investigation, followed by psychiatric referral. There are problems with this, however. Firstly, it draws out the investigation process, with the risk of increasing any iatrogenic aggravation of the underlying problem. Secondly, it reflects the sequential pursuit of a unicausal model, rather than the interactive model set out above: and thirdly, it makes it more likely that psychiatric referral will be resisted and resented by the patients, because it is introduced as a last resort. In these circumstances patients often feel disbelieved and dismissed. For such a referral to work, it is important to "prepare" the patient and to explain the reasons for referral. If this stage is not "negotiated" by the cardiologist it is likely that the patient will not accept the referral. A suitable opening gambit could be:

"I think it is possible that emotional factors or stress could be aggravating or contributing to your chest pain/breathlessness/fatigue, etc. I have a colleague who works in this hospital who has a lot of experience in helping patients with this type of problem. Would you like me to arrange for him/her to make you an appointment?"

Two other factors need to be addressed before psychiatric treatment can begin. These are (a) providing a plausible alternative explanation for the pain; and (b) withdrawing cardiac medication. The first is necessary because the patient will want to know the rationale for psychiatric referral. The explanation should be congruent with the patient's socio–cultural background and should provide new information, not merely explain to the patient that "the angiogram was normal so there is nothing to worry about". To be most effective reassurance needs to be both *negative*, removing a major threat ("your heart is fine") and *positive*, suggesting a non-threatening and treatable alternative cause ("It's cramp in your chest wall muscles, an abnormal breathing pattern/ spasm in your esophagus.") Patients are most likely to believe such alternative explanations, and therefore be reassured, if they can be presented with evidence, such as a breath-holding test which provokes the usual chest pain, a positive hyperventilation provocation test or abnormal capnograph recording, or abnormalities on esophageal manometry.

If the patient with non-cardiac chest pain has been taking anti–anginal medication before referral to the psychiatrist or psychologist, then this medication should be gradually withdrawn. This phase of management requires skillful handling, especially if the patient has been prescribed nitrates or calcium–channel blockers for months (or years) before referral. In effect, the therapist is inviting the patient to negotiate the transition from a "sick" to a "healthy" mode of living. This may be difficult for the patient who has already adjusted to the life of an invalid. Attempting to "undiagnose" angina is beset with problems [83]: prolonged unemployment and receipt of welfare payments increase the chance of the patient remaining in a sick role.

Mayou *et al* [75] have argued against a sequential referral, and for a greater integration of psychological and medical approaches from the outset of assessment. The relative emphasis will vary from patient to patient, and management needs to be flexible to reflect the psychological and organic heterogeneity referred to above. Thus a proportion of patients in cardiac clinics (perhaps 30% to 50%) will respond positively to simple reassurance after initial negative investigation. They will generally have minor symptoms of shorter duration. Those undergoing angiography tend to have longer lasting symptoms of greater severity. They are more likely to have been told they have angina, and to be on cardiac medication. These patients require preparation *before* angiography, especially where clinical features and risk factor profiles indicate a low likelihood of CAD. Preparation should include explicit discussion of the possibility that angiography will prove normal, and that psychological factors may be relevant. If this does prove to be the case, further discussion is required at the time of the negative findings, and at follow-up after six weeks or so. A cursory discussion, without follow-up, in an unprepared patient hours after a normal angiogram is likely to be incompletely and inaccurately recalled, misunderstood and ineffective. Indeed it is possible that misunderstandings may heighten the patient's anxiety and worsen the problem.

Even with careful discussion before, at the time of, and after angiography, some patients will continue to experience pain and other symptoms, and will remain disabled. It is this group for whom entry into a formal CBT program is likely to be most beneficial. It has to be recognized, however, that there some patients who will not engage with any attempt at psychological treatment, or for whom it proves ineffective. Where such patients pose continuing demands on medical services, by calling out their general practitioner, presenting to emergency services, and returning to cardiac clinics, a collaborative approach to management, involving the cardiologist, liaison psychiatrist and GP will be required, to limit repeated unnecessary admissions and investigations.

Chambers [81] makes a case for a multidisciplinary chest pain clinic, involving a cardiologist, psychologist or psychiatrist, and a gastro-enterologist. This may the best way of delivering the kind of flexible, stepped approach set out above, but, in practice, resource constraints make it more of a future development than a present reality.

Summary

There is no doubt that patients with NCA have high rates of psychiatric morbidity at the time of angiography, and that psychological and social problems continue after angiography in concert with disability and continuing chest pain in a substantial number of patients. In as many as 30% of cases these patients have a treatable psychiatric disorder, and another 30% have psychological problems which probably contribute to the continuing symptomatology. These psychological problems interact with a number of organic factors such as esophageal spasm/reflux, muscular tension and, in a small minority, microvascular angina. These interactions lead to the experience of chest pain and consulting behavior. Even in a patient without conspicuous psychiatric morbidity, the belief that the pain is coming from the heart (despite negative tests) can lead to excessive bodily preoccupation and maintenance of chronic pain.

We believe that studies that focus solely on an organic cause of NCA are likely to be unsatisfactory as well as costly. For example, in a study in which an organic diagnosis was established in only 11% of primary care patients presenting with chest pain [84], the estimated cost of establishing an organic diagnosis in each of the patients was US $4354. This figure is consistent with findings by Kaski et al [85] in patients with cardiac "syndrome X". A more plausible explanation, borne out by recent experimental findings, is that mechanisms of pain production overlap and interact. For this reason it is important to look for positive evidence of psychiatric disorder or abnormal psychological processes and address them early [86]: we have already emphasized that abnormal beliefs and illness worries can act as maintaining factors in patients with NCA whatever the initial etiology.

Psychological treatment is more likely to be effective if it is begun as soon after the negative angiogram as possible. If symptoms become persistent and the patient is allowed to develop chronic handicaps then the likelihood of responding to psychological intervention is reduced. We recommend that an assessment by carried out four to six weeks after negative angiography: some patients will have been reassured by the negative angiogram but others will not. Those with continuing physical symptoms and psychological problems may then benefit from the effects of psychological treatment before chronic and intractable problems develop. The benefits of early intervention are likely to lead to less distress and disability, as well as fewer iatrogenic complications and reduced utilization of costly medical resources.

References

1. Hartshorne H. On heart disease in the army. Am J Med Sci 1864;48:89-92.
2. DaCosta JM. On irritable heart: a clinical study of a form of functional cardiac disorder and its consequences. Am J Med Sci 1871;61:17-52.
3. Maclean WC. Diseases of the heart in the British army: the cause and the remedy. BMJ1867;i:161-164.
4. Mackenzie J. The soldier's heart. BMJ1916;i:117-119.
5. Freud S. On the grounds for detaching a particular syndrome from neurasthenia under the description "anxiety neurosis". In: The Standard Edition of the Complete Psychological Works of Sigmund Freud. Vol III Early Psychoanalytical publications 1894. London: Hogarth Press, 1962;90-115.
6. Lewis T. The soldier's heart and the effort syndrome. London: Shaw and Sons, 1918;
7. Culpin M. The psychological aspect of the effort syndrome. Lancet 1920;ii:184-186.
8. Wood P. Da Costa's syndrome (or effort syndrome). BMJ1941;i:767-851.
9. Jones M, Lewis A. Effort syndrome. Lancet 1941;i:813-818.
10. Craig HR, White PD. Etiology and symptoms of neurocirculatory asthenia. Analysis of 100 cases, with comments on prognosis and treatment. Arch Intern Med 1934;53:633-648.
11. Waxler EB, Kimbiris D, Dreifus LS. The fate of women with normal coronary arteriograms and chest pain resembling angina pectoris. Am J Cardiol 1971;28:25-32.
12. Bass C, Wade C. Chest pain with normal coronary arteries: a comparative study of psychiatric and social morbidity. Psychol Med 1984;14:51-61.
13. Katon W, Hall ML, Russo J, et al. Chest pain: relationship of psychiatric illness to coronary arteriographic results. Am J Med 1988;84:1-9.
14. Beitman BD, Mukerji V, Lamberti JW, et al. Panic disorder in patients with chest pain and angiographically normal coronary arteries. Am J Cardiol 1989;63:1399-1403.
15. Carney RM, Freedland KE, Ludbrook PA, Saunders RD, Jaffe AS. Major depression, panic disorder, and mitral valve prolapse in patients who complain of chest pain. Am J Med 1990;89:757-761.

16. Eifert GH, Hodson SE, Tracey DR, Seville JL, Gunawardene K. Heart-focussed anxiety, illness beliefs and behavioral impairment: comparing healthy heart-anxious patients with cardiac and surgical inpatients. Journal of Behavioral Medicine 1996; 19 (4): 385-399.

17. Serlie AW, Duivenvoorden HJ, Passchier J, ten Cate FJ, Deckers JW, Erdman RA. Empirical psychological modeling of chest pain: a comparative study. Journal of Psychosomatic Research 1996; 40 (6): 625-635.

18. Alexander PJ, Prabhu SG, Krishnamoorthy ES, Halkatti PC. Mental disorders in patients with non-cardiac chest pain. Acta Psychiatrica Scandinavica 1994; 89(5): 291-293.

19. Tennant C, Mihailidou A, Scott A, et al. Psychological symptom profiles in patients with chest pain. Journal of Psychosomatic Research 1994; 38(4): 365-371.

20. American Psychiatric Association . Diagnostic And Statistical Manual of Mental Disorders, Fourth Edition. Washington: American Psychiatric Association, 1994;

21. PSVT misdiagnosed as panic attack. Arch Intern Med 1997; 157: 537-543.

22. Fleet RP, Dupuis G, Burelle D, Arsenault A, Beitman BD. Panic disorder in emergency department chest pain patients: prevalence comorbidity, suicidal ideation, and physician recognition. American Journal of Medicine 1996; 101(4): 371-380.

23. Fleet RP, Beitman BD. Unexplained chest pain: when is it panic disorder? Clinical Cardiology 1997; 20(3): 187-194.

24. Yingling KW, Wulsin LR, Arnold LM, Rouan GW. Estimated prevalence of panic disorder and depression among consecutive patients seen in an emergency department with chest pain. J Gen Int Med 1993; 8(5): 231-235.

25. Katon W. Panic disorder: relationship to high medical utilization, unexplained physical symptoms, and medical costs. Journal of Clinical Psychiatry 1996; 57 suppl 10: 11-18.

26. Yasue H, Nagao M, Omote S, Tazikawa A, Miwa K, Tanaka S. Coronary arterial spasm amd Prinzmetal's variant of angina induced by hyperventilation and Tris-buffer infusion. Circulation 1978;58:56-62.

27. Bohlen HG. Arteriolar closure mediated by hyper-responsiveness to norepinephrine in hypertensive rats. Am J Physiol 1979;236:H157-H164.

28. Bass C, Cawley R, Wade C, et al. Unexplained breathlessness and psychiatric morbidity in patients with normal and abnormal coronary arteries. Lancet 1983;i:605-609.

29. Saisch SG, Wessely S, Gardner WN. Patients with acute hyperventilation presenting to an inner-city emergency department. Chest 1996; 110(4): 952-957.

30. Magarian GJ. Hyperventilation syndromes: infrequently recognised common expressions of anxiety and stress. Medicine 1982;61:219-236.

31. Rasmussen K, Ravnbaek J, Funch-Jensen P. Esophageal spasm in patients wih coronary artery spasm. Lancet 1986;i:174-176.

32. Chauhan A, Mullins PA, Taylor G, Petch MC, Schofield PM. Effect of hyperventilation and mental stress on coronary blood flow in syndrome X. Br Heart J 1993; 69(6): 516-524.

33. Chambers JB, Kiff PJ, Gardner W, Jackson G, Bass C. Value of measuring end tidal partial pressure of carbon diaxide as an adjunct to treadmill exercise testing. BMJ1988;296:1281-1285.

34. Lary D, Goldschlager N. Electrocardiographic changes during hyperventilation resembling myocardial ischemia in patients with normal coronary arteriograms. Am Heart J 1974;87:383-390.

35. Chambers JB, Bass C. Chest pain with normal coronary anatomy. In: Jackson G, ed. Difficult cardiology. Practical management and decision-making. London: Martin Dunitz, 1990;301-350.

36. Wise CM, Semble EL, Dalton CB. Musculoskeletal chest wall syndromes in patients with noncardiac chest pain: a study of 100 patients. Arch Phys Med Rehabil 1992;73:147-149.

37. Bass C. Unexplained chest pain and breathlessness. Med Clin North Am 1991;75:1157-1173.

38. Evans DW, Lum LC. Hyperventilation: an important cause of pseudoangina. Lancet 1977;i:155-157.

39. Bass C, Chambers JB, Gardner WN. Hyperventilation provocation in patients with chest pain and a negative treadmill exercise test. J Psychosom Res 1991;35:83-89.

40. Lindsay S, Saqi S, Bass C. The test-retest reliability of the hyperventilation provocation test. J Psychosom Res 1991;35:155-162.

41. Young LD. The effect of psychological and environmental stressors on peristaltic esophageal contractions in healthy volunteers. Psychophysiology 1987;24:132-141.

42. Richter JE, Bradley LC. Pathophysiological reactions in esophageal diseases. Seminars in Gastrointestinal Disease 1996; 7(4): 169-184.

43. Carter CS, Servan-Schreiber D, Perlstein WM. Anxiety disorders and the syndrome of chest pain with normal coronary arteries: prevalence and pathophysiology. Journal of Clinical Psychiatry 1997; 58

suppl 3: 70-73.

44. Peters L, Maas L, Petty D, *et al*. Spontaneous noncardiac chest pain: evaluation by 24-hour ambulatory esophageal motility and pH monitoring. Gastroenterology 1988;94:878-886.

45. Richter JE, Dalton CB, Bradley LA. Oral nifedipine in the treatment of non-cardiac chest pain in patients with the nutcracker oaesophagus. Gastroenterology 1987;93:21-24.

46. Clouse RE, Lustman PJ, Eckert TC. Low dose trazodone for symptomatic patients with esophageal contraction abnormalities: a double-blind placebo-controlled trial. Gastroenterology 1987;92:1027-1031.

47. Cannon RO, Camici PG, Epstein SE. Pathophysiological dilemma of syndrome X. Circulation 1992;85:883-896.

48. Alban Davies H. Anginal pain of esophageal origin: clinical presentation, prevalence, and prognosis. Am J Med 1992;92 (suppl. 5A):5S-11S.

49. Anonymous . The oesophagus and chest pain of uncertain cause. Lancet 1992;339:583-584.

50. Cooke RA, Chambers JB, Anggiansah A, Henderson RA, Sowton E, Owen W. Chest pain and normal coronary arteries: a clinical evaluation with esophageal function tests, exercise ECG, end-tidal CO_2 measurement and psychiatric scores. Eur Heart J 1991;12 (suppl):103.

51. Von Korff M, Dworkin SF, Le Resche L, Kruger A. An epidemiological comparison of pain complaints. Pain 1988;32:173-183.

52. Hannay DR. Symptom prevalence in the community. J R Coll Gen Pract 1978;28:492-499.

53. Savage DD, Devereux RB, Garrison RJ, *et al*. Mitral valve prolapse in the general population.2. Clinical features: The Framingham study. Am Heart J 1983;106:577-581.

54. Costa PT, Zonderman AB, Engel BT, Baile WF, Brimlow, DL, Brinker J. The relationship of chest pain symptoms to angiographic findings of coronary artery stenosis and neuroticism. Psychosom Med 1985;47:285-293.

55. Frasure-Smith N. Levels of somatic awareness in relation to angiographic findings . J Psychosom Res 1987;31:545-554.

56. Mayou RA. Patients fears of illness: chest pain and palpitations. In: Creed F, Mayou R, Hopkins A, eds. Medical symptoms not explained by organic disease. London: Royal College of Psychiatrists and Royal College of Physicians, 1992;

57. Clark DM. A cognitive approach to panic. Behav Res Ther 1986;24:461-470.

58. Lantinga LJ, Sprafkin RP, McCroskery JH, Baker MT, Warner RA, Hill NE. One-year psychosocial follow-up of patients with chest pain and angiographically normal coronary arteries. Am J Cardiol 1988;62:209-213.

59. Potts SG, Bass C. Psychological morbidity in patients with chest pain and normal coronary arteries: a long-term follow-up study. Psychological Medicine 1995; 25:339-347.

60. Potts SG, Bass C. Psychosocial outcome and medical resource use in patients with chest pain and normal coronary arteries: a long-term follow-up study. Quarterly Journal of Medicine 1993; 86: 583-593.

61. Bass C, Wade C, Hand D, Jackson G. Angina with normal and near-normal coronary arteriograms: clinical and psychosocial state 12 months after angiography. BMJ1983;ii:1505-1508.

62. Weilgosz AT, Fletcher RH, McCants CB, McKinnis RA, Haney TL, Williams RB. Unimproved chest pain patients with minimal or no coronary disease: a behavioural phenomenon. Am J Cardiol 1984;108:67-72.

63. Beitman BD, Kushner MG, Basha I, Lamberti J, Mukerji V, Bartels K. Follow-up status of patients with angiographically normal coronary arteries and panic disorder. JAMA 1991;265:1545-1549.

64. Derogatis LR, Lipman RS, Covi L. The SCL-90: an out-patient psychiatric rating scale. Psychopharmacol Bull 1973;9:13-28.

65. Spitzer RL, Williams JR. Structured clinical interview for DSM-III. New York: New York State Psychiatric Institute, 1983;

66. Tew R, Guthrie EA, Creed FH, Cotter L, Kiseley S, Tomenson B. A long-term follow-up study of patients with ischemic heart disease versus patients with non-specific chest pain. Journal of Psychosomatic Research 1995; 39: 977-985.

67. Mayou R, Bryant B, Forfar C, Clark D. Non-cardiac chest pain and benign palpitations in the cardiac clinic. Br Heart J 1994; 72: 548-553.

68. Klimes I, Mayou RA, Pearce MJ, Coles L, Fagg JR. Psychological treatment for atypical non-cardiac chest pain: a controlled evaluation. Psychol Med 1990;20:605-611.

69. Salkovskis P. Psychological treatment of non-cardiac chest pain: the cognitive approach. Am J Med

1992;92 (suppl 5A):114S-121S.

70. de Guire S, Gervitz R, Kawahara Y, Maguire W. Hyperventilation syndrome and the assessment and treatment of functional cardiac symptoms. Am J Cardiol 1992;70:673-677.

71. Van Peski-Oosterbaan AS, Spinhoven P, van Rood Y, Van der Does AJW, Bruschke AVG. Cognitive behavioural therapy for unexplained non-cardiac chest pain: a pilot study. Behavioural and Cognitive Psychotherapy 1997; 25: 339-350.

72. Potts SG Lewin, R Fox KAA, Johnstone EC Cay EL. Group psychological treatment for chest pain with normal coroanry arteries: a controlled trial. Submitted

73. Mayou RA, Bryant BM, Sanders D, Bass C, Klimes I, Forfar C. A controlled trial of cognitive behavioral therapy for non-cardiac chest pain. Psychological Medicine 1997; 27: 1021-1031.

74. Sanders D, Bass C, Mayou RA, Goodwin S, Bryant BM, Tyndel S. Non-cardiac chest pain: why was a brief intervention apparently ineffective? Psychological Medicine 1997; 27: 1933-1040.

75. Mayou R, Bass C, Bryant B. Treatment of non-cardiac chest pain: from research into clinical practice. Heart (in press) 1997;

76. Cannon RO, Quyyumi AA, Mincemoyer R, Stine AM, Gracely RH, Smith WB. Imipramine in patients with chest pain despite normal cornary angiograms. N Engl J Med 1994; 330: 1411-1417.

77. Rosen SD, Paulesu E, Camicii PG. Brain activation during chest pain. Data presented to Syndrome X summit,London 1997;

78. Cox ID, Hann CM, Kaski JC. Low dose imipramine improves chest pain but not quality of life in patients with angina and normal coronary angiograms. Eur Heart J 1998; 19: 250-254.

79. Cannon RO. The problem of myocardial iscaemia and strategies for chest pain management. Data presented to Syndrome X summit,London 1997;

80. Beitman BD, Basha I, Trombka LH, Jayaratna MA, Russell B, Tarr SK. Alprazolam in the treatment of cardiology patients with atypical chest pain and panic disorder. J Clin Psychopharmacol 1988;8:127-130.

81. Chambers J. Chest pain: heart, body or mind? J Psychosom Res 1997; 43 (2): 161-165.

82. Cooke RA, Smeeton N, Chambers JB. A comparative study of chest pain characteristics in patients with normal and abnormal coronary angiograms. Heart 1997; 78:142-146.

83. Dart AM, Alban Davies T, Griffith T, Henderson A. Does it help to undiagnose angina? Eur Heart J 1983;4:461-462.

84. Kroenke K, Mangelsdorff D. Common symptoms in ambulatory care: incidence, evaluation, therapy and outcome. Am J Med 1989;86:262-267.

85. Kaski JC, Rosano GM, Collins P, Nihoyannopoulos P, Maseri A, Poole-Wilson PA. Cardiac syndrome X: Clinical characteristics and left ventricular function. Long-term follow-up study. J Am Coll Cardiol 1995; 25:807-814.

86. Chambers JB, Bass C. Towards a confident diagnosis of non-cardiac chest pain. In: Creed F, Mayou R, Hopkins A, eds. Medical symptoms not explained by organic disease. London: Royal College of Psychiatrists and Royal College of Physicians, 1992.

Chapter 3

ESOPHAGEAL CHEST PAIN

John S de Caestecker

Esophageal chest pain has come under critical scrutiny recently [1]. Motility disorders in particular have fallen out of favor as a cause of chest pain [1-3], to the extent that chest pain of uncertain origin has now become a rare indication for esophageal manometry in the United States [4]. The reasons for this include changing perceptions about the relevance of the commonest manometric diagnosis, the so called "nutcracker esophagus" [2,3,5], the effect of stress on manometric parameters [2,6], the lack of response of chest pain to motility modifying drugs [7] and the finding in several studies employing prolonged ambulatory motility recording that chest pain events in patients with chest pain of uncertain origin are rarely accompanied by disturbances of esophageal motility [8-10]. Gastro-esophageal reflux (GOR) remains the single commonest disorder resulting in atypical chest pain [11,12], but it will continue to remain unrecognized and untreated without appropriate investigation: indeed, the importance of carrying out 24 hour esophageal pH monitoring in all such individuals, even those with manometric abnormalities, though proposed more than 12 years ago [11,12], has only gradually received acceptance [13,14]. Abnormal esophageal sensory perception is an emerging concept, with new conditions of hypersensitive, hyper-reactive [15] or irritable esophagus [16] being proposed. The value of provocation with esophageal acid perfusion [17] and pharmacological agents such as edrophonium [18] has been called into question. There is however a danger of allowing the pendulum to swing too far: it is premature to dismiss provocation tests and motility disorders entirely. The aim of this review is to provide a balanced overview with particular emphasis on the value of gastroenterological investigations in patients with chest pain of uncertain origin.

Who should have gastroenterological investigations?

It remains likely that "it is difficult to rescind a diagnosis of heart disease once it has been made" [19]. Thus, some investigators have taken the approach of carrying out ambulatory esophageal motility and pH studies in patients admitted to a coronary care unit (after a myocardial infarction has been excluded) [20] or early in the investigation of referrals to a cardiology clinic for recurrent chest pain [21]. The problem with the acute chest pain patients is, firstly, that the high incidence of apparently abnormal esophageal motility could simply reflect patient distress and anxiety at an early stage of an acute admission [6] and secondly, that it is recognized that many of these patients will only ever have a single episode of chest pain [22], so further investigation may not be appropriate. In the second case, although a high proportion of patients were found to have unsuspected esophageal abnormalities (particularly GOR) [21], some also had coexistent coronary artery disease and indeed one patient had a myocardial infarction during his ambulatory esophageal monitoring study! Nevertheless, the study highlights a fact established in earlier studies [12,23] that a carefully taken history including inquiry into specific esophageal symptoms is poorly predictive of the final diagnosis (cardiac or esophageal). Surprisingly, this is true even for highly specific esophageal symptoms such as dysphagia or odynophagia [12,23]. The reason for this may be that GOR is common among patients with coronary artery disease [24] and indeed both nitrates and calcium channel blockers used in treatment of ischemic heart disease (IHD) may increase it [24,25].

Can symptoms provide any guide? Certain symptoms are predictive of an esophageal disorder, such as pain severe in onset and continued as a background ache for several hours, variation in the degree of exercise producing pain, pain commencing up to 10 minutes after exercise has ceased and pain awaking patients from sleep at night [23]. However, the predictive value is imperfect [23]. In my view, it continues to be true that cardiological investigation should precede gastroenterological evaluation in most cases [26,27] though the intensity of cardiological testing must be governed by the degree of clinical suspicion. The pattern of further investigation is then best guided by the clinical features: there are many potential extracardiac causes of chest pain. The high incidence of specific abnormalities (to the apparent exclusion of others) found by enthusiasts highlighting a particular type of disorder, though likely a phenomenon of selection [28], should not deter the clinician from taking a wide and balanced view. Thus, musculoskeletal causes, including cervical [29] and thoracic [30] spine disorders, thoracic inlet syndromes [31] and chest wall pain [32] can usually be excluded by appropriate history and examination, while atypical presentations of common gastrointestinal conditions such as peptic ulcer [33], gallstones [34,35] and colonic (splenic flexure) gas entrapment [36] can be suggested by features in the clinical history, such as relationship to eating or to passage of stool and flatus, radiation of the pain to the back, and night waking.

In patients with no particular clinical clues, an esophageal diagnosis is still the commonest extracardiac disorder to be considered [37]. The symptom pattern will still guide investigation: for instance, where dysphagia is a prominent symptom, a structural esophageal problem or a motility disorder require exclusion.

What gastroenterological investigation is appropriate?

Endoscopy and barium radiology

In most cases, an upper gastrointestinal endoscopy will be appropriate. Not only can esophagitis be detected (though relatively uncommon among patients with chest pain and GOR [11,12] but other lesions such as peptic ulceration (which can present atypically with chest pain) may be seen. However, mere detection of esophagitis does not prove a "cause and effect" relationship with chest pain: it may simply be an "innocent bystander", as in the case shown in Figure 1. Nevertheless, such a finding would normally prompt a therapeutic trial of acid suppression. A hiatus hernia on its own is of no diagnostic value [38]. Barium radiology is not a particularly sensitive method of detecting GOR [39], but may be helpful where a motility disorder is strongly suspected. Although not as sensitive as esophageal manometry at detecting a motility disorder, demonstration of an abnormality by more than one technique strengthens the diagnosis [40]. The investigation must be carried out in a manner appropriate to examining esophageal motility (usually a video barium swallow in the prone position with swallows of liquid barium and a solid bolus such as bread [41]).

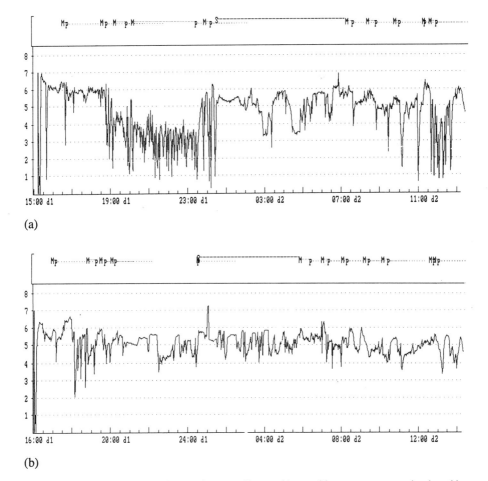

Figure 1. Two 24-hour esophageal pH tracings on a 43-year-old man with recurrent non-exertional crushing central chest pain. *x axis:* time of day in hours; *y axis:* pH scale; M = meal, p.... = postprandial period, S = sleep. Exercise electrocardiography was negative to stage 6 of the modified Bruce protocol. He had Savary Miller grade 2 esophagitis at endoscopy and trace (a) confirms excess acid reflux (% daytime pH<4 = 18.3%; % night-time pH<4 = 9.2%). However, his pain was unchanged on omeprazole. Trace (b) confirms that omeprazole has successfully abolished acid reflux, suggesting that his pain is not due to GOR.

Static esophageal manometry

Because motility disorders are not now thought to be an important cause of chest pain where this is an isolated symptom, esophageal manometry is not essential to the investigation of these patients [1]. However, it is still the best way to determine the lower esophageal sphincter location, essential to accurate placement of a 24-hour pH monitoring catheter [42]. Where dysphagia forms part of the symptomatology, manometry may still play a role. Some investigators believe that performing manometry during eating of bread aids diagnosis of motility disorders causing dysphagia [43]. Although recent doubts [44] have been cast on the value of accepted criteria for diagnosing diffuse esophageal spasm during static manometry tests [45] and the value of a diagnosis of "nutcracker" esophagus has been questioned [2-7], it should be recognized that manometric abnormalities such as the nutcracker esophagus may be a marker for a more marked abnormality such as diffuse esophageal spasm [5]. In general, the criteria proposed by Cohen some years ago for accepting a diagnosis of an esophageal motility disorder have much to recommend them [40]. These are summarized in Table 1.

Table 1. Criteria for diagnosis of esophageal motility disorder during manometry (after Cohen [40])

The motility event must be a major alteration in esophageal physiology, not a minor variation.

The motility change must be associated with a clinical symptom(s) of esophageal disease and be observed in temporal relationship with it.

The abnormality of esophageal function must be confirmed by some other independent measurement.

The symptoms or signs of esophageal abnormality must be improved if the esophageal abnormality is corrected.

Prolonged ambulatory esophageal motility recording

Prolonged recording of esophageal motility is not necessary in the majority of patients with chest pain of uncertain origin. The reasons for this are firstly that disordered motility detected by this method is uncommonly observed during episodes of spontaneous pain [8-10], and secondly that the abnormalities of motility are relatively minor, generally identified by observing values outside a reference range. The reference range can be that established by studying healthy controls, although it is clear that parameters for ambulant esophageal motility are very variable and dependent on posture, sleep, meals and drinks [46]. The alternative is to use asymptomatic periods from each patient as a control for the motility pattern observed during symptoms [47]. There are 2 provisos: the control period (meal period, postprandial, night-time etc.) should be appropriate to the period of symptom occurrence, and the optimum time window for examining the motility pattern related to symptoms is 2 minutes before the onset of chest pain ending at the onset of pain [48]. This is to reduce the likelihood that the pain itself influences the motility pattern through a stress response [2,6,49]. Using shorter baseline periods, such as 5 minute periods each hour on the hour or 10 minute periods immediately preceding the painful event have been tried, but the fact that the estimates of abnormal motility related to pain vary by a factor of 2.5 depending on which method is used does not encourage their adoption [50].

Recent evidence suggests that ambulatory motility monitoring is the best way of identifying diffuse esophageal spasm [44]. Barlow and colleagues propose stringent criteria for the establishment of this diagnosis [44] and report that the majority (13 of 16) of patients they found to have diffuse esophageal spasm also had dysphagia, with only 3 having chest pain as the sole symptom. It would therefore seem reasonable to withhold this test in all except those with additional dysphagia. These 16 patients were from among a group of 390 patients who underwent the test; 55 had diffuse spasm diagnosed by conventional manometry of which only 3 were confirmed by ambulatory monitoring. This implies a poor sensitivity and specificity for the criteria proposed for diagnosis of diffuse spasm during static manometry [45].

Provocation tests

Three established tests are still used, namely the acid perfusion test, the edrophonium test and esophageal balloon distension. All are subjective and depend on the patient recognizing the similarity of any provoked symptoms to those occurring spontaneously. Methods of performing the tests and their drawbacks have been reviewed elsewhere [51]. In my view, these tests remain useful at present in helping to both identify and specify an esophageal cause of chest pain although not all agree with this view [1]. It is usual to performed 12-lead ECG monitoring before and during all these tests.

Esophageal acid perfusion can identify an acid sensitive esophagus. This may be useful in 2 situations: firstly, among patients with proven GOR (either on the basis of endoscopic esophagitis or abnormal 24 hour esophageal pH monitoring), some may not develop symptoms during the period of monitoring to allow a correlation between pain and reflux events [52]. Others may only have 1 or 2 episodes of pain which makes a conclusion about the relevance of GOR to symptoms difficult (see below). Secondly, esophageal acid perfusion may identify an "irritable esophagus" [16] in patients without abnormal GOR [52]. For these reasons, I do not believe that this test has outlived its usefulness as some have contended [17].

The edrophonium test was originally introduced because it provoked abnormal motility in the same patients as ergonovine (ergometrine) [51]. With the recognition that the degree of motility change overlapped considerably with those found in healthy volunteers, it has been suggested that provocation of typical symptoms with the active agent but not saline should be the endpoint of the test without the requirement for changes in motility [53]. Work using balloon distension has suggested a mechanism of action of edrophonium through reducing esophageal wall compliance [54]. Doubt has been cast on the validity of the edrophonium test: firstly, some studies find a low yield of positive tests [9,10] and secondly there is evidence that the likelihood of a positive result is influenced by the patients' expectations [18]. Nevertheless, patients with a positive edrophonium test often have a positive acid perfusion test [55,56] and lowered esophageal sensory thresholds [57]. This is because a positive edrophonium test probably identifies some patients with an irritable esophagus [16] and may therefore have some value despite the limitations alluded to.

The balloon distension test was revived about 12 years ago [58,59] after a 30 year interlude resulting from the observation that patients with ischemic heart disease could not differentiate their spontaneous angina from the pain of esophageal balloon distension [60]. This objection is probably less of an issue once coronary artery disease has been excluded, but in the context of patients with chest pain of uncertain origin, it emphasizes the need for concomitant ECG monitoring. The technique and reproducibility of this provocation test has been clarified and fully reviewed [61]. The sensory endpoints, as for the acid perfusion and edrophonium tests, are subjective, but using this technique the concept, now widely accepted, of abnormal esophageal sensory perception has been proposed as a cause of chest pain [59]. Objectivity may be improved by observing failure of the normal inhibition of esophageal motor activity distal to balloon distension [15, 62] or by recording evoked cerebral potentials by EEG [63]. The latter technique in particular is difficult to perform and requires additional expensive equipment. Furthermore, although some differences have been reported between healthy controls and patients with chest pain of uncertain origin [64] the value of these observations to clinical practice has not been established.

Rao and colleagues [15] have used a modified balloon inflation technique termed impedance planimetry to calculate changes in electrical resistance through a weak saline solution with which the balloon is distended. Using this, they are able to calculate the diameter of the distending balloon (and therefore of the esophagus) and to measure esophageal wall tension and compliance. This technique has demonstrated a weakness of the balloon technique, namely that the diameter of the esophagus varies from patient to patient and therefore simple measurement of inflation volume required for the sensory endpoint is liable to be inaccurate [15]. This paper has also suggested mechanisms for chest pain: reduced sensory thresholds were accompanied by reduced esophageal wall compliance and greater reactivity (increased contraction at the level of the balloon distension) [15]. One interesting study has proposed that patients with chest pain provoked by balloon distension have an abnormally high belch threshold, such that esophageal distension with air which they are unable to dispel by belching, gives rise to their pain [65].

In summary, the acid perfusion test, edrophonium test and balloon distension test have all been criticized but I believe they still have an important role in the investigation of patients with chest pain of uncertain origin. The balloon distension test in particular may require modification in view of the findings discussed above.

Prolonged esophageal pH monitoring and other tests for GOR

There has been recent interest in the "omeprazole test" for diagnosing reflux-induced chest pain. This involves giving a high dose of a proton pump inhibitor, such as omeprazole 40-80 mg daily, for 1-2 weeks and observing the effect on symptoms. This test, using 60 mg of omeprazole for 7 days with crossover to placebo, has been reported to have a sensitivity of 82% and a specificity of 90% in patients with chest pain of uncertain origin [66]. However, there must remain some suspicion about the specificity of the test, since patients with functional upper GI disorders are known to have a high placebo response to treatment (30-60% in patients with functional dyspepsia) [67]. Furthermore, a proportion of patients (estimated at 10-30%) with proven GOR disease fail to suppress gastric acid production even on high doses of proton pump inhibitors [68-70]. For these reasons, and because patients requiring long-term acid inhibition (as many do) should have objective determination of GOR, the therapeutic trial is of limited value. Indeed it has been proposed that a longer period of 2-3 months is more appropriate for "diagnostic" treatment of patients with atypical GOR symptoms [27], which reduces the cost benefit of such an approach over esophageal pH monitoring.

Exercise-induced reflux has been shown to be associated with chest pain of noncardiac origin [71]. However, a recent careful study of 50 patients with exertional chest pain and normal coronary angiograms has found GOR-associated pain to be uncommon during esophageal pH testing with exercise [72].

Prolonged 24-hour esophageal pH monitoring remains the most sensitive tool for proving the relevance of GOR to chest pain and is in my view the single most valuable test a gastroenterologist can carry out in these patients. It will detect GOR in patients in whom barium radiology and endoscopy have been normal, as they frequently are in this group of patients [11,12]. Some recent studies have found a relatively low proportion of GOR among patients with chest pain of uncertain origin, but these have involved small numbers of patients [9,73] who may well have reduced their activities because the test was carried out on an inpatient basis [10,73]. Moreover, the method of relating GOR to pain events in the largest study [10] has been criticized [74]: time of acid exposure and reflux-symptom association were given as group rather than individual data, making it difficult to assess how many individuals did have GOR-associated symptoms. Other investigators emphasize the importance of carrying out this test [11-14, 20,21,56].

Twenty four-hour esophageal pH monitoring is best carried out on ambulant outpatients on a near normal diet. The data can be analyzed for the period of exposure of the distal esophagus to pH<4, using well-accepted control values to establish whether excess reflux has occurred [75,76]. The sensitivity of the test is improved by assessing the day and night-time separately [75]. Fortunately, most patients either have clearly normal or abnormal reflux, and an exact dividing line between normal and abnormal reflux is not critical [77]. The few patients who have values close to the upper limit of normal cannot be categorized solely on the basis of quantitation of GOR. In patients who develop no symptoms during the period of monitoring, the finding of excess reflux should lead to a trial of antireflux therapy (Figure 2).

The test also allows correlation of symptoms with reflux events. Where many chest pain events occur during the period of monitoring, it is possible to derive a "symptom index" to express the degree of association (or not) of reflux and symptoms. The temporal relationship between the symptom and the reflux event is crucial to this determination, and work of a group from the Netherlands suggests that the pain should occur during or within 2 minutes of the start of a reflux event [48]. The exact point at which a symptom index becomes significant is debatable, though a cutoff of a 50% association seems reasonable [78]; there exists evidence to support this cut off in respect of patients with heartburn, but a distinction is less clear in patients with chest

40

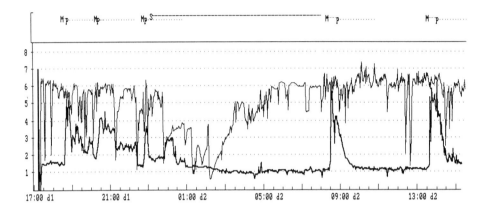

Figure 2. pH tracing from a 55-year-old man with anginal quality chest pain waking him from sleep. *x axis:* time of day in hours; *y axis:* pH scale; M = meal, p.... = postprandial period, S = sleep. The dark line is intragastric pH and the lighter line intra-esophageal pH. Dipyridamole thallium scan and endoscopy both normal. He had no symptoms but excess night-time GOR (% night-time pH<4 = 42%). His symptoms were abolished by use of a proton pump inhibitor.

pain [79]. If only 1 or 2 pain events occur, particularly if there are very frequent reflux episodes, it is difficult to be sure whether any observed association (or not) is simply due to chance. Therefore, some investigators have proposed statistical methods of relating symptoms to GOR which take into account these variables [56,80,81]. An example of the use of this technique is shown in Figure 3, which also illustrates the concept of the "acid hypersensitive esophagus" [82], characterized by acid-induced symptoms in the face of normal quantities of GOR. Statistical associations do not prove clinical relevance [83]: no-one has as yet validated any of the methods of determining symptom-reflux association against the results of acid suppression. My preference is to perform an acid perfusion test in addition to 24-hour pH monitoring in the situation where few or no symptoms occur during monitoring.

The concept of "linked" angina is addressed elsewhere in this book, but it should be noted that 24 hour pH monitoring frequently shows GOR to be a cause of atypical symptoms in patients with proven IHD [84,85]. Furthermore, it appears that reflux is not only common in patients with typical angina from IHD (perhaps in part due to the refluxogenic potential of anti-anginal medication [24,25]) but that GOR may contribute to the "pain burden" in these patients since some of them mistake the pain of reflux for their angina [24].

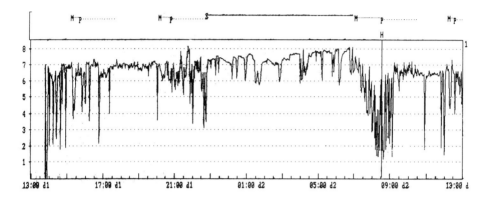

Figure 3. pH tracing from a 38 year old man with reflux-like symptoms but a normal endoscopy. *x axis:* time of day in hours; *y axis:* pH scale; M = meal, p.... = postprandial period, S = sleep. The amount of acid reflux is within the normal range (% daytime pH<4 = 4.8%; % night-time pH<4 = 0%). He developed his usual symptom once (marked "H") corresponding with a reflux event. The binomial symptom index [80] was 0.05, suggesting the association is not simply due to chance.

Summary: which tests?

I believe an endoscopy should be the initial investigation, supplemented by video barium swallow radiology and upper abdominal ultrasound in selected cases. The most important esophageal test to perform is 24-hour esophageal pH monitoring. In selected cases (usually with dysphagia) 24-hour motility studies can be carried out concomitantly. Static manometry appears to offer little benefit in these patients other than to localize the lower esophageal sphincter for accurate placement of the pH probe. Carrying out provocation testing is controversial, although I continue to believe that acid perfusion testing is a useful adjunct to 24 hour pH monitoring, and that both this and the edrophonium test may identify patients with an irritable esophagus, a diagnosis which has therapeutic consequences. Balloon distension testing may also identify such patients, but the accuracy of the technique as currently performed is questionable.

Treatment of esophageal chest pain

It is clear from recent follow up studies that the mere diagnosis of an esophageal abnormality does not reduce the long-term morbidity in patients with chest pain of uncertain origin [86,87]. In other studies, improvement in terms of less use of medical facilities and ability to return to work was confined either to small patient subgroups [88,89] or to highly selected patient populations [7]. It is clear that many patients do not accept or remember that an esophageal cause of chest pain has been found [87,88] or that, having accepted that an esophageal abnormality is present they still perceive their pain as cardiac in origin [86].

The targets for treatment have been aptly summed up by Goyal [1]: the chest pain may be caused by a true noxious occurrence in the esophagus itself, by a decrease in the threshold of the esophageal pain receptors or by disordered central processing in the nociceptive pathways - or ".... the sounding of a fire alarm in the case of a real fire, a sensitive alarm activated by smoke without fire, or a defective alarm, respectively". Candidate noxious occurrences in the esophagus include motility disorders and GOR. Treatment of abnormalities of motility such as nutcracker esophagus [7] and diffuse esophageal spasm [90] using calcium channel antagonists have been shown in controlled trials to be ineffective in the relief of chest pain. There is now one published controlled trial of the efficacy of proton pump inhibitors in patients with atypical chest pain due to GOR [91], other than one placebo controlled study of omeprazole as a diagnostic test [66]. Since proton pump inhibitors are the most potent suppressors of gastric acid secretion and the most effective agents in patients with typical GOR disease, there seems no a priori reason to believe this should not also be the case in those presenting with chest pain. Omeprazole is effective in patients without esophagitis [91], which is pertinent to most patients with GOR and chest pain. It should not however be assumed that failed response in a patient with proven GOR disease means that the symptoms are not due to reflux. Adequate suppression of GOR should be documented by performing additional pH monitoring on treatment (Figure 1) [68].

Abnormal sensory perception has been documented in the esophagus [15,59] and heart [92,93]. It is presently unclear to what extent these coincide in individual patients or whether the abnormality is one of defective central processing of sensory information from esophagus, heart or both. There is evidence that patients with lowered esophageal pain thresholds may have a generalized reduction in visceral but not cutaneous pain thresholds [92,95]. Some evidence has been produced to support the concept of altered central processing of sensory information from the esophagus [64,94]. There are no specific methods of altering nociceptor thresholds within the esophagus, although the recent demonstration that esophageal stretch receptors can be sensitized to painful distension by prior acid perfusion in patients without abnormal quantities of GOR [57] raises the as yet unanswered question of whether in some patients acid suppression could reverse this process. Other potential ways of modulating visceral afferent function are beginning to emerge. The specific peripheral opioid κ agonist, fedotozine appears to act directly on peripheral pain receptors to reduce the pain of gut distension [96]. Granisitron, a 5HT$_3$ antagonist, reduces rectal sensation to stretch in patients with irritable bowel syndrome [97]. Fedotozine is effective in reducing symptoms from gastric distension [98] unlike the 5HT$_3$ antagonist alosetron [99], implying that the former but not the latter may have therapeutic potential in painful functional foregut disorders. Both await evaluation in patients with functional chest pain.

Patients with chest pain of undetermined origin, some of whom have evidence of esophageal disorders, may respond to low dose antidepressant therapy [100,101]: in one trial, a high placebo response rate was noted and the beneficial effect on pain reduction did not appear to be associated with any measurable psychometric change, making a drug effect on pain perception possible [100]. This is presumed to be a central effect. In the other, improvement was associated with reduction in cardiac hypersensitivity [101]. Alternative therapies, such as gut-directed hypnotherapy which has been reported to have impressive effects in some patients with refractory irritable bowel syndrome [102], are beginning to be explored in patients with chest pain of undetermined origin [103]. There is clearly potential for some exciting therapeutic developments in the area of altering visceral sensory thresholds. Controlled clinical trials in both this area and the more traditional area of acid suppression in patients with chest pain would be welcome.

References

1. Goyal RK. Changing focus on unexplained esophageal chest pain. Ann Intern Med 1996;124:1008-1011.
2. Valori RM. Nutcracker, neurosis or sampling bias? Gut 1990; 31: 736-737.
3. Kahrilas PJ. Nutcracker esophagus: an idea whose time has gone? Am J Gastroenterol. 1993; 88:167-169.
4. Alrakawi A, Clouse RE. Change in esophageal manometric patterns over a 10year period parallels a change in referral indication. Gastroenterology 1997; 112: A57.
5. Dalton CB, Castell DO, Richter JE. The changing faces of the nutcracker esophagus. Am J Gastroenterol 1988; 83: 623 - 628.
6. Anderson KO, Dalton CB, Bradley LA, Richter JE. Stress induces alteration of esophageal pressures in healthy volunteers and non-cardiac chest pain patients. Dig Dis Sci 1989; 34: 83 - 91.
7. Richter JE, Daiton CB, Bradley LA, Castell DO. Oral nifedipine in the treatment of noncardiac chest pain in patients with the nutcracker esophagus. Gastroenterology 1987; 93: 21 - 28.
8. Peters L, Maas L, Petty D et al. Spontaneous noncardiae chest pain: evaluation by 24-hour ambulatory esophageal motility and pH monitoring. Gastroenterology 1988; 94: 878 - 886.
9. Soffer EE, Scalabrini P, Wingate DL. Spontaneous non-cardiac chest pain: value of ambulatory esophageal pH and motility monitoring. Dig Dis Sci 1989; 34: 1651-1655.
10. Frobert 0, Funch-Jensen P, Bagger JP. Diagnostic value of esophageal studies in patients with angina-like chest pain and normal coronary arteriograms. Ann Intern Med 1996; 124: 959-969.
11. Demeester TR, O'Sullivan GC, Bermudez G et al. Esophageal function in patients with angina-type chest pain and normal coronary angiograms. Ann Surg 1982; 196: 488 - 498.
12. de Caestecker JS, Blackwell JN, Brown J, Heading RC. The oesophagus as a cause of recurrent chest pain: which patients should be investigated and which tests used? Lancet 1985; ii: 1143 -1146.
13. Hewson EG, Sinclair JW, Dalton CB, Richter JE. Twenty four hour esophageal pH monitoring: the most useful test for evaluating noncardiac chest pain. Am J Med 1991; 90: 576-583.
14. Achem SR, Kolts BE, Wears R, Burton L, Richter JE. Chest pain associated with the nutcracker esophagus: a preliminary study of the role of gastroesophageal reflux. Am J Gastroenterol 1993; 88: 187-192.
15. Rao SSC, Gregersen H, Hayek B, Summers RW, Christensen J. Unexplained chest pain: the hypersensitive, hyperreactive, and poorly compliant esophagus. Ann Intern Med 1996; 124: 950-958.
16. Vantrappen G, Janssens J, Ghillebert G. The irritable esophagus - a frequent cause of angina-like pain. Lancet 1987; i: 1232 - 1234.
17. Hewson EG, Sinclair JW, Dalton CB et al. Acid perfusion test: does it have a role in the assessment of non-cardiac chest pain? Gut 1989; 30: 305 - 3 10.
18. Rose S, Achkar E, Falk GW, Fleshler B, Revta R. Interaction between patient and test administrator may influence the results of edrophonium provocative testing in patients with noncardiac chest pain. Am J Gastroenterol 1993; 88: 20-24.
19. Dart AM, Alban Davies H, Griffith T, Henderson AH. Does it help to undiagnose angina? Eur Heart J 1983; 4: 461 - 462.
20. Lam HGT, Dekker W, Kan G et al. Acute noncardiac chest pain in a coronary care unit: evaluation by 24-hour pressure and pH recording of the esophagus. Gastroenterology 1992; 102: 453-460.

44

21. Voskuil JH, Cramer J, Breumelhof R, Timmer R, Smout AJPM. Prevalence of esophageal disorders in patients with chest pain newly referred to a cardiologist. Chest 1996; 109: 1210-1214.

22. Wilcox RG, Roland JM, Hampton JR. Prognosis of patients with "chest pain ? cause". Br Med J 1981; 282: 431-433.

23. Alban Davies H, Jones DB, Rhodes J, Newcombe RG. Angina-like esophageal pain: differentiation from cardiac pain by history. J Clin Gastroenterol 1985; 7: 477 - 481.

24. Mehta AJ, de Caestecker JS, Camm AJ, Northfield TC. Gastro-esophageal reflux in patients with coronary artery disease: how common is it and does it matter? Eur J Gastroenterol Hepatol 1996; 8: 973-978.

25. Mehta A, de Caestecker JS , Northfield TC. Effect of nifedipine and atenolol on gastro-esophageal reflux. Eur J Gastroenterol Hepatol 1993; 5: 627 629.

26. de Caestecker JS. Chest pain with normal coronary arteriograms: esophageal abnormalities. The gastroenterologist's view. In: "Angina Pectoris with normal coronary arteries: Syndrome X" ed. J-C Kaski. Kluwer Academic Publishers, 1994; p 31-64.

27. Richter JE. Angina-like chest pain: heart, esophagus, or something else? Chest 1996; 109: 1139-1140.

28. Cannon RO. Causes of chest pain in patients with normal coronary angiograms: the eye of the beholder. Am J Cardiol 1988; 62: 306-308.

29. Wells P. Cervical angina. Am Fam Phys 1997; 55: 2262-2264.

30. Hamberg J, Lindahl O. Angina pectoris caused by thoracic spine disorders: clinical examination and treatment. Acta Med Scand 644 1981; Suppl.: 84 - 86.

31. Urschel HC, Razzuk MA, Hyland JW et al. Thoracic outlet syndrome masquerading as coronary artery disease (pseudoangina). Ann Thorac Surg 1973; 16: 239 - 248.

32. Brand DL. Chest pain of esophageal origin. In: Diseases of the esophagus. Eds Cohen S, Soloway RD. Pub Churchill Livingstone 1982; p. 137 - 159.

33. Long WB, Cohen S. The digestive tract as a cause of chest pain. Am Heart J 1980; 100: 567 - 572.

34. Ravdin IS, Fitz-Hugh T, Wolferth CC, Barbier EA, Ravdin RG. Relation of gallstone disease to angina pectoris. Arch Surg 1955; 115: 1055 - 1062.

35. Hampton AG, Beckwith JR, Wood JE. The relationship between heart disease and gallbladder disease. Ann Intern Med 1959; 50: 1135 - 1148.

36. Dworken HJ, Biel FJ, Machella TE. Supradiaphragmatic reference of pain from the colon. Gastroenterology 1952; 22:222-231.

37. Bennett JR. Chest pain: heart or gullet? Br Med J 1983; 286: 1231 - 1232.

38. Dyer NH, Pridie RB. Incidence of hiatus hernia in asymptomatic subjects. Gut 1968; 9: 696 - 699.

39. Sellar RJ, de Caestecker JS, Heading RC. Barium radiology: a sensitive test for gastro-esophageal reflux. Clin Radiol 1987; 38: 303 - 307.

40. Cohen S. Esophageal motility disorders and their response to calcium channel antagonists: the sphinx revisited. Gastroenterology 1987; 93: 201-203.

41. Alban Davies H, Evans KT, Butler F, McKirdy H, Williams GT, Rhodes J. Diagnostic value of "bread-barium" swallow in patients with esophageal symptoms. Dig Dis Sci 1983; 28: 1094-1100.

42. Mattox HE, Richter JE, Sinclair JW, Price JE, Case LD. Gastroesophageal pH step-up inaccurately locates the proximal border of lower esophageal sphincter. Dig Dis Sci 1992; 37: 1185-1191.

43. Howard PJ, Pryde A, Heading RC. Esophageal manometry during eating in the investigation of patients with chest pain or dysphagia. Gut 1989; 30: 1179-1186.

44. Barham CP, Gotley DC, Fowler A, Mills A, Alderson D. Diffuse esophageal spasm: diagnosis by 24 hour manometry. Gut 1997; 41: 151-155.

45. Richter JE, Castell DO. Diffuse esophageal spasm: a re-appraisal. Ann Intem Med 100: 242-245.

46. Smout AJPM, Lam HGTH, Breumelhof R. Clinical application of 24-hour ambulatory esophageal pH and pressure monitoring. Scand J Gastroenterol 1992; 27 (Suppl 194): 30-37.

47. Emde C, Armstrong D, Castiglione F, Cilluffo T, Riecken EO, Blum AL. Reproducibility of long-term ambulatory esophageal pH-manometry. Gastroenterology 1991; 100: 1630-1637.

48. Lam HGT, Breumelhof R, Roelofs JMM, Van Berge Henegouwen GP, Smout AJPM. What is the optimum time window in the symptom analysis of 24-hour esophageal pressure and pH data? Dig Dis Sci 1994; 39: 402-409.

49. Ayres RCS, Robertson DA, Naylor K, Smith CL. Stress and esophageal motility in normal subjects and patients with irritable bowel syndrome. Gut 1989; 30:1540 - 1-543.

50. Richter JE, Castell DO. 24 hour ambulatory oesophageal motility monitoring: how should motility data be analysed? Gut 1989; 30: 1040-1047.

51. de Caestecker JS. Esophageal provocation tests-techniques and interpretation. In: Clinical measurements in Gastroenterology - Vol. 1: Esophagus. Eds, Evans D, Buckton G. Blackwell Science Ltd, Oxford 1997; 10: 233-244.

52. de Caestecker JS, Heading RC. Acid perfusion in the assessment of non-cardiac chest pain. Gut 1989; Gut 30: 1795 -1796.

53. Richter JE, Hackshaw BT. Wu WC, Castell DO. Edrophonium: a useful provocative test for esophageal chest pain. Ann Intem Med 1985;. 103: 14 - 21.

54. deCaestecker JS, Pryde A, Heading RC. Site and mechanism of pain perception with esophageal balloon distension and intravenous edrophonium in patients with esophageal chest pain. Gut 1992; 33: 580 -586.

55. de Caestecker JS, Pryde A, Heading RC. Comparison of intravenous edrophonium and esophageal acid perfusion during esophageal manometry in patients with non-cardiac chest pain. Gut 1988; 29: 1029 -1034.

56. Ghillebert G, Janssens J, Vantrappen G, Nevens F, Piessen J. Ambulatory 24 hour intraesophageal pH and pressure recordings v. provocation tests in the diagnosis of chest pain of esophageal origin. Gut 1990;31: 738 -744.

57. Mehta AJ, de Caestecker JS, Camm AJ, Northfield TC. Sensitisation to painful distension and abnormal sensory perception in the esophagus. Gastroenterology 1995; 108: 311-319.

58. Barish CF, Castell DO, Richter JE. Graded esophageal balloon distension: a new provocative test for noncardiac chest pain. Dig Dis Sci 1986; 31: 1292 1298.

59. Richter JE, Barish CF, Castell DO. Abnormal sensory perception in patients with esophageal chest pain. Gastroenterology 1986; 91: 845 - 852.

60. Kramer P, Hollander W. Comparison of experimental esophageal pain with clinical pain of angina pectoris and esophageal disease. Gastroenterology 1955; 29: 719 - 743.

61. Johnston BT, Castell DO. Intra-esophageal balloon distension and esophageal sensation in humans. Eur. J. Gastroenterol. Hepatol. 1995; 7: 1221-1230.

62. Deschner WK, Maher KA, Cattau EL, Benjamin SB. Intraesophageal balloon distension versus drug provocation in the evaluation of non-cardiac chest pain. Am J Gastroenterol 1990; 85: 938 - 943.

63. DeVault KR, Castell DO. Esophageal balloon distension and cerebral evoked potential recording in the evaluation of unexplained chest pain. Am J Med 1992; 92 (Suppl 5A): 20S -26S.

64. Smout AJPM, DeVore MS, Dalton CD, Castell DO. Cerebral potentials evoked by esophageal distension in patients with noncardiac chest pain. Gut 1992; 33: 298 -302.

65. Gignoux C, Bost R, Hostein J et al. Role of upper esophageal reflex and belch reflex dysfunctions in noncardiac chest pain. Dig Dis Sci 1993; 38: 1909-1914:

66. Fas R, Fennerty MB, Yalam JM, Camargo L, Garewal H, Sampliner RE. Evaluation of the "omeprazole test" in patients with noncardiac chest pain. Gastroenterology 1997; 112: A730.

67. Talley NJ. Non-ulcer dyspepsia: myths and realities. Aliment. Phannacol. Therap. 1991; 5: 145-162.

68. Castell DO. Omeprazole works best when used properly. Eur J Gastroenterol Hepatol 1996; 8: 413-414.

69. Hendel J, Hendel L, Hage E, Hendel J, Aggestrup S, Nielsen OH. Monitoring of omeprazole treatment in gastro-esophageal reflux disease. Eur J Gastroenterol Hepatol 1996; 8: 417-420.

70. Katzka DA, Paoletti V, Leite L, Castell DO. Prolonged ambulatory pH monitoring in patients with persistent gastroesophageal reflux disease symptoms: testing while on therapy identifies the need for more aggressive anti-reflux therapy. Am J Gastroenterol 1996; 91: 2110-2113.

71. Schofield PM, Bennett DH, Whorwell PJ et al. Exertional gastro-oesophageal reflux : a mechanism for symptoms in patients with angina pectoris and normal coronary angiograms. Br Med J 1987; 294: 1459 - 1461.

72. Cooke RA, Anggiansah A, Smeeton NC, Owen WJ, Chambers JB. Gastroesophageal reflux in patients with angiographically normal coronary arteries: an uncommon cause of exertional chest pain. Br Heart J 1994; 72: 231-236.

73. Paterson WG, Abdollah H, Beck IT, Da Costa LR. Ambulatory esophageal manometry, pH-metry and Holter EKG monitoring in patients with atypical chest pain. Dig Dis Sci 1993; 38: 795-802.

74. Katz PO, Katzka DA, Castell DO. Chest pain and the esophagus. Ann Intern Med 1997; 126: 740.

75. Schindlbeck NE, Heinrich C, Konig A et al. Optimal thresholds, sensitivity and specificity of long term pH-metry for the detection of gastroesophageal reflux disease. Gastroenterology 1987; 93: 85 - 90.

76. Richter JE, Bradley LA, DeMeester TR, Wu WC. Normal 24-hr ambulatory pH values: influence of study center, pH electrode, age and gender. Dig Dis Sci 1992; 37: 849-856.

77. Schindlbeck NE, Ippisch H, Klauser AG, Muller-Lissner SA. Which pH threshold is best in esophageal pH monitoring? Am J Gastrocnterol 1991; 86: 1138-1141.
78. de Caestecker JS, Heading RC. Esophageal pH monitoring: what use and what limitations? Eur J Gastroenterol Hepatol 1991; 3: 285-287.
79. Singh S, Richter JE, Bradley LA, Haile JM. The symptom index: differential usefulness in suspected acid-related complaints of heartburn and chest pain. Dig Dis Sci 1993; 38: 1402-1408.
80. Johnston BT, Collins JSA, McFarland RJ, Love AHG. Are esophageal symptoms reflux-related? A study of different scoring systems in a cohort of patients with heartburn. Am J Gastroenterol 1994; 89: 497-502.
81. Weusten BLAM, Roelops JMM, Akkermans LMA, Van Berge-Henegouwen GP, Smout AJPM. The symptom-association probability: an improved method for symptom analysis of 24-hour esophageal pH data. Gastroenterology 1994; 107: 1741-1745.
82. Galmiche JP, Scarpignato C. Esophageal sensitivity to acid in patients with non-cardiac chest pain: is the esophagus hypersensitive? Eur J Hepatol Gastroenterol 1995; 7: 1152-1159.
83. Orr WC. The physiology and philosophy of cause and effect. Gastroenterology 1994; 107: 1898-1901.
84. Garcia PJ, Patel PH, Hunter WC, Douglas JE, Thomas E. Esophageal contribution to chest pain in patients with coronary artery disease. Chest 1990; 98: 806 -810.
85. Singh S, Richter JE, Hewson EG, Sinclair JW, Hackshaw BT. The contribution of gastroesophageal reflux to chest pain in patients with coronary artery disease. Ann Int Med 1992; 117: 824 -830.
86. de Caestecker JS, Bruce GM, Heading RC. Follow-up of patients with chest pain and normal coronary arteriography: the impact of esophageal investigations. Eur J Gastroenterol Hepatol 1991; 3:899 -905.
87. Rose S, Achkar E, Easley KA. Follow up of patients with noncardiac chest pain: value of esophageal testing. Dig. Dis. Sci. 1994; 39: 2063-2068.
88. Ward BW, Wu WC, Richter JE, Hackshaw BT, Castell DO. Long term followup of symptomatic status of patients with non-cardiac chest pain: is diagnosis of esophageal etiology helpful? Am J Gastroenterol 1987; 82: 215 - 218.
89. Lee CA, Reynolds JC, Ouyang A, Baker L, Cohen S. Esophageal chest pain value of high-dose provocative testing with edrophonium chloride in patients with normal esophageal manometries. Dig Dis Sci 1987; 32: 682 - 688.
90. Alban Davies FIA, Lewis MJ, Rhodes J, Henderson AH. Trial of nifedipine for prevention of oesophageal spasm. Digestion 1987; 36: 81 - 83.
91. Achem SR, Kolts BE, MacMath T, Richter J, Mohr D, Burton L, Castell DO. Effects of omeprazole versus placebo in treatment of non-cardiac chest pain and gastroesophageal reflux. Dig Dis Sci 1997;42:2138-2145.
92. Cannon RO, Quyyumi AA, Schenke WH *et al.* Abnormal cardiac sensitivity in patients with chest pain and normal coronary arteries. J Am Coll Cardiol 1990; 16: 1359 -1366.
93. Chauhan A, Mullins PA, Thuraisingham SI, Taylor G, Petch MC, Schofield PM. Abnormal cardiac pain perception in syndrome X. J Am Coll Cardiol 1994; 24:329-335.
94. Frobert O, Arendt-Nielsen L, Bak P, Funch-Jensen P, Bagger JP. Pain perception and brain evoked potentials in patients with angina despite normal coronary angiograins. Heart 1996; 75: 436-441.
95. Trimble KC, Farouk R, Pryde A, Douglas S, Heading RC. Heightened visceral sensation in functional gastrointestinal disease is not site-specific: evidence for a generalised disorder of gut sensitivity. Dig Dis Sci 1995; 40: 1607-1613.
96. Junien JL, Riviere P. Review article: the hypersensitive gut - peripheral kappa agonists as a new pharmacological approach. Alim Pharmacol Therap 1995; 9: 117-126.
97. Prior A, Read NW. Reduction of rectal sensitivity and postprandial motility by granisitron, a 5HT$_3$ receptor antagonist, in subjects with irritable bowel syndrome (IBS). Aliment Phannacol Therap 1993; 7: 175-180.
98. Coffin B, Bouhassira D, Chollet R *et al.* Effect of the kappa agonist fedotozine on perception of gastric distension in healthy humans. Aliment Pharmacol Therap 1996; 10: 919-926.
99. Zerbib F, Bruley des Varannes S, Oriola RC *et al.* Alosetron does not affect the visceral perception of gastric distension in healthy subjects. Aliment PharTnacol Therup 1994; 8: 403-407.
100. Clouse RE, Lustman PJ, Eckert TC, Ferney DM, Griffith LS. Low dose trazidone for symptomatic patients with esophageal contraction abnormalities: a double-blind, placebo-controlled trial. Gastroenterology 1987; 92: 1027 -1036.
101. Cannon RO, Quyyumi AA, Mincemoyer R *et al.* Imipramine in patients with chest pain despite normal coronary angiograms. New Eng J Med 1994; 330: 1411 1417.

102. Houghton LA, Francis CY. Use of hypnotherapy in gastrointestinal disorders. Eur J Gastroenterol Hepatol 1996; 8: 525-529.
103. Pace F, Molteni P, Bollani S, Bianchi Porro G. Hypnotherapy in the treatment of noncardiac chest pain: report of three cases. Gastroenterology 1997; 112: A249.

Chapter 4

ESOPHAGEAL ABNORMALITIES AND "LINKED-ANGINA" IN SYNDROME X

Anoop Chauhan

Approximately 10-30% of patients undergoing coronary angiography for the investigation of chest pain have normal coronary arteries [1-3]. Patients with angina pectoris and normal coronary angiogram who also have a positive exercise test are often defined as "syndrome X". The spectrum of current controversy regarding the pathophysiology of syndrome X is wide [4,5]. Many syndrome X patients have an abnormal coronary flow reserve (microvascular angina) which provides support for an ischemic basis for this syndrome. However, many patients also have esophageal dysfunction. Esophageal abnormalities, which have been commonly reported in patients with chest pain and normal coronary arteries [6-8], can cause symptoms that closely mimic the chest pain produced by coronary artery disease, due to the common innervation of the heart and the esophagus. This chapter will focus on the relationship between cardiac and esophageal chest pain. The content of this work will be based on a prospective study that we carried out to ascertain the relative prevalence of abnormalities of esophageal function (motility and reflux disorders) and coronary flow reserve in strictly characterized syndrome X patients.

Esophageal dysfunction and coronary blood flow reserve study

We studied 32 syndrome X patients, defined as typical anginal chest pain, normal coronary arteriograms and a positive ECG response to exercise testing. All patients underwent esophageal manometry tests, 24 hour pH monitoring, and coronary flow reserve studies. The left ventricle and the coronary arteries were completely normal on angiography and this was confirmed by two independent observers. Patients with hypertension, diabetes mellitus and valvular heart disease were excluded from the study. Echocardiographic assessment was also performed in all patients. Cross sectional and M mode assessment of the left ventricular posterior wall and septal thickness was made. Patients with a diastolic septal or posterior wall thickness of more than 11 mm were excluded from the study to minimize any effect of left ventricular hypertrophy on coronary flow measurements.

Cardiac catheterization protocol

All the patients were fasted overnight for their cardiac catheter study and all cardiac medications were stopped for at least 48 hours. Coronary angiography was performed by the Judkins technique through the right femoral artery in all patients and coronary blood flow measurements were obtained as detailed in our previous studies [9,10]. A 3.6F 20 Mega Hertz Doppler-tipped catheter (Schneider, UK) was positioned in the proximal segment of the left anterior descending coronary artery and was connected to a Millar velocimeter (Model MDV-20, Millar Instruments, Houston, Texas). Baseline mean resting and phasic coronary blood flow velocity were then recorded. After an initial 2 mg intracoronary test dose of papaverine hydrochloride through the guide catheter, further injections of up to 14 mg of papaverine (2 mg per ml in 0.9% saline) were given in 2 mg increments until maximum flow was achieved. The hyperemic response was recorded in the form of maximum mean and phasic blood flow velocity.

Coronary Flow Reserve

Coronary flow reserve was defined as the ratio of mean flow velocity achieved at peak hyperemia to the mean resting flow velocity. An impaired coronary flow reserve was defined as < 3.0.

Esophageal function tests

A multi-sensor catheter (Gaeltec, Scotland, diameter 2.5 mm) was passed into the esophagus. This probe has six mounted microtransducers spaced at 5 cm intervals from the tip. This was connected to a GR 800 analyzing station and signals were displayed on a screen and stored in the computer for analysis. Peristaltic activity was assessed with 5 wet and dry swallows, each separated by a 30-second interval. Patients were asked to report any chest pain and to distinguish whether the pain was typical or atypical of their usual pain. After the baseline study, edrophonium hydrochloride (80µg/Kg) was administered intravenously followed immediately by 5 wet swallows. Manometric responses were recorded for later analysis. Criteria for abnormal esophageal function were defined as:
1) Achalasia: aperistalsis of the esophageal body with incomplete lower esophageal sphincter relaxation and elevated lower esophageal sphincter pressure equal to or greater than 26 mmHg;
2) Nutcracker Esophagus: mean peristaltic amplitude, measured with the catheter lumen 3 or 8 cm above the lower esophageal sphincter, of equal to or greater than 180 mmHg averaged over 5 wet swallows;
3) Diffuse esophageal spasm: repetitive, spontaneous, non-peristaltic contractions in at least 30% of contractions, with otherwise normal peristalsis;
4) Non-specific motility disorder: prolonged duration of esophageal contraction (greater than 7 seconds) and/or isolated repetitive contractions after wet swallows.

Esophageal pH monitoring

Twenty-four hour pH monitoring of the distal esophagus was performed following the manometry in all patients. An ambulatory pH recorder unit (Gaeltec Research, type PH100) was connected to the pH replay unit (GR 800 system, Gaeltec Research, Ross-shire, Scotland). The pH electrode was positioned 5 cms above the lower esophageal sphincter the position of which had been determined during the manometry study and recording was commenced.

Gastro-esophageal reflux was defined as a fall in distal esophageal pH to less than 4 for more than 10 seconds. Abnormal reflux during 24 hour recording period was present when esophageal pH was < 4 for more than 5.5% of the study period [11]. A "pH score" was also calculated as described by Johnson and DeMeester.12 A score greater than 21.3 was considered abnormal [6,12].

Treadmill exercise testing

Patients underwent symptom-limited treadmill exercise testing (Bruce protocol) during esophageal pH monitoring. The onset and termination of the exercise test was recorded and it was determined whether or not gastro-esophageal reflux (pH less than 4) occurred during exercise testing. It was noted whether or not the patients experienced chest pain during treadmill exercise testing and whether this pain was typical of their usual pain. It was also noted if there were any ECG changes.

Results

Coronary flow reserve study

The coronary flow reserve was normal in 19 patients (4.3 ± 1.1). The coronary flow reserve was < 3.0 in 13 patients (41%). There were no significant changes in heart rate and mean arterial pressure before and after intracoronary papaverine injections.

Esophageal manometry

Table 1. Esophageal manometry abnormalities in syndrome X patients *

Manometric abnormality	Number of patients
Nutcracker esophagus	4
Repetitive contractions	7
Simultaneous contractions	3
Prolonged duration of contractions	5
Hypertensive lower esophageal sphincter	1
Positive edrophonium challenge	6
No other abnormality	2
Prolonged duration	1
Simultaneous contractions	1
Nutcracker esophagus	2

* Total of 12 patients out of 32 with esophageal dysmotility

Twelve (38%) syndrome X patients had esophageal manometric abnormalities (Table 1). The commonest abnormality observed was repetitive contractions which occurred in 7 (22%) patients. Figure 1 demonstrates an example of nutcracker esophagus developing in response to wet swallows in a syndrome X patient.

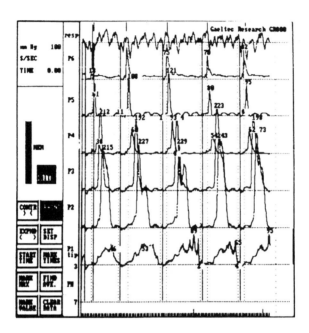

Figure 1. An example of nutcracker esophagus on manometry after wet swallows. This produced symptoms typical of angina. The mean amplitude of contraction in the lower esophagus was 237.4 mmHg.

Esophageal pH studies

Table 2 shows the results of the 24 hour pH score and the results of the treadmill test. Seven out of the 32 syndrome X patients (group 1) had an abnormally high 24 hour esophageal pH score. Six of these demonstrated gastro-esophageal reflux during treadmill exercise testing which was associated with their usual chest pain. A further 10 patients demonstrated exercise-induced gastro-esophageal reflux but did not reflux significantly at other times (group 2). The remaining 15 patients (group 3) had a normal 24 hour esophageal pH score and did not have gastro-esophageal reflux during exercise testing.

The 17 patients in groups 1 and 2 were considered to have gastro-esophageal reflux disease. The mean lower esophageal sphincter pressure of patients in group 3 (20.3 ± 9.9 mmHg) was significantly higher than that of patients in group 1 and 2 (13.3 ± 2.5; p <0.01). There was no difference in the mean lower esophageal sphincter pressure between patients in group 1 (14 ± 2.4 mmHg) and group 2 (12.8 ± 2.6).

Table 2. 24 hour pH score and exercise-induced gastro-esophageal reflux in syndrome X patients

	Group 1 n = 7	Group 2 n = 10	Group 3 n = 15
24 hour pH score	61.9 ± 22.4 *	14.9 ± 8.2	15.8 ± 8.7
Exercise test			
No chest pain / no reflux	0	0	4
Chest pain / no reflux	1	0	11
No chest pain / reflux	0	0	0
Chest pain / reflux	6	10	0

Group 1 = Patients with abnormally high 24 hour esophageal pH score
Group 2 = Normal esophageal pH score. Exertional gastro-esophageal reflux coincident with chest pain
Group 3 = Normal esophageal pH score. No exertional gastro-esophageal reflux
* significantly different from groups 2 and 3 (p<0.01)

Coronary flow reserve and esophageal dysfunction

Table 3 shows the prevalence of esophageal motility disorders and gastro-esophageal reflux in syndrome X patients with an impaired coronary flow reserve and in patients with a normal flow reserve. There was no significant difference in the prevalence of esophageal disorders in patients with impaired coronary flow reserve and patients with a normal coronary flow reserve.

Table 3. Coronary flow reserve and esophageal disorders in syndrome X

	Impaired CFR n = 13	Normal CFR n = 19
Motility abnormality	4	8
Abnormal pH score	2	5
GOR disease	7	10
Abnormal motility and GOR disease	3	5
Normal motility and pH study	5	6
Total no. of patients with esophageal abnormality	8 (62%)	13 (68%)

CFR = coronary flow reserve (Normal ≥ 3.0)
GOR = gastro-esophageal reflux disease (patients with a high 24 hour pH score or exertional reflux

Esophagus and syndrome X

This study demonstrated that approximately 41% of syndrome X patients had an impaired coronary flow reserve indicating microvascular dysfunction and 66% had an abnormality of esophageal function indicating that the esophagus may be an important source of pain in these patients. Twenty six (81%) of the 32 syndrome X patients in this study had either an abnormal coronary flow reserve or an esophageal abnormality. This was the first study to compare coronary flow reserve, esophageal motility, and esophageal reflux in the same syndrome X patients. The findings of our study suggest that an impaired coronary flow reserve, abnormal esophageal motility, or gastro-esophageal reflux disease may provide a pathophysiological basis for chest pain in over 80% of the syndrome X patients investigated in this study, thus highlighting the heterogeneous nature of this syndrome.

Syndrome X and "linked angina"

Clinicians have long suspected that esophageal disease may aggravate myocardial ischemia. Smith and Papp [13], coined the term "linked angina" which implies that gastrointestinal factors can bring on attacks of genuine angina in patients with established coronary artery disease. A high prevalence of esophageal abnormalities in syndrome X raises the possibility that myocardial ischemia may occur as a result of "linked angina". This may be of particular importance in patients who have an impaired coronary flow reserve. Figure 2 demonstrates an example of the possible association of esophageal reflux and ECG changes in a syndrome X patient associated with symptoms of typical angina and lends support to this hypothesis.

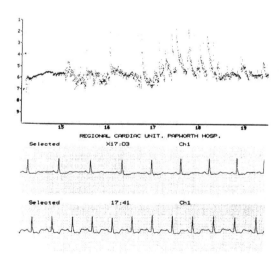

Figure 2. An example of esophageal reflux producing typical angina and ECG changes in a syndrome X patient. A) 24 hour pH recording. Frequent episodes of esophageal reflux associated with typical anginal chest pain developed during 1700 and 1830 hours. B) The ECG at 1703 hours was unchanged as compared to the baseline recording. C) the ECG tracing at 1741 hours is clearly ischemic.

We have shown previously that esophageal acid stimulation can produce typical angina in syndrome X patients which is associated with a reflex decrease in coronary blood flow [9]. We therefore further investigated the hypothesis that esophageal acid stimulation reduces coronary blood flow in syndrome X patients as a result of the presence of a cardio-esophageal reflex which may provide a mechanism for "linked angina".

Patients

The effect of esophageal stimulation on coronary blood flow was studied in 35 patients with syndrome X (14 males) and 24 patients (21 males) with heart transplants. All syndrome X patients gave a history of chest pain typical of angina pectoris and had a positive exercise electrocardiogram with completely normal coronary arteries on angiography as confirmed by two independent observers. All transplant patients were more than one year after their heart transplant operation. None of these patients had chest pain. There were no ischemic changes on exercise testing in these patients. Coronary flow studies were performed at the time of their routine follow-up cardiac catheter. In all transplant patients the coronary angiograms were also reviewed prior to the study by two independent observers and only patients with completely normal coronary arteries were included in the study. Patients with hypertension, diabetes mellitus, valvular heart disease or left ventricular hypertrophy were excluded from the study.

Patients were fasted overnight for their cardiac catheter. All cardiac medications had been stopped for 48 hours. A soft, fine bore nasogastric tube was introduced through the nose after the nasopharynx had been sprayed with Lignocaine. The distal tip of the tube was positioned at a distance of 35 cm from the nose. Coronary blood flow velocity was measured using a monorail 3.6F 20 Mega Hertz Doppler-tipped catheter (Schneider, UK) positioned in the proximal segment of the left anterior descending coronary artery as described previously [9,10]. Baseline mean resting and phasic coronary blood flow velocity were then recorded. Patients were instructed before the study to report any chest pain.

Esophageal stimulation protocol

After the baseline recording of resting coronary flow velocity had been performed, esophageal stimulation with 0.1M hydrochloric acid was commenced through the previously positioned nasogastric tube. A volume of 60 ml was given over 5 minutes. After the infusion, coronary flow velocity was measured again. It was noted whether the patients experienced any chest pain and if this was typical of their usual pain (syndrome X group). As required by the protocol, the infusion was stopped immediately if patient's typical chest pain occurred or if the coronary blood flow velocity decreased by > 50%. Quantitative coronary angiography was performed immediately before and after the esophageal infusions in all patients once the coronary flow measurements had been recorded.

Results

Twenty (57%) patients in the syndrome X group experienced their typical chest pain on esophageal acid stimulation. No patient in the transplant group reported any chest pain with acid esophageal stimulation. There were no significant changes in heart rate, the systolic arterial pressure, and the rate pressure product on esophageal stimulation in both groups. Esophageal acid stimulation in the syndrome X group produced a significant reduction in coronary blood flow from 78.9 ± 36.4 to 50.8 ± 32.9 ml/min (p $= 0.0001$, Figure 3). In the transplant group the resting coronary blood flow was unaffected by the acid infusion (Figure 3).

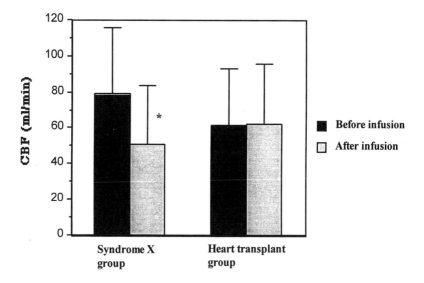

Figure 3. The effect of acid infusion on coronary blood flow in syndrome X and heart transplant patients. CBF, coronary blood flow. *p = 0.0001

The group of syndrome X patients who had chest pain with acid esophageal stimulation were then compared to those syndrome X patients who did not experience their typical anginal chest pain. Twenty patients experienced their typical chest pain on acid infusion. There were no significant differences in systemic hemodynamics. The coronary flow decreased from 85.3 ± 34.3 to 35.7 ± 16 ml/min (p = 0.0001, Figure 4). Fifteen patients did not experience any chest pain on acid infusion. There were no significant changes in heart rate, systolic arterial pressure, and the rate pressure product. The coronary flow also did not alter significantly (Figure 4).

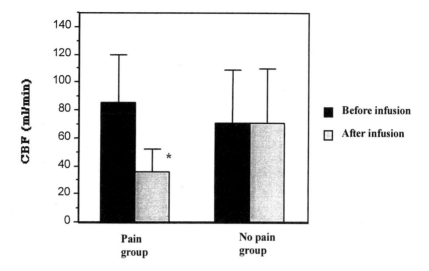

Figure 4. The effect of acid infusion on coronary blood flow in syndrome X patients with and without chest pain during acid infusion. CBF, coronary blood flow. *p = 0.0001

"Linked angina"?

The esophagus is a notorious mimic of cardiac pain as discussed by J. de Caestecker in another chapter of this book [14]. Esophageal pain may be indistinguishable from cardiac pain and may lead to a mistaken diagnosis of "angina". The relation between cardiac and esophageal pain is complicated by the high rate of electrocardiographic abnormalities in some group of patients with esophageal disease [15,16]. The observations that esophageal stimulation can produce cardiovascular effects complicates matters further [17-21]. Instillation of acid into the esophagus has been shown to significantly reduce the exertional angina threshold in patients with coronary artery disease [22]. There is also evidence that patients with angina brought on by esophageal stimulation with acid are especially likely to proceed to myocardial infarction [18].

The esophagus and the heart share a common innervation and there does exist a possibility that esophageal stimulation may exert an influence on the coronary circulation. Evidence for an association between esophageal disorders, vagal tone, and cardiac effects in support of a cardio-esophageal reflex is also provided by several studies [23-26]. Although a resting parasympathetic coronary vasodilator tone had not been demonstrated in humans, previous studies had suggested that coronary arteries may be constricted by vasomotor nervous impulses transmitted by the vagus nerve. It has been shown in dog experiments that coronary flow may be reduced by distension of the stomach or abdominal cavity [27]. This reduction in flow does not occur after vagal section or after the administration of atropine suggesting reflex coronary vasoconstriction initiated by vagal irritation in the gastrointestinal tract. Gilbert *et al* [28], have shown that, despite a small increase in blood pressure, flow through the circumflex coronary artery in the dog decreased by a quarter when a balloon was inflated in the gastro-esophageal area. This effect could be abolished by atropine or vagotomy. We have previously shown that esophageal stimulation with acid can produce their typical angina pain associated with a reduction in coronary blood flow in patients with chest pain and normal coronary arteries on angiography [9]. The mechanism for the above observation was not clear but the presence of a cardio-esophageal reflex in humans was suggested. The results of this study have demonstrated that esophageal acid stimulation can reduce coronary blood flow in syndrome X patients although the coronary blood flow remained unaffected in the transplant group. This reduction in coronary blood flow is associated with typical angina pain and occurs in the absence of any significant change in the epicardial coronary artery diameter. This study provides direct evidence for the presence of a cardio-esophageal reflex in humans affecting coronary blood flow which has not been demonstrated before.

This study supports the hypothesis that esophageal acid stimulation can reduce coronary blood flow in humans as a result of the presence of a cardio-esophageal reflex. The results suggest that stimulation of this reflex produces an increase in microvascular resistance in some patients, since the reduction in coronary blood flow occurred in the absence of significant changes in the epicardial coronary artery diameter. The increase in microvascular resistance may have been due to a release of vasoconstrictor substances, either locally at the level of the coronary microcirculation or systemically. In the absence of such measurements this possibility can not be ruled out. However, the absence of any hemodynamic changes during the study make the release of any substances in to the systemic circulation unlikely. Evidence for inappropriate constriction of the small diameter distal vessels as a cause of myocardial ischemia is accumulating [29,330]. Vasoconstrictor substances such as neuropeptide Y and endothelins have also been identified recently which produce ischemia predominantly by small vessel coronary constriction [31,32]. Increased constriction of coronary microvasculature causing a reduction in coronary blood flow has also been proposed as a possible mechanism for myocardial ischemia in syndrome X [33,34].

The absence of any effect on coronary blood flow in the heart transplant group gives support to the presence of a cardio-esophageal reflex in humans which is disrupted in the transplant patients as a result of their surgery. The reflex may either increase the tone of the microcirculation directly or produce the same effect by causing the release of vasoconstrictor substances locally. This study can not distinguish between the two mechanisms.

It may be argued that the chest pain experienced by syndrome X patients in our study was of esophageal origin, thus simulating angina, although a reflex may be elicited that results in a drop in coronary blood flow. This still demonstrates a novel reflex which has not been demonstrated in humans before. Furthermore, as a majority of syndrome X patients have been shown to have an abnormality of coronary flow reserve and/or esophageal disease [35,36], the activation of such a reflex in the presence of an impaired vasodilatory capacity of the microcirculation may be an important factor in the production of chest pain in a proportion of these patients.

Conclusion

Despite over two decades of investigations syndrome X remains a heterogeneous syndrome and it is now a general belief that it encompasses several pathophysiological disease entities. Esophageal abnormalities are common in syndrome X patients and esophageal stimulation, which may occur during daily activities, may produce chest pain associated with a reflex decrease in coronary blood flow ("linked angina") in a proportion of syndrome X patients. This suggests that other factors must also be important in patients who do not experience chest pain on acid infusion. An abnormal pain perception [37,38], a significant reduction in coronary blood flow on hyperventilation and mental stress [33], an impaired coronary flow reserve [4,10], a heightened sympathetic tone [33,39], and insulin resistance [40,41] have all been reported in syndrome X and may contribute to the pathophysiology of this syndrome.

References

1. Dart AM, Alban Davies H, Dalal J, Ruttley M, Henderson AH. "Angina" and normal coronary arteriograms: a follow-up study. Eur Heart J 1980; 1: 97-100.
2. Kemp HG,Vokonas PS, Cohn PF, Gorlin R. The anginal syndromes associated with normal coronary arteriograms: Report of a six year experience. Am J Med 1973; 54: 735-742.
3. Kemp HG, Kronmal EA, Vlietsra RE, et al. Seven year survival of patients with normal or near normal coronary arteriograms: A CASS registry study. J Am Coll Cardiol 1986; 7: 479-483.
4. Cannon RO, Camici PG, Epstein SE. Pathophysiological dilemma of syndrome X. Circulation 1992; 85: 883-892.
5. Chauhan A. Syndrome X: Angina and Normal Coronary Angiography. Postgraduate Medical J 1995; 71: 341-345
6. DeMeester TR, O'Sullivan GC, Bermudez G, et al. Esophageal function in patients with angina-type chest pain and normal coronary angiograms. Ann Surg 1982; 196: 488-498.
7. Schofield PM, Brooks NH, Colgan S, et al. Left ventricular function and esophageal function in patients with angina pectoris and normal coronary angiograms. Br Heart J 1987; 58: 218-214.
8. Brand DC, Martin D, Pope C. Esophageal manometrics in patients with angina-like chest pain. Dig Dis Sci 1977; 22: 300-304.
9. Chauhan A, Petch MC, Schofield PM. Esophageal stimulation can affect coronary blood flow. Lancet 1993; 341: 1309-1310.
10. Chauhan A, Mullins PA, Petch MC, Schofield PM. Is coronary flow reserve in response to papaverine really normal in syndrome X? Circulation 1994; 89: 1998-2004.
11. Richter JE, Bradley LA, DeMeester TR, Wu WC. Normal 24 hour ambulatory esophageal pH values. Influence of study center, pH electrode, age, and gender. Dig Dis Sci 1992; 37: 849-56.
12. Johnson LF, DeMeester TR. Twenty-four hour pH monitoring of the distal esophagus: A quantitative measure of gastroesophageal reflux. Am J Gastroenterol 1974; 62: 325-332.
13. Smith KS, Papp C. Episodic, postural and linked angina. Br Med J 1962; ii: 1425-30.
14. Evans W. Faults in the diagnosis of cardiac pain. Br Med J 1959; 1: 249-254.
15. Dart AM, Alban Davies H, Lowndes RH, Dalal J, Ruttley M, Henderson AH. Esophageal spasm and angina: diagnostic value of ergometrine provocation. Eur Heart J 1980; 1; 91-95.
16. Koch KL, Curry RC, Feldman RL, et al. Ergonovine induced esophageal spasm in patients with chest pain resembling angina pectoris. Dig Dis Sci 1982; 27: 1073-1080.
17. Bexton JR, Nathan AW, Hellestrand KJ, Camm AJ. Paroxysmal atrial tachycardia provoked by swallowing. Br Med J 1981; 282: 952
18. Serebro HA. The prognostic significance of the viscerocardiac reflex phenomenon. S Afr Med J 1976; 50: 769-772.

60

19. Mellow MH, Simpson AG, Watt L, Schoolmeester L, Haye OL. Esophageal acid perfusion in coronary artery disease. Induction of myocardial ischemia. Gastroenterology 1983; 85: 306-12.
20. Bennett JR, Atkinson M. Esophageal acid perfusion in the diagnosis of precordial pain. Lancet 1966; ii: 1150-1152.
21. Morrison LM, Swalm WA. Role of the gastrointestinal tract in production of cardiac symptoms. JAMA 1940; 114: 217-223.
22. Alban Davies II, Page Z, Rush EM, Brown EM, Lewis MJ, Petch MC. Esophageal stimulation lowers exertional angina threshold. Lancet 1985; i: 1011-14.
23. Kenigsberg K, Griswold PG, Buckley B, Gootman N, Gootman P. Cardiac effects of esophageal stimulation: Possible relationship between gastroesophageal reflux (GER) and Sudden Infant Death Syndrome (SIDS). J Paed Surg 1983; 18: 542-545.
24. Fontan JP, Heldt GP, Heyman MB, Marin MS, Tooley WH. Esophageal spasm associated with apnoea and bradycardia in an infant. J Pediatr 1984; 73: 52-55.
25. Herbst JJ, Minton SD, Book LS. Gastroesophageal reflux causing respiratory distress and apnea in newborn infants. J Pediatr 1979; 95: 763.
26. Bortolotti M, Cirignotta F, Labo G. Atrioventricular block induced by swallowing in a patient with diffuse esophageal spasm. JAMA 1982; 248: 2297-2299.
27. Von Bergmann G. Das "epiphrenale Syndrome", Seine Beziehung zur Angina Pectoris und zum Kardiospasms. Deutch Med Wschr 1932;58: 605-09
28. Gilbert NC, LeRoy GV, Fenn GK. The effect of distension of abdominal viscera on the blood flow in the circumflex branch of the left coronary artery of the dog. Am Heart J 1940; 20: 519-24.
29. Wilson RF, Laxson DD, Lesser JR, White CW. Intense microvascular constriction after angioplasty of acute thrombotic coronary arterial lesions. Lancet 1989; i: 807-11.
30. Pupita G, Maseri A, Kaski JC, et al. Myocardial ischemia caused by distal coronary artery constriction in stable angina pectoris. N Eng J Med 1990; 323: 514-20.
31. Clarke JG, Davies GJ, Kerwin R, et al. Coronary artery infusion of neuropeptide Y in patients with angina pectoris. Lancet 1987; 1: 1057-59.
32. Larkin SW, Clarke JG, Keogh BE, et al. Intracoronary endothelin induces myocardial ischemia by small vessel constriction in the dog. Am J Cardiol 1989; 64: 956-8.
33. Chauhan A, Mullins P, Taylor G, Petch MC, Schofield PM. The effect of hyperventilation and mental stress on coronary blood flow in Syndrome X patients. British Heart Journal 1993; 69(6): 516-524.
34. Kaski JC, Crea F, Nihoyannopoulos P, Hackett D, Maseri A. Transient myocardial ischemia during daily life in patients with syndrome X. Am J Cardiol 1986; 58: 1242-1247.
35. Cannon RO, Cattau EL, Yakshe PN, et al. Coronary flow reserve, esophageal motility, and chest pain in patients with angiographically normal coronary arteries. Am J Cardiol 1990; 88: 217-222.
36. 36.Chauhan A, Mullins PA, Gill R, Taylor G, Petch MC, Schofield PM. Esophageal dysfunction and coronary flow reserve in syndrome X. Postgraduate Medical J 1996;72:99-104.
37. Cannon RO, Quyyumi AA, Schenke WH et al. Abnormal cardiac sensitivity in patients with chest pain and normal coronary arteries. J Am Coll Cardiol 1990; 16: 1359-1366.
38. Chauhan A, Mullins PA, Thuraisingham SI, Taylor G, Petch MC, Schofield PM. Abnormal cardiac pain perception in syndrome X. J Am Coll Cardiol 1994; 24: 329-335.
39. Rosano GMC, Ponikowski P, Adamopoulos S, Collins P, Poole-Wilson PA, Coats A, Kaski JC. Abnormal autonomic control of the cardiovascular system in syndrome X. Am J Cardiol 1994; 73: 1174-1179.
40. Dean JD, Jones CJ, Hutchison SJ, Peters JR, Henderson AH. Hyperinsulinaemia and microvascular angina ("syndrome X"). Lancet 1991; 337: 456-457.
41. Chauhan A, Foote J, Petch MC, Schofield PM. Hyperinsulinaemia, coronary artery disease and syndrome X. J Am Coll Cardiol 1994; 23: 364-368.

Chapter 5

ABNORMAL PAIN PROCESSING IN SYNDROME X

Ole Frøbert, Lars Arendt-Nielsen and Jens Peder Bagger

Several pathophysiological explanations have been suggested for the pains in patients with angina pectoris despite normal coronary angiograms and without any specific cardiac, esophageal, musculo-skeletal, or psychiatric disorders. There are many clues indicating that this anginal syndrome is in fact many different syndromes giving rise to a similar symptomatology. However, a general abnormality of nociception could incorporate many of the results from previous studies [1].

It has been postulated that pain, as other sensory modalities, is, at least in part, a learned experience [2]. This is in line with the observation that angina pectoris is more common in subjects with other diseases in the same anatomical region [3]. Several studies have demonstrated that angina-like chest pain may be provoked by nociceptive stimulation of various thoracic organs. Some of these studies have also measured brain responses to painful stimuli. This chapter will briefly review the possible mechanisms and organs which may contribute to abnormal pain perception in syndrome X.

Neural pathways signaling visceral pain in the thorax

The thoracic viscera are innervated by sensory afferents, either free nerve endings or polymodal receptors, which anastomose in sympathetic and parasympathetic ganglia [1,4]. Nociceptive impulses travel in the dorsal columns of the medulla spinalis or via the vagus nerve to the central nervous system [5]. Although visceral afferent fibers represent a small proportion of the total afferent inflow to the spinal cord these fibers can activate many neurons through functional divergence [4]. The expanding neural activation may feed back on neighboring organs and augment their excitability, increase muscle tone and cause profound cardiovascular alterations such as rise of pulse and blood pressure. Neural convergence of visceral and somatic input in the spinal cord furthermore makes anatomical discrimination of pain stimuli difficult [6]. The complexity increases as the sensory input is conducted to central brain structures which may modulate the impulses via efferents. The thalamus seems together with other nuclei to play a key role as a gate in pain processing from the heart and neighboring organs [7]. Cortical activation and the possible gating role of thalamus as indicated by the measurement of regional cerebral blood flows will be discussed by Stuart Rosen in this book.

The heart

Shapiro and co-workers were the first to report altered cardiac sensitivity in syndrome X patients during cardiac catheterization [8]. Six of seven patients with positive stress tests and four of four patients with typical angina but negative exercise tests experienced short-lived episodes of their typical chest pain during catheter movements within the proximal 3-5 cm of the superior vena cava and the right atrium. Patients with atherosclerotic coronary artery disease and patients with mitral valve disease were insensitive to manipulations with the catheter. The inferior vena cava, right ventricle, pulmonary artery, and coronary sinus were not sensitive to catheter manipulations in any subject. In another open-label study, Cannon *et al* [9] demonstrated that right ventricular pacing provoked the usual chest pain in 81% of 36 patients with chest pain and normal coronary arteries (only four of whom had a positive exercise ECG). Catheterization procedures in the right ventricle produced chest pain in less than 40% of the same group and no patient experienced chest pain during stimulation of the left heart chambers by a pigtail catheter. Chauhan *et al* [10] extended these findings by investigating subjective pain responses to right atrial and ventricular catheter manipulation in 36 patients with syndrome X. Thirty (83%) patients reported chest pain during atrial stimulation and 34 (94%) patients experienced pain during ventricular stimulation; there were no coronary flow changes associated with the chest pain. Injection of contrast medium into the left coronary artery induced chest pain in 50% of patients. Intracardiac stimulation elicited pain in less than 20% of a control group of patients with mitral valve disease and in none of a control group of heart transplant recipients.

Adenosine is a well known messenger for angina pectoris in both healthy volunteers [11] and patients with ischemic heart disease [12]. It is a local vasodilator that is released in large quantities in the coronary circulation during ischemia. The lowest dose of adenosine resulting in chest pain and the maximally tolerated dose of adenosine have both been found to be lower in patients with angina pectoris and normal coronary angiograms than in either healthy volunteers or patients with coronary artery disease [13]. Intravenous dipyramidole infusion (0.56 mg/kg) caused angina in 21 of 29 syndrome X patients and in no controls [14].

These studies provide clear evidence to support the existence of increased cardiac sensitivity to right heart catheter manipulations and left coronary artery adenosine infusion in syndrome X [8,13]. However, the mechanism(s) responsible for the facilitation of cardiac pain in syndrome X remain obscure, a fact which is hardly surprising since the mechanisms responsible for classical anginal pain in obstructive coronary disease are still unresolved [5]. Nevertheless, it seems possible that a variable relationship between cardiac ischemia and pain perception could lead to a spectrum of clinical entities with syndrome X at one end and patients with obstructive coronary disease and silent ischemia at the other [1]. Equally, it remains possible that syndrome X represents a disease of pain unrelated to myocardial ischemia.

The esophagus

The esophagus has been suspected of being the source of angina-like chest pain in symptomatic patients with normal coronary arteriograms. Several previous studies have shown a high incidence (23 to 80 %) of spontaneous esophageal abnormalities in patients with so-called non-cardiac chest pain [15-19]. However, the cardiological evaluation of patients in many such studies has been criticized and the extent to which esophageal abnormalities can be linked in a cause-effect fashion to the chest pain episodes remains controversial [20]. We examined the esophagus in a consecutive population of patients with chest pain in whom coronary artery disease, coronary artery spasm, cardiac wall motion abnormalities, valvular heart disease, cardiomyopathy, or ischemic myocardial metabolism had been excluded [21,22]. Approximately half of the patients had a positive ECG exercise stress test and the remainder had typical angina but a negative exercise test. Upper gastrointestinal endoscopy was performed in 49 patients with findings similar to healthy controls [21]. Twenty-four hour 3-channel esophageal manometry and 2-channel pH-monitoring were performed in 63 patients and showed no pain-related changes and no differences compared to a healthy control group (n=22).

Esophageal pain provocation with various algogenic substances has been widely used but the interpretation is uncertain since myocardial function may be influenced by the majority of these tests. Pain has been reported in 10% to 36% of angina patients during esophageal acid instillation [22-29]. However, esophageal acid installation may itself influence coronary blood flow [30,31]. The commonly used cholinesterase inhibitor and esophageal spasmomimetic edrophonium chloride has been shown, in uncontrolled studies, to provoke chest pain symptoms in 4.5% to 55 % of non-atherosclerotic angina patients [22,25,27,28,32-34]. However, when edrophonium chloride and saline have been administered in a double blind fashion to patients none of them experienced more chest pain after edrophonium [29,35]. It further complicates the interpretation of these findings that cholinergic stimulation may dilate normal coronary arteries but may constrict atherosclerotic vessels. The last of the three classical esophageal pain provocation tests - balloon distension - may also cause coronary vasoconstriction as shown in a recent study [36].

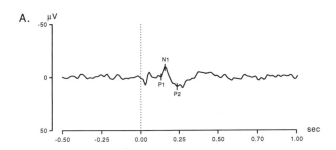

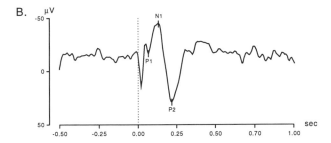

Figure 1. Brain evoked potentials following electrical stimulation of the esophageal mucosa at 1.3 times the pain threshold. (A) Female patient with a 6 year history of chest pain despite a normal coronary angiogram. (B) Female control person with similar pain threshold as A. Reproduced with permission from Heart, ref. 37.

We evaluated visceral pain in 10 patients with chest pain mimicking angina pectoris and normal coronary angiograms and in 10 controls, using electrical stimulation of the esophageal mucosa [37]. Angina pectoris was provoked in 7 patients following continuous esophageal electrical stimulation and distant projection of pain occurred in 4 patients. However, none of 10 controls experienced chest pain. The patients had higher esophageal pain thresholds to repeated stimuli than the controls but there were no inter-group differences in thresholds to single stimuli. Repeated stimulation elicits temporal summation which is an integrative mechanism in the nociceptive system. It has been shown that when central hyperexcitability occurs, temporal summation of stimuli is facilitated. In the patients with angina-like pain the opposite situation has been demonstrated; these patients appear to have a hypoexcitability which could be caused by increased descending control of spinal cord nociceptive neurons [37]. Electrical esophageal stimulation in these patients did not alter the pulse frequency, the blood pressure, or resulted in ST-segment changes. Brain evoked potentials, which are regarded as the summated electrical fields of a large number of neuronal membranes acting in synchrony [38] and facilitate a quantitative measure of the central responses [39], were substantially reduced in amplitude in patients compared with controls despite similar pain thresholds. We concluded from these findings that there is an altered central nervous system response to visceral nociceptive input in patients with angina and normal coronary angiograms.

The musculo-skeletal system and the skin as the source of chest pain

Chest wall abnormalities believed to mimic angina pectoris include osteoarthritis of the cervicodorsal spine, muscle strain, chest wall fibrositis, costosternal syndromes, scoliosis, disc space narrowing, and trauma to the chest [40-44]. In addition, a myofascial origin of pain has been suggested [45]. A chest wall mechanism in angina pectoris has been described in early studies [40] with a classical description by Davis and Ritvo of osteoarthritis of the cervicodorsal spine simulating coronary artery disease [42]. More recent studies have also dealt with this subject in case reports [43,46]. In a study of 100 patients with chest pain and normal coronary angiography, 69 were found to have chest wall "tenderness" compared with none of 25 control patients with arthritis and no symptoms of chest pain [47]. No information of other cardiac investigations was given in this report and the physical examination was limited to a few palpatory maneuvers of the spine and anterior chest wall. However, the angina-like pain could be reproduced by palpation in only a minority of the chest pain patients. A controlled, blinded study should be carried out to establish whether the musculo-skeletal system plays a role as the cause of chest pain in syndrome X.

A few studies have dealt with the assessment of cutaneous pain thresholds in syndrome X and the results are controversial. Turiel et al [48] found a significantly lower threshold and tolerance for electrical skin stimulation in 12 syndrome X patients compared with 10 controls. In the study by Cannon et al [9] thermal pain sensitivity was investigated by means of 72 thermal staircase stimuli of 3 seconds duration delivered to a volar thermode. Patients with chest pain and normal coronary arteries required a higher temperature to produce the same level of subjective responses compared with controls (hypertrophic cardiomyopathy and coronary artery disease). We did not find any differences in thresholds of perception or pain to single and repeated electrical sternal skin stimuli between syndrome X patients and controls [37]. However, the syndrome X patients had substantially reduced brain evoked potential amplitudes after single skin stimuli despite the similar pain thresholds.

General considerations on chest pain in syndrome X

Syndrome X patients perceive that their symptoms originate from the heart. As described above abnormal processing of nociceptive input with inappropriate feedback to neighboring organs may exist in these patients. However, the question remains whether organs other than the heart could be the primary source of pain or minor events in the heart initiate a cascade of afferent impulses from other organs. The nociceptive system in syndrome X patients may be sensitized in such a way that minimal activity, not normally perceived as pain, suddenly becomes painful due to hyperexcitability of specific neuronal pathways. A theory that encompasses all the positive findings in studies of patients with angina and normal coronary angiograms may be somewhat speculative. However, one could propose a working hypothesis that repeated nociceptive stimuli from the periphery to the central nervous system gives rise to a condition of chronic pain. A vicious circle between the periphery and central nervous system may be established. The activation of visceral nociceptors evokes persistent increases in muscle tone, changes in viscero-motor and viscero-secretory reflexes and profound cardiovascular alterations [49] (including increased sympathetic drive [50]) and a strong aversive sensation of pain [4]. In this way, what began as a single organ disorder ends up with the involvement of multiple anatomical regions. This spread of pain due to ongoing barrage of nociceptive input has been reported experimentally with continuous electrical stimulation of the gut [51]. As time progresses the referred pain involves larger and larger territories. A recent study with spinal cord stimulation seems to support a multiple-organ involvement. Twelve syndrome X patients were treated with a spinal cord stimulator at the T1-T2 level; on subsequent exercise testing the time to angina, exercise tolerance, and the time to ST-segment depression increased [52]. Although the authors suggest that the responsible mechanism of spinal cord stimulation is related to an anti-ischemic effect, the outcome could also be explained by interference of a vicious circle of afferent and efferent neuronal stimuli.

There are of course several good reasons to interpret syndrome X as a disease of the heart. However, chest pain in syndrome X may be triggered by dysfunctions in other organs and result in perturbation of the nociceptive system. When syndrome X patients have electrocardiographic ST segment depressions, concomitant pain is more often the exception than the rule. Kaski et al [53] demonstrated that 52 % of Holter ST segment depression episodes in syndrome X patients were asymptomatic and we have found that the proportion of silent ST depression may be up to 90 % in similar studies [22]. We also observed that the heart rate rarely increased during pain episodes which is in line with the lack of deterioration in left ventricular function during ST-segment depression [54]. The positive exercise test result is probably responsible for the fact that syndrome X patients are seen mainly by cardiologists. There may be less focus on the larger group of patients with normal exercise ECG's, normal coronary arteries and a similar symptomatology. Do these patients suffer from other diseases or is the positive exercise ECG just an epiphenomenon that has been used to separate a group of patients with the same complexity of underlying disorders?

Conclusion

The etiology of chest pain in syndrome X remains a puzzle. It is not even certain which organ(s) are involved. The statement by Reid and De Witt Andrus in 1925 (quoted in [5]): "Nobody believes that all pain originating in and around the heart is always due to the same cause" still remains unchallenged.

References

1. Cannon RO, Benjamin SB. Chest pain as a consequence of abnormal visceral nociception. Dig Dis Sci 1993;38:193-6.
2. Melzack R. The puzzle of pain. Harmondsworth: Penguin; 1973.
3. Procacci P, Maresca M. Clinical aspects of heart pain. Advances in Pain Research and Therapy 1987;10:127-33.
4. Cervero F. Vecchiet L, Albe-Fessard D, Lindblom U, Giamberadino MA, editors.New trends in referred pain and hyperalgesia. Elsevier Science Publishers B.V. 1993; 4, Pathophysiology of referred pain and hyperalgesia from viscera. p. 35-46.
5. Malliani A, Lombardi F. Consideration of the fundamental mechanisms eliciting cardiac pain. Am Heart J 1982;103:575-8.
6. Ness TJ, Gebhart GF. Visceral pain: a review of experimental studies. Pain 1990;41:167-234.
7. Rosen SD, Paulesu E, Frith CD, Frackowiak RSJ, Davies GJ, Jones T, Camici PG. Central nervous pathways mediating angina pectoris. Lancet 1994;344:147-50.
8. Shapiro LM, Crake T, Poole Wilson PA. Is altered cardiac sensation responsible for chest pain in patients with normal coronary arteries? Clinical observation during cardiac catheterization. Br Med J Clin Res Ed 1988;296:170-1.
9. Cannon RO, Quyyumi AA, Schenke WH, Fananapazir L, Tucker EE, Gaughan AM, Gracely RH, Cattau EL, Epstein SE. Abnormal cardiac sensitivity in patients with chest pain and normal coronary arteries. JACC 1990;16:1359-66.
10. Chauhan A, Mullins PA, Thuraisingham SI, Taylor G, Petch MC, Schofield PM. Abnormal cardiac pain perception in syndrome X. JACC 1994;24:329-35.
11. Sylven C, Beermann B, Jonzon B, Brandt R. Angina pectoris-like pain provoked by intravenous adenosine in healthy volunteers. Br Med J Clin Res Ed 1986;293:227-30.
12. Lagerqvist B, Sylven C, Beermann B, Helmius G, Waldenstrom A. Intracoronary adenosine causes angina pectoris like pain - an inquiry into the nature of visceral pain. Cardiovasc Res 1990;24:609-13.
13. Lagerqvist B, Sylven C, Waldenstrom A. Lower threshold for adenosine-induced chest pain in patients with angina and normal coronary angiograms. Br Heart J 1992;68:282-5.
14. Rosen SD, Uren NG, Kaski JC, Tousoulis D, Davies GJ, Camici PG. Coronary vaodilator reserve, pain perception, and sex in patients with syndrome X. Circulation 1994;90:50-60.
15. De-Caestecker JS, Blackwell JN, Brown J, Heading RC. The esophagus as a cause of recurrent chest pain: which patients should be investigated and which tests should be used? Lancet 1985;2:1143-6.
16. Brand DL, Martin D, Pope II CE. Esophageal manometrics in patients with angina-like chest pain. Digestive Diseases 1977;22:300-4.
17. Janssens J, Vantrappen G, Ghillebert G. 24-hour recording of esophageal pressure and pH in patients with noncardiac chest pain. Gastroenterology 1986;90:1978-84.
18. Lam HG, Dekker W, Kan G, Breedijk M, Smout AJ. Acute noncardiac chest pain in a coronary care unit. Evaluation by 24-hour pressure and pH recording of the esophagus. Gastroenterology 1992;102:453-60.
19. Peters L, Maas L, Petty D, Dalton C, Penner D, Wu W, Castell DO, Richter J. Spontaneous noncardiac chest pain. Evaluation by 24-hour ambulatory esophageal motility and pH monitoring. Gastroenterology 1988;94:878-86.
20. Cohen S. Noncardiac chest pain. The crumbling of the sphinx. Dig Dis Sci 1989;34:1649-50.
21. Frøbert O, Funch-Jensen P, Jacobsen NO, Kruse A, Bagger JP. Upper endoscopy in patients with angina and normal coronary angiograms. Endoscopy 1995;27:365-70.
22. Frøbert O, Funch-Jensen P, Bagger JP. Diagnostic value of esophageal studies in patients with angina-like chest pain and normal coronary angiograms. Ann Intern med 1996;11:959-69.
23. Hewson EG, Sinclair JW, Dalton CB, Wu WC, Castell DO, Richter JE. Acid perfusion test: does it have a role in the assessment of non cardiac chest pain? Gut 1989;30:305-10.
24. Hewson EG, Dalton CB, Richter JE. Comparison of esophageal manometry, provocative testing, and ambulatory monitoring in patients with unexplained chest pain. Dig Dis Sci 1990;35:302-9.

25. De-Caestecker JS, Pryde A, Heading RC. Comparison of intravenous edrophonium and esophageal acid perfusion during esophageal manometry in patients with non-cardiac chest pain. Gut 1988;29:1029-34.
26. Cannon RO, Cattau ELJ, Yakshe PN, Maher K, Schenke WH, Benjamin SB, Epstein SE. Coronary flow reserve, esophageal motility, and chest pain in patients with angiographically normal coronary arteries. Am J Med 1990;88:217-22.
27. Nevens F, Janssens J, Piessens J, Ghillebert G, De Geest H, Vantrappen G. Prospective study on prevalence of esophageal chest pain in patients referred on an elective basis to a cardiac unit for suspected myocardial ischemia. Dig Dis Sci 1991;36:229-35.
28. Ghillebert G, Janssens J, Vantrappen G, Nevens F, Piessens J. Ambulatory 24 hour intraesophageal pH and pressure recordings v provocation tests in the diagnosis of chest pain of esophageal origin. Gut 1990;31:738-44.
29. Soffer EE, Scalabrini P, Wingate DL. Spontaneous noncardiac chest pain: value of ambulatory esophageal pH and motility monitoring. Dig Dis Sci 1989;34:1651-5.
30. Mellow MH, Simpson AG, Watt L, Schoolmeester L, Haye OL. Esophageal acid perfusion in coronary artery disease. Induction of myocardial ischemia. Gastroenterology 1983;85:306-12.
31. Chauhan A, Petch MC, Schofield PM. Effect of esophageal acid instillation on coronary blood flow. Lancet 1993;341:1309-10.
32. Schofield PM, Whorwell PJ, Brooks NH, Bennett DH, Jones PE. Esophageal function in patients with angina pectoris: a comparison of patients with normal coronary angiograms and patients with coronary artery disease. Digestion 1989;42:70-8.
33. Breumelhof R, Nadorp JH, Akkermans LM, Smout AJ. Analysis of 24-hour esophageal pressure and pH data in unselected patients with noncardiac chest pain. Gastroenterology 1990;99:1257-64.
34. Richter JE, Hackshaw BT, Wu WC, Castell DO. Edrophonium: a useful provocative test for esophageal chest pain. Ann Intern med 1985;103:14-21.
35. Limburg AJ, Beekhuis H, Van Dijk RB, Kleibeuker JH. Noncardiac chest pain : Is the esophagus really a frequent source? Scand J Gastroent 1990;25:793-8.
36. Gayheart PA, Gwirtz PA, Bravenec JS, Longlet N, Jones CE. An alpha-adrenergic coronary constriction during esophageal distention in the dog. J Cardiovasc Pharmacol 1991;17:747-53.
37. Frøbert O, Arendt-Nielsen L, Bak P, Funch-Jensen P, Bagger JP. Pain perception and brain evoked potentials in patients with angina despite normal coronary angiograms. Heart 1996;75:436-41.
38. Chudler EH, Dong WK. The assessment of pain by cerebral evoked potentials. Pain 1983;16:221-44.
39. Frøbert O, Arendt-Nielsen L, Bak P, Andersen OK, Funch-Jensen P, Bagger JP. Electrical stimulation of the esophageal mucosa: Perception and brain evoked potentials. Scand J Gastroenterol 1994;29:776-81.
40. Nachlas IW. Pseudo-angina pectoris originating in the cervical spine. JAMA 1934;103:323-5.
41. Allison DR. Pain in the chest wall simulating heart disease. Br Med J 1950;1:332-6.
42. Davis D, Ritvo M. Osteoarthritis of the cervicodorsal spine (radiculitis) simulating coronary-artery disease. Clinical and roentgenologic findings. N Engl J Med 1948;238:857-66.
43. Arroyo JF, Jolliet P, Junod AF. Costovertebral joint dysfunction: another misdiagnosed cause of atypical chest pain. Postgrad Med J 1992;68:655-9.
44. Wolf E, Stern S. Costosternal syndrome: its frequency and importance in differential diagnosis of coronary heart disease. Arch Intern Med 1976;136:189-91.
45. Travell J, Rinzler SH. The myofascial genesis of pain. Postgraduate Medicine 1952;11:425-34.
46. Epstein SE, Gerber LH, Borer JS. Chest wall syndrome. A common cause of unexplained chest pain. JAMA 1979;241:2793-7.
47. Wise CM, Semble EL, Dalton CB. Musculoskeletal chest wall syndromes in patients with noncardiac chest pain: a study of 100 patients. Arch Phys Med Rehabil 1992;73:147-9.
48. Turiel M, Galassi AR, Glazier JJ, Kaski JC, Maseri A. Pain threshold and tolerance in women with syndrome X and women with stable angina pectoris. Am J Cardiol 1987;60:503-7.
49. Sampson JJ, Cheitlin MD. Pathophysiology and differential diagnosis of cardiac pain. Progr Card Dis 1971;13:507-31.
50. Frøbert O, Mølgaard H, Bøtker HE, Bagger JP. Autonomic balance in patients with angina and normal coronary angiogram. Eur Heart J 1995;16:1356-60.
51. Arendt-Nielsen L, Drewes AM, Hansen JB, Tage-Jensen U. Gut pain reactions in man: an experimental investigation using short and long duration transmucosal electrical stimulation. Pain 1997;69:255-62.
52. Eliasson T, Albertsson P, Hardhammar P, Emanuelsson H, Augustinsson LE, Mannheimer C. Spinal cord stimulation in angina pectoris with normal coronary arteriograms. Coron Artery Dis 1993;4:819-27.
53. Kaski JC, Crea F, Nihoyannopoulos P, Hackett D, Maseri A. Transient myocardial ischemia during daily life in patients with syndrome X. Am J Cardiol 1986;58:1242-7.
54. Levy RD, Shapiro LM, Wright C, Mockus L, Fox KM. Syndrome X: the hemodynamic significance of ST segment depression. Br Heart J 1986;56:353-7.

Chapter 6

INSIGHTS INTO THE PATHOPHYSIOLOGY OF SYNDROME X OBTAINED USING POSITRON EMISSION TOMOGRAPHY (PET)

Stuart D Rosen and and Paolo G Camici

In the last five years, many studies have been performed to try to improve understanding of the clinical condition of syndrome X (anginal quality chest pain, ischemic-like changes on the stress ECG yet a normal coronary arteriogram). In this chapter, we review advances in knowledge of the pathophysiology of this condition which have been obtained by means of positron emission tomography (PET). The context in which the PET studies have been performed, i.e. several invasive studies and a number of non-PET nuclear cardiological investigations, is also outlined. Finally, we attempt to arrive at a conclusion more substantive than the somewhat vague and mysterious closing comments about a "heterogeneous disorder" with which many authors on the subject have taken leave of their readers.

Definition

The starting point of any survey of this subject must commence with a definition. A clinically homogenous entity can be identified which comprises typical angina [1], >0.1mV rectilinear or downsloping ST segment depression on the exercise ECG [without left bundle branch block (LBBB) at rest or on exercise], angiographically normal coronary arteries, without even minimal luminal irregularities; exclusion of epicardial arterial spasm, exclusion of valve disease (including mitral valve prolapse) and of left ventricular hypertrophy; exclusion of hypertension and diabetes. Even if a single, all-encompassing pathogenetic mechanism for this condition may not exist, we feel that such a rigorous definition offers the advantage of removing a considerable number of confounding factors, which dogged a fair amount of research in the 1970s and early 1980s.

Myocardial ischemia and blood flow

For obvious reasons - the anginal quality of the pain and the stress ECG changes – myocardial blood flow (MBF) and lactate release during stress have been frequent objects of attention in attempts to establish whether myocardial ischemia is the cause of the chest pain in these patients [2-8]. In the 1980s, use of both invasive and non-invasive techniques, particularly argon washout [3] and coronary sinus thermodilution

[4], appeared to report a reduction in coronary vasodilator reserve (CVR, i.e. MBF during maximal hyperemia/MBF at rest). In the present decade there have been several further studies, both invasive, using the Doppler catheter technique [9-15] and non-invasive studies, principally using nuclear cardiology techniques [16-31] to measure respectively coronary blood flow velocity (from which actual flow is derived) and to assess regional changes in MBF distribution

Although from the combination of quantitative angiography and the measured epicardial flow velocity, flow can be derived, the Doppler catheter method has a number of limitations [54]: a) The mass of myocardium supplied by the artery under study cannot be defined precisely; b) measurements in the different regions of the heart cannot be made simultaneously; c) ethical considerations rule out the study of true normal controls. With the foregoing provisos, several studies deserve mention. Holdright *et al* [14] reported a comparison of three of the commonest vasodilator stressor agents used, intravenous (iv) dipyridamole, intracoronary (ic) adenosine and ic papaverine. The latter has to date been assumed to produce maximal coronary vasodilatation. The main findings were that the syndrome X patients achieved a flow reserve >4 with both papaverine and adenosine; dipyridamole achieved a slightly lower value ($\approx$3.5). There were no differences between subjects who had a positive stress ECG and those with a negative stress ECG. In contrast, Chauhan *et al* [13] have described a reduction in CVR after papaverine, with a mean value in 53 subjects of 2.72±1.39. This value was well below the 5.22±1.26 which they described for heart transplant subjects, although how appropriate this control group is might be queried in the light of more recent non-invasive studies which suggest that the effect of denervation of the heart should be to increase hyperemic MBF [32]. The same group has subsequently reported yet further reductions of CVR in syndrome X patients after oesophageal acid instillation [12], hyperventilation and mental stress [15]. An increase in CVR after transcutaneous nerve stimulation has also been found [11].

In parallel with the catheter-based techniques just outlined, a number of radionuclide imaging techniques have been applied to patients with syndrome X for the non-invasive assessment of regional myocardial blood flow distribution [16-31]. It must be acknowledged, though, that quantitative measurements of regional MBF have not generally been feasible with these methods because of the technical limitations of the available radionuclide imaging systems, not least due to attenuation of the emitted photons by body tissues, a particular problem when the principal energy level of emission is low as it is in the case of [201]Tl [33]. In addition, although in principle these methods have the distinct advantage that true matched control populations can be studied as well as patients, the high doses of radiation involved (other than with PET) also impose ethical restrictions. Overall, the majority of thallium and SPECT studies performed in syndrome X populations have reported regions of 'impaired perfusion' [17,19-23,27,34,35]. The highest prevalence of Tl abnormalities is probably in the study of Tweddel *et al* [27]. In their paper, 98/100 patients with typical angina, normal arteriograms and no other cardiovascular abnormality, who underwent gated planar thallium scans at peak exercise, showed defects of thallium uptake. However, no consistent pattern and no significant correlation existed between the extent of thallium defect, the presence of a positive exercise test or the level of exercise tolerance. Similar results were reported by Kao and colleagues [22] who performed exercise ^{201}Tl single photon emission tomography (SPET) studies in 28 patients, adhering to a strict definition of syndrome X. Three patients (11%) had a normal ^{201}Tl SPET scan whereas

25 (89%) had an abnormal scan. Again, the results of the exercise ECGs did not correlate with the perfusion defects observed on the thallium scans. More recently, Fragasso *et al* [17] presented stress-redistribution ^{201}Tl myocardial perfusion scintigraphy data on 25 syndrome X patients and compared the findings to those of 32 patients with atypical chest pain and a negative exercise test. The thallium stress images revealed 40 hypoperfused segments in 27 patients (77%); after 4 hours, 16 segments had completely normalized, 10 were unchanged, in 6 there was partial reperfusion and 8 worsened. Twenty-four patients (69%) exhibited thallium reverse redistribution in 33 segments. Of these 24 patients, eight also underwent stress-rest ^{99m}Tc-MIBI SPECT. Six showed reduced tracer uptake at rest, which normalized on the stress images, in the same segments which showed thallium reverse redistribution. In contrast, there were seven controls (22%) with at least one hypoperfused myocardial segment in one of the two scintigraphic phases. The authors suggested that it was due to inhomogeneous perfusion, with the hyperemic response induced by exercise masking resting hypoperfusion of certain areas.

More recently, Inobe and colleagues [19] performed myocardial scintigraphy with ^{201}Tl in 26 patients with angina and 'normal coronary arteries' (in this study 'normal' included coronary stenoses of <25% of luminal diameter). They compared the findings after exercise ± intravenous aminophylline or saline solution with those after adenosine. The effects of adenosine and dobutamine infusions on hemodynamics at cardiac catheterization were also examined. Exercise evoked abnormalities of Tl uptake in 14 of 26 patients. Intravenous infusion of aminophylline was reported to suppress the scintigraphic perfusion defect and to prolong the time to 1-mm ST segment depression. Intravenous infusion of adenosine was reported to induce a defect in the same myocardial area where the perfusion defect was observed at exercise in 7 of the 14 patients. At cardiac catheterization, patients with syndrome X with abnormal exercise scintigrams had lower flow reserve, greater frequency of myocardial lactate production and ST segment depression in response to the infusions of adenosine and dobutamine than the patients with normal scintigraphic appearances. It was concluded that a heterogeneous response to endogenous adenosine might contribute to the scintigraphic perfusion abnormalities observed.

There is a great need, however, for a critical appraisal of these studies [28]. Thus, amongst other considerations, it is important to remember that what is actually being determined in the above studies is a comparison of counts recovered from the myocardial regions with the highest number of counts to those with the lowest. The latter are then assumed to have impaired perfusion, although the same appearances would occur in the presence of normal absolute values of MBF with mild regional heterogeneity [16,18]. Although, as illustrated above, abnormalities of Tl and ^{99m}Tc-MIBI SPECT scans have frequently been reported, it is noteworthy that similar patterns of heterogeneous perfusion with areas of apparent hypoperfusion, often inconstant both temporally and spatially, are demonstrable in the normal heart, at least in animal studies [37].

Positron emission tomography

Although not as widely available as the investigative tools so far described, PET is a technique which for a range of technical reasons (including tomographic acquisition, the use of high energy photons and accurate attenuation correction) permits absolute quantification of MBF with a high degree of spatial resolution [33]. In 1990, using PET and $H_2^{15}O$, Geltman *et al* [29] reported a comparison of MBF, between 17 patients with angina and angiographically normal coronary arteries (but including CAD with <50% reductions in luminal diameter) and 16 normal controls (who were significantly younger than the patients). That study [29] revealed no difference in MBF between patients and controls either at rest or after dipyridamole; however, the imposition of an arbitrary cut off of 2.5 for CVR seemed to establish a sub group of patients with abnormally low coronary flow reserve, although two of the controls also had results in this range. It has subsequently been shown [36] that many normal individuals have a CVR <2.5. This is particularly true for older subjects - flow reserve is reasonably well preserved up to the age of about 60 years, then it steadily declines after this, due chiefly to a limitation of hyperemic MBF [36].

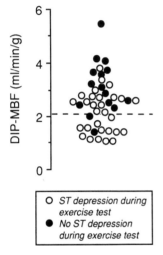

Figure 1. The plot shows individual values of myocardial blood flow (MBF) after dipyridamole infusion (DIP). Although the occurrence of ST depression during exercise shows a good sensitivity (86%) for identifying a low coronary vasodilator reserve, the specificity is poor (45%). From Camici *et al* [30].

In a further study [30] in 1992, Camici *et al* assessed MBF and CVR using PET and $^{13}NH_3$ in a large group of patients (n=45) with a history of chest pain and a normal coronary arteriogram, with or without ischemic-like changes in the stress ECG. No normal controls were studied. The data indicated that MBF values following dipyridamole were widely dispersed and analysis of the frequency of distribution suggested that a subgroup of patients could be identified with a lower CVR. It was, however, noted that there was no correspondence between the flow data and ECG changes on exercise (Figure 1).

In a smaller series of patients Galassi *et al* [26] used PET with $H_2^{15}O$ to compare 13 syndrome X patients, 7 normals and 8 patients with single vessel coronary artery disease. MBF at rest was slightly higher in the syndrome X group but there were no differences after dipyridamole (apart from the expected blunting of hyperemic MBF in the CAD patients in the territory of the stenosed artery). In this study, there were marked differences between the syndrome X patients and the normal controls in terms of age (means of 54 and 30 respectively) and gender of the subjects studied (11/13 syndrome X were female; all 7 controls were male). Also there was no correction for the higher RPPs in syndrome X patients. This group also reported greater heterogeneity of flow in the syndrome X patients, by employing a method of drawing ROIs of small size. However, their data are somewhat difficult to interpret since the size of ROIs was close to the resolution of the scanner and no data were presented to quantify noise in the measurements. Smaller ROIs are more susceptible to the confounding effects of motion artifact, which may well be more likely due to the greater heart rate response to dipyridamole in this patient group. In addition, the distribution of heterogeneous areas of flow (whether greater or less than the mean) was not constant over time (the latter may also simply reflect normal variability [37]). Similar findings with respect to heterogeneity of flow were reported more recently by Meeder et al [16,18].

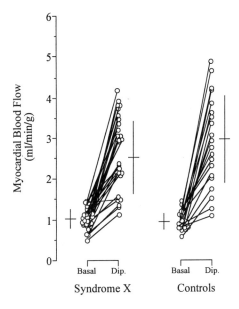

Figure 2. Myocardial blood flow at rest and after dipyridamole for syndrome X patients and normal controls (Dip.=dipyridamole). From Rosen et al [25].

A further study from our group [25], published in 1994, is germane to this discussion. We investigated myocardial blood flow in a series of 29 syndrome X patients and, uniquely in syndrome X research to date, 20 matched true normal controls. It was found that both whole heart and regional MBF at rest and after dipyridamole were comparable in patients and controls [25] (Figures 2 and 3). The coefficient of variation of flow did not differ between patients and controls and was comparable to that in Galassi et al's study [26], although the ROI size was certainly larger. In addition, as in Camici et al's study [30], no relationships were demonstrable amongst MBF, chest pain and ECG changes during stress.

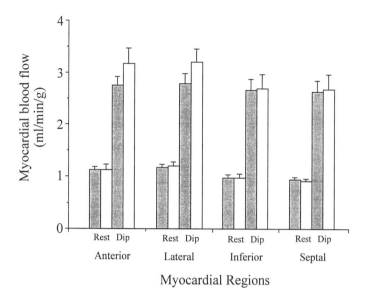

Figure 3. Regional myocardial blood flow at rest and after dipyridamole for syndrome X patients (hatched columns) and normal controls (white columns). Columns represent mean (SEM). (Dip.=dipyridamole). From Rosen *et al* [25].

Myocardial blood flow and sympathetic activation in patients with syndrome X

Because in Camici *et al*'s 1992 study, increased adrenergic activity had been hypothesized in syndrome X patients, it was suggested that limitation of the MBF response to dipyridamole, observed in some syndrome X patients, might be due to α_1 mediated coronary vasoconstriction. A preliminary open study [55] was then performed to measure the effect of the α_1 antagonist doxazosin in the subgroup of patients with CVR at the lower end of the range. Doxazosin was indeed shown to increase MBF following dipyridamole. However, in seven out of ten patients dipyridamole-induced chest pain persisted despite a significant improvement of CVR. It should also be noted that both the resting values of MBF and those after dipyridamole were widely distributed.

Subsequently, [32], in an investigation of normal volunteers using PET with ^{15}O labeled water, during control conditions and selective α_1 blockade with doxazosin, we discovered that α_1-mediated vasoconstriction limits MBF at rest and during pharmacological vasodilatation with dipyridamole (Figure 4). Following on from this, a series of syndrome X patients has been studied to investigate [38], in a double bind protocol, the effects of α_1-blockade upon MBF at rest and after dipyridamole in patients with syndrome X. No significant differences were demonstrable between patients treated with doxazosin and normal controls given the drug, with respect to resting MBF, MBF after dipyridamole, or CVR (Figure 4). We concluded that the data did not support the case for α_1-mediated vasoconstriction having an etiologic role in the chest pain of syndrome X.

Syndrome X patients treated with doxazosin

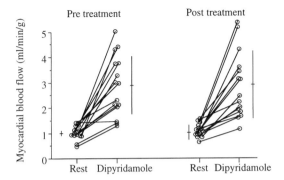

Syndrome X patients treated with placebo

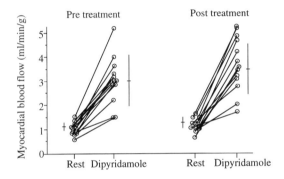

Control subjects treated with doxazosin

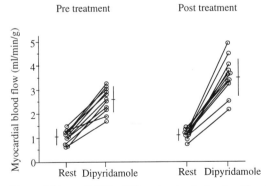

Figure 4. Myocardial Blood Flow, at rest and after dipyridamole, before and after treatment, for Syndrome X patients treated with doxazosin (top panel), for Syndrome X patients given placebo (middle panel) and for Control subjects treated with doxazosin (lower panel).

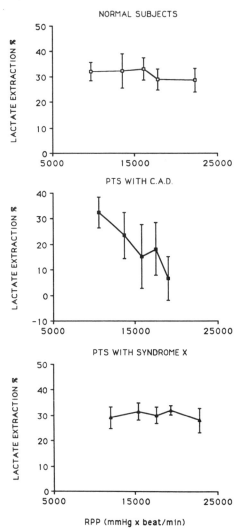

Figure 5. Lactate extraction during atrial pacing in normal subjects (upper panel) patients with coronary artery disease (CAD, middle panel) and patients with syndrome X (lower panel). The abscissa shows the prevailing rate pressure product (RPP; heart rate x systolic blood pressure).

A very important observation from several of the above studies is that regardless of how one interprets the flow data, *there is little or no relationship amongst MBF, chest pain and ischemic-like ECG changes.* This, when combined with 1) the repeated demonstration of normal left ventricular function at rest, after exercise [39], pacing [40] or pharmacological stress and transthoracic [39] or transesophageal echocardiography [41]; 2) the absence of any unequivocal demonstration of lactate [40] or hydrogen ion release [42] during stress in patients with syndrome X (Figure 5), fundamentally undermine the case for an ischemic etiology of chest pain in the vast majority of syndrome X patients.

Abnormal pain perception

Clinical observations

The case for abnormal visceral pain perception being a crucial aspect of syndrome X is becoming well established. Evidence for this comes from studies of direct stimulation of the heart at cardiac catheterization [43,44] and by pharmacological means with epinephrine [45] and dipyridamole [25]. A lowered pain threshold to somatic stimuli has also been suggested on the basis of electrical stimulation or forearm ischemia experiments [46].

Functional imaging of the brain in patients experiencing myocardial ischemia

We have recently described a new approach to the investigation of the pathways mediating visceral pain perception [47,48]. Positron emission tomography (PET) with $H_2^{15}O$, which has been employed to measure regional cerebral blood flow (rCBF) as an index of neuronal activation in a number of neurological studies [49,50], was applied to the study of pharmacologically induced angina pectoris in patients with coronary artery disease. Although angina pectoris is a common example of visceral pain, its central nervous pathways had never previously been demonstrated in vivo in man. We applied a well established neurological use of PET - the measurement of changes in regional cerebral blood flow (rCBF) as an index of altered synaptic activity - to examine the central neural correlates of i) angina due to coronary artery disease [47], ii) silent myocardial ischemia [48] and, most recently, iii) the chest pain of syndrome X [51].

Angina pectoris in patients with coronary disease

Initially [47], 12 patients with stable angina pectoris and angiographically proven coronary artery disease were studied under baseline conditions and during angina induced by intravenous dobutamine. Angina was induced in all patients. Compared to baseline, angina was associated with increased rCBF in the hypothalamus, periaqueductal grey, bilaterally in the thalamus and lateral prefrontal cortex and left inferior anterocaudal cingulate cortex.

Silent ischemia in patients with coronary disease

Subsequently [48], 9 coronary artery disease patients were investigated; all had reproducible myocardial ischemia, but no angina (none was diabetic nor had any other systemic disease). During ischemia in these patients, both thalami were activated, but cortical activation was limited to the right frontal region. Significant differences were found between angina and silent ischemia with respect to activation of the basal frontal cortex, ventral cingulate cortex and left temporal pole. In both coronary artery disease patient groups, thalamic rCBF remained increased after the symptoms and signs of myocardial ischemia had ceased.

PET neuroimaging during the chest pain of syndrome X

Finally, we studied 9 patients with syndrome X [51]. Compared to the patients with angina due to coronary artery disease, the syndrome X patients showed greater rCBF increases in the midbrain, right thalamus and right insular cortex and bilaterally in the frontal and prefrontal cortices. The chest pain in syndrome X occurred in the absence of correlates of myocardial ischemia such as left ventricular wall motion abnormality. We suggest on the basis of these data that the brain areas activated in syndrome X, but not in coronary artery disease, might represent the central neural substrate of abnormal pain perception in syndrome X. Rather than use of drugs which have been of value in the treatment of coronary disease patients with angina but which have been generally unsuccessful in patients with syndrome X, the most appropriate therapy for syndrome X patients might be drugs which specifically target the central nervous pathways identified [52,53].

References

1. Rose G, McCartney P, Reid DD. Self-administration of a questionnaire on chest pain and intermittent claudication. Br J Prevent Soc Med 1977; 31:42-48.
2. Green LH, Cohn PF, Holman BL, Adams DF, Markis JE. Regional myocardial blood flow in patients with chest pain syndromes and normal coronary arteriograms. Br Heart J 1978; 40: 242-249.
3. Opherk D, , Zebe H, Weihe E, Mall G, Dürr C, Gravert B, Mehmal HC, Schwartz F, Kubler W. Reduced coronary dilatory capacity and ultrastructural changes in the myocardium in patients with angina pectoris but normal coronary arteriograms. Circulation 1981; 63: 817-825.
4. Cannon RO, Schenke WH, Leon MB, Rosing DR, Urqhart J, Epstein SE. Limited coronary flow reserve after dipyridamole in patients with ergonovine-induced coronary vasoconstriction. Circulation 1987; 75: 163-174.
5. Crake T, Canepa-Anson R, Shapiro L, Poole-Wilson PA. Continuous reading of coronary sinus oxygen saturation during atrial pacing in patients with coronary artery disease or syndrome X. Br Heart J 1988; 59: 31-38.
6. Epstein SE, Cannon RO. Site of increased resistance to coronary flow in patients with angina pectoris and normal epicardial coronary arteries. J Am Coll Cardiol 1986; 8: 459-461.
7. Kemp HG, Elliott WC, Gorlin R. The anginal syndrome with normal coronary arteriography. Trans Assoc Am Physicians 1967; 80: 59-70.
8. Arbogast R, Bourassa MG. Myocardial function during atrial pacing in patients with angina pectoris and normal coronary arteriograms. Comparison with patients having significant coronary artery disease. Am J Cardiol 1973; 32:257-263.
9. Holdright DR. Chest pain with normal coronary arteries. Br J Hosp Med 1996; 56: 347-50.
10. Chauhan A, Mullins PA, Gill R, Taylor G, Petch MC, Schofield PM. Coronary flow reserve and oesophageal dysfunction in syndrome X. Postgrad Med J 1996; 72: 99-104.
11. Sanderson JE, Woo KS, Chung HK, Chan WW, Tse LK, White HD. The effect of transcutaneous electrical nerve stimulation on coronary and systemic haemodynamics in syndrome X. Coron Artery Dis 1996; 7: 547-52.
12. Chauhan A, Petch MC, Schofield PM. Cardio-oesophageal reflex in humans as a mechanism for "linked angina' Eur Heart J 1996; 17: 407-13.
13. Chauhan A, Mullins PA, Petch MC, Schofield PM. Is coronary flow reserve in response to papaverine really normal in syndrome X? Circulation. 1994; 89: 1998-2004.
14. Holdright DR, Lindsay DC, Clarke D, Fox K, Poole-Wilson PA, Collins P. Coronary flow reserve in patients with chest pain and normal coronary arteries. Br Heart J. 1993; 70: 513-9.
15. Chauhan A, Mullins PA, Taylor G, Petch MC, Schofield PM. Effect of hyperventilation and mental stress on coronary blood flow in syndrome X. Br Heart J 1993; 69: 516-24.
16. Meeder JG, Blanksma PK, van der Wall EE, Willemsen AT, Pruim J, Anthonio RL, de Jong RM, Vaalburg W, Lie KI Coronary vasomotion in patients with syndrome X: evaluation with positron emission tomography and parametric myocardial perfusion imaging. Eur J Nucl Med. 1997; 24: 530-7.
17. Fragasso G, Rossetti E, Dosio F, Gianolli L, Pizzetti G, Cattaneo N, Fazio F, Chierchia SL. High prevalence of the thallium-201 reverse redistribution phenomenon in patients with syndrome. Eur Heart J 1996; 17: 1482-7.
18. Meeder JG, Blanksma PK, Crijns HJ, Anthonio RL, Pruim J, Brouwer J, de Jong RM, van der Wall EE, Vaalburg W, Lie KI. Mechanisms of angina pectoris in syndrome X assessed by myocardial perfusion dynamics and heart rate variability. Eur Heart J 1995; 16: 1571-7.

19. Inobe Y, Kugiyama K, Morita E, Kawano H, Okumura K, Tomiguchi S, Tsuji A, Kojima A, Takahashi M, Yasue H. Role of adenosine in pathogenesis of syndrome X: assessment with coronary hemodynamic measurements and thallium-201 myocardial single-photon emission computed tomography. J Am Coll Cardiol 1996; 28: 890-6.

20. Kao CH, Wang SJ, Ting CT, Chen YT. ^{99m}Tc sestamibi myocardial SPECT in syndrome X. Clin Nucl Med 1996; 21: 280-3.

21. Palleschi L, Gianni W, De Vincentis G, Banci M, Sottosanti G, Ierardi M, Scopinaro F, Marigliano V. Dipyridamole technetium-99m Sestamibi imaging in the diagnosis of syndrome X. Angiology. 1996; 47: 369-73.

22. Kao CH, Wang SJ, Ting CT, Chen YT. Thallium-201 myocardial SPET in strictly defined syndrome X. Nucl Med Commun 1995; 16: 640-6.

23. Thorley PJ, Ball J, Sheard KL, Sivananthan UM. Evaluation of ^{99m}Tc-tetrofosmin as a myocardial perfusion agent in routine clinical use. Nucl Med Commun 1995; 16: 733-40.

24. Rosano GM, Peters NS, Kaski JC, Mavrogeni SI, Collins P, Underwood SR, Poole-Wilson PA. Abnormal uptake and washout of thallium-201 in patients with syndrome X and normal-appearing scans. Am J Cardiol 1995; 75: 400-2.

25. Rosen SD, Uren NG, Kaski J-C, Tousoulis D, Davies GJ, Camici PG. Coronary Vasodilator Reserve, Pain Perception and Gender in Patients with Syndrome X. Circulation 1994; 90: 50-60.

26. Galassi AR, Crea F, Araujo LI, Lammertsma AA, Pupita G, Yamomoto Y, Rechavia E, Jones T, Kaski J-C, Maseri A. Comparison of regional myocardial blood flow in syndrome X and one-vessel coronary artery disease. Am J Cardiol 1993; 72: 134-139.

27. Tweddel AC, Martin W, Hutton I. Thallium scans in syndrome X. Br Heart J 1992; 68: 48-50.

28. Rosen SD, Camici PG. Syndrome X: radionuclide studies of myocardial perfusion in patients with chest pain and normal coronary arteriograms [editorial] Eur J Nucl Med 1992; 19: 311-4.

29. Geltman EM, Henes CG, Sennef MJ, Sobel BE, Bergman SR. Increased myocardial perfusion at rest and diminished perfusion reserve in patients with angina and angiographically normal coronary arteries. J Am Coll Cardiol 1990; 16: 586-595.

30. Camici PG, Gistri R, Lorenzoni R, Sorace O, Michelassi C, Bongiorni MG, Salvadori PA, L'Abbate A. Coronary reserve and exercise ECG in patients with chest pain and normal coronary angiograms. Circulation 1992; 86: 179-186.

31. Galassi AR, Kaski J-C, Pupita G, Vejar M, Crea F, Maseri A. Lack of evidence for alpha-adrenergic receptor-mediated mechanisms in the genesis of ischemia in syndrome X. Am J Cardiol 1989; 64: 264-269.

32. Lorenzoni R, Rosen SD, Camici PG. Effect of selective α_1 blockade on resting and hyperemic myocardial blood flow in normal humans. Am J Physiol 1996; 271: H1302-H1306.

33. Camici PG, Rosen SD. Does positron emission tomography contribute to the management of clinical cardiac problems? Eur Heart J 1996; 17: 174-181.

34. Baig MW, Sheard K, Thorley PJ, Rees MR, Tan LB. The use of dobutamine stress thallium scintigraphy in the diagnosis of syndrome X. Postgrad Med J 1992; 68 Suppl 2: S20-4.

35. Kataoka T, Shih WJ. False-positive myocardial perfusion scintigraphy in syndrome X. Semin-Nucl-Med. 1997; 27: 186-9.

36. Uren NG, Camici PG, Melin JA, Bol A, de Bruyne B, Radvan J, Olivotto I, Rosen SD, Impallomeni M and Wijns W. The effect of ageing on the coronary vasodilator reserve in man. J Nucl Med 1995; 36: 2032-2036.

37. Hoffman JIE. Heterogeneity of myocardial blood flow. Bas Res Cardiol 1995; 90: 103-111.

38. Rosen SD, Boyd H, Lorenzoni R, Kaski J-C, Camici PG. Effects of a_1 blockade on myocardial blood flow in patients with cardiac syndrome X. Circulation 1997; 96: I-625.

39. Nihoyannopoulos P, Kaski JC, Crake T, Maseri A. Absence of myocardial dysfunction during pacing stress in patients with syndrome X. J Am Coll Cardiol 1991;18:1463-1470.

40. Camici PG, Marraccini P, Lorenzoni R, Buzzigoli G, Pecori N, Perissinotto A, Ferrannini E, L'Abbate A, Marzilli M: Coronary hemodynamics and myocardial metabolism in patients with syndrome X: response to pacing stress. J Am Coll Cardiol 1991;17:1461-1470.

41. Panza JA, Laurienzo JM, Curiel RV, Unger EF, Quyyumi AA, Dilsizian V, Cannon RO. Investigation of the mechanism of chest pain in patients with angiographically normal coronary arteries using transesophageal dobutamine stress echocardiography. J Am Coll Cardiol 1997; 29: 293-301.

42. Rosano GM, Kaski JC, Arie S, Pereira WI, Horta P, Collins P, Pileggi F, Poole-Wilson PA. Failure to demonstrate myocardial ischemia in patients with angina and normal coronary arteries. Evaluation by continuous coronary sinus pH monitoring and lactate metabolism. Eur Heart J 1996; 17: 1175-80.

43. Shapiro LM, Crake T, Poole-Wilson PA. Is altered cardiac sensation responsible for chest pain in patients with normal coronary arteries? Clinical observation during cardiac catheterization. Br Med J 1988; 296: 170-171.
44. Cannon RO, Quyyumi AA, Schenke WH, Fananapazir L, Tucker EE, Gaughan AM, Gracely RH, Cattau EL, Epstein SE. Abnormal cardiac sensitivity in patients with chest pain and normal coronary arteries. J Am Coll Cardiol 1990; 16: 1359-1366.
45. Eriksson B, Svedenhag J, Martinsson A, Sylvén C. Effect of epinephrine infusion on chest pain in syndrome X in the absence of signs of myocardial ischemia. Am J Cardiol. 1995; 75: 241-245.
46. Turiel M, Galassi AR, Glazier JJ, Kaski JC, Maseri A: Pain threshold and tolerance in women with syndrome X and women with stable angina pectoris. Am J Cardiol 1987; 60:503-507.
47. Rosen SD, Paulesu E, Frith CD, Jones T, Davies GJ, Frackowiak RSJ, Camici PG. Central neural correlates of angina pectoris as a model of visceral pain. Lancet 1994; 344: 147-150.
48. Rosen SD, Paulesu E, Nihoyannopoulos P, Tousoulis D, Frackowiak RSJ, Frith CD, Jones T and Camici PG. Silent ischemia as a central problem: regional brain activation compared in silent and painful myocardial ischemia. Ann Int Med 1996; 124: 939-949.
49. Raichle M. Circulatory and metabolic correlates of brain function in normal humans In: Mountcastle VB, Plum F, Geiger SR eds. Handbook of Physiology. Section 1: The nervous system. Vol V Higher functions of the brain Part 2, Chapter 16. Bethesda Md, USA: American Physiological Society, 1987: 643-674.
50. Friston KJ, Frackowiak RSJ. Imaging functional anatomy. In: Lassen NA. Ingvar DH, Raichle ME, Friberg L eds. Brain work and mental activity, Alfred Benzon symposium vol 31, Copenhagen, Munksgaard 1991: 267-279.
51. Rosen SD, Paulesu E, Frackowiak RSJ, Camici PG. Regional Brain Activation Compared in Angina Pectoris and Syndrome X. Circulation 1995; 92: I-651.
52. Cannon RO, Quyyumi AA, Mincemoyer R, Stine AM, Gracely RH, Smith WB, Geraci MF, Black BC, Uhde TW, Waclawiw MA, et al. Imipramine in patients with chest pain despite normal coronary angiograms. N Engl J Med 1994; 330: 1411-7.
53. Cannon RO. The sensitive heart. A syndrome of abnormal cardiac pain perception [clinical conference] J Am Med Assoc 1995; 273: 883-7.
54. Marcus ML, Wilson RF, White CW. Methods of measurement of myocardial blood flow in patients: A critical review. Circulation 1987; 76: 245-53.
55. Camici PG, Marraccini P, Gistri R, Salvadori PA, Sorace O, L'Abbate A. Adrenergically mediated coronary vasoconstriction in patients with syndrome X. Cardiovasc Drugs Ther. 1994; 8: 221-6.

Chapter 7

MYOCARDIAL METABOLISM IN CARDIAC SYNDROME X

Jens Peder Bagger

Patients with normal coronary arteries who experience chest pain have constituted an enigma for many years. As some of these patients have ischemia-like ST segment depression in response to exercise stress testing attempts have been made to ascertain whether the syndrome has an ischemic etiology. Measurement of cardiac metabolite exchange in response to pacing stress is one of the methods used to investigate ischemia in these patients. Ischemia increases the myocardial carbohydrate-lipid utilization ratio and the change in cardiac lactate exchange from uptake to output, due to enhanced anaerobic glycolysis, has been the most frequently used metabolic index of ischemia. Despite that initial studies had demonstrated cardiac ischemia in patients with chest pain and normal coronary arteries, using metabolic markers, abnormal lactate findings in these patients have declined in recent studies. Thus, the findings of myocardial lactate production during stress in up to 40% of patients in the early studies have almost "vanished" in recent studies.

This review will discuss changes in metabolism that can be observed in the ischemic heart and will specially focus on findings in syndrome X.

Metabolism in the normal myocardium

Free fatty acids (FFA) and carbohydrates are two major, and competitive, cardiac energy sources [1]. In the fasting state the arterial concentration of FFA is high and positively related to cardiac FFA uptake [2]. Within the cell FFA may be oxidized or synthesized to triglycerides or other complex lipids [3]. In case of oxidation, FFA combine to CoA to form long-chain acyl CoA that is transported across the mitochondrial membrane by means of carnitine [4]. Within the mitochondria acyl CoA is converted to acetyl-CoA by means of beta-oxidation and this end product enters the Krebs-cycle [3,4]. FFA oxidation suppresses that of carbohydrates due to intracellular accumulation of citrate, acetyl-CoA and NADH [3,5]. Cytosolic citrate is one of the main inhibitors of phosphofructokinase, a rate-controlling enzyme of glucose breakdown [6]. Citrate is released by both the normal and ischemic human myocardium and transmyocardial citrate gradients are positively related to arterial FFA concentration and negatively to cardiac glucose extraction [7]. Intra-mitochondrially produced acetyl-CoA and NADH decrease carbohydrate utilization by inhibiting pyruvate dehydrogenase activity and thereby retard pyruvate entry into the Krebs-cycle [8]. Glycolysis is controlled mainly at the steps of phosphofructokinase and glyceraldehyde 3-P dehydrogenase [3,5] (Figure 1). After meals and in the presence of insulin, glucose uptake and activity of phosphofructokinase are increased and

82

glyceraldehyde 3-P dehydrogenase becomes rate limiting for glucose breakdown [3,5]. Reoxidation of cytosolic NADH is necessary for the continuous glucose and lactate utilization [3,5,9]. NADH is oxidized indirectly via the malate-aspartate cycle [10]. Activity of this cycle is in part linked to the cytosolic concentration of glutamate and requires uptake of glutamate from the circulation [10]. Glutamate may furthermore contribute to aerobic and anaerobic cardiac metabolism or it can be transaminated with pyruvate to form alanine [11,12]. The findings in patients with and without coronary artery disease that myocardial glutamate uptake is positively related to uptake of glucose and lactate and to the release of alanine, support the existence of an interrelationship between these amino acids and carbohydrate metabolism [13,14,15].

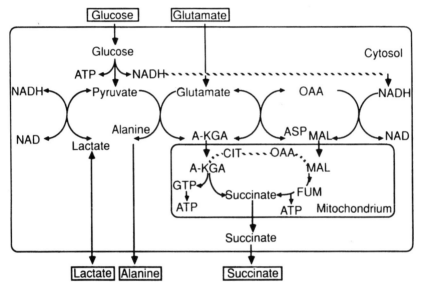

Figure 1. Coupling glutamate metabolism with reactions of the Krebs cycle and glycolysis indicating the pathways of anaerobic energy formation. Abbreviations: A-KGA: alfa-ketoglutarate; ASP: aspartate; ADP, ATP: adenosine di- and triphosphate; CIT: citrate; FUM: fumarate; GDP, GTP: guanosine di- and triphosphate; MAL: malate; NAD, NADH: oxidized and reduced nicotinamide adenine dinucleotide; OAA: oxaloacetate.

Metabolism in the ischemic myocardium

FFA utilization requires more oxygen than that of carbohydrates for the release of a given amount of energy [16]. In an attempt to approach normal energy charge the ischemic heart shifts towards a preference for carbohydrates at the expense of FFA [1,3,5,17] (Figure 2). The attempt to maintain energy production is met primarily by increased breakdown of glucose from the circulation and from cardiac glycogen stores [1,3,5]. Oxidation of NADH produced by glycolysis and from lactate to pyruvate conversion is necessary for continued glucose utilization due to its inhibition of glyceraldehyde 3-P dehydrogenase [18]. As a consequence, the malate-aspartate shuttle activity would be expected to accelerate. Consistent with this, increased glutamate extraction has been found both

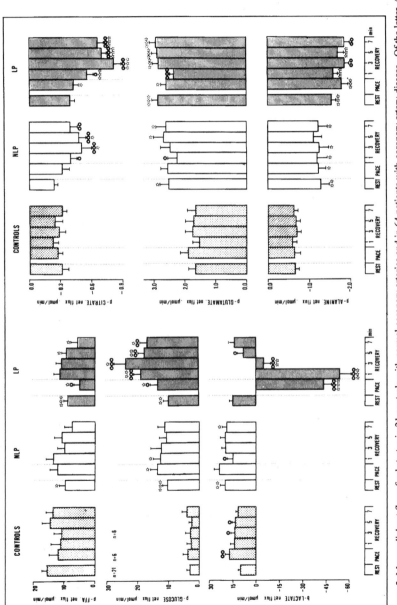

Figure. 2. Myocardial net flux of substrates in 21 controls with normal coronary arteries and in 64 patients with coronary artery disease. Of the latter, 40 showed cardiac lactate production (LP) and 24 no lactate production (NLP) during pacing. Positive and negative values correspond to cardiac uptake or release of substrates, respectively. Data are expressed as mean ± SEM. FFA = free fatty acids. Differences are shown by single (p<0.05), double (p<0.01) or triple (p<0.001) asterisks. Differences within groups are shown by asterisks within circles in the same way. With permission from Am J Cardiol, ref. 17.

globally and in regions with reduced blood flow in coronary artery disease [19,20]. The increased cardiac alanine production seen in patients with ischemic heart disease probably reflects the augmented glucose and glutamate metabolism that takes place in these patients [14,15,19]. However, the more ischemic the tissue, the less effectively operates the malate-aspartate cycle and NADH oxidation becomes increasingly dependent on pyruvate to lactate conversion [9]. Although glycolytic flux is increased within certain limits of reduced blood flows, accumulation of lactate, hydrogen and ammonium ions depress the action of glycolytic enzymes [5,21]. Consequently, the initial increase in glycolytic flux during severe ischemia is followed by a decreased rate of glycolysis, depending on the operational state of the mitochondria and/or the rate at which toxic metabolites can be washed out [3,5,21]. Although the glycolytically produced pyruvate can be shunted to alanine [11,22], thus lowering the amount of pyruvate converted to lactate (and thereby lactate accumulation?), the importance of this mechanism for the maintenance of glycolytic flux is not known. The recovery phase after an episode of ischemia is characterized by a short-lasting wash-out of lactate and a longer lasting period of increased cardiac uptake of glucose to re-build glycogen stores [23-25]. The fact that cardiac citrate release is increased for several minutes after an episode of severe ischemia supports the fact that glucose taken up by the heart is directed towards glycogen repletion instead of glycolysis [23].

Cardiac lactate exchange as a metabolic marker of ischemia

Although cardiac lactate production has been employed as a metabolic marker of ischemia in many studies there are limitations to the use of lactate exchange for this purpose. Thus, myocardial lactate release is not seen during stress provocation in up to 50% of patients with documented coronary artery disease [26-28]. There are various reasons for that. The coronary sinus mainly drains areas in the left ventricle supplied by the left coronary arteries. Efflux from an ischemic zone might be obscured by dilution with blood emerging from normally perfused areas or ischemia may be so mild that no detectable anaerobic glycolysis occurs. Furthermore, decreased lactate escape does not always reflect lesser ischemia because lactate accumulation itself hampers the anaerobic glycolysis and thereby retards further lactate production [3,5,21]. A fall in global lactate extraction short of production could reflect the net result of efflux from an area with lactate production vs continuous uptake in the remaining myocardium. It could also reflect spontaneous variations [29], changes in coronary blood flow [30] or the effect of substrate competition [1,3,5]. Therefore, reduced lactate uptake should not be regarded to represent a reliable marker of myocardial ischemia. Even a net shift in cardiac lactate exchange from uptake to production may not necessarily represent ischemia if the absolute A-Cs differences are small and near the analytical precision of the method used for detection of this metabolite.

Early studies of cardiac metabolism in syndrome X

In the early studies where lactate exchange was used as a marker of ischemia, cardiac lactate production was found in 13-38% of the patients in response to pacing or pharmacological stress [28,31-36]. Patients with hypertension or a history of hypertension, diabetes, left bundle branch block, and irregularities of the vessel wall were included to various degrees in these studies. A history of angina pectoris, normal coronary arteries and a positive exercise stress test was suggested by some as a diagnostic criterium for syndrome X in an attempt to confine the disease to the heart and to identify a subgroup of patients. However, in large consecutive series of patients with angina pectoris and normal coronary arteries only 11-20 % had a positive exercise test [31,37]. In most of the studies the pain characteristics and severity did not differ between patients with abnormal or normal stress tests. Furthermore, the symptoms were indistinguishable from those in coronary artery disease in some studies, and were atypical in other studies. Chest pain was reported in 60-88% of patients during pacing. Two of the studies of cardiac metabolism in patients with chest pain and normal coronary angiogram comprised consecutive patients. In 200 patients (50% men) with anginal pain that was indistinguishable from that in patients with coronary artery disease 20% had a positive exercise stress test and 22% (out of 100 patients) showed cardiac lactate production in response to pacing or pharmacologically provoked stress [31]. In the study of Boudoulas *et al.* of 29 consecutive patients, 14% of these had a positive exercise test and 48% showed post-pacing ST-depression [33]. Nine of these patients (31%) showed cardiac lactate production during pacing. All 9 had chest pain and post-pacing electrocardiographic signs of ischemia. Only one of the 9 patients with cardiac lactate production had a positive exercise test vs 3 of 20 patients who showed no lactate production. However, patients with lactate production had a higher degree of ST depression in response to pacing than patients with continuous lactate extraction. Bemiller *et al.* [32] found no correlation between positive exercise stress testing or pacing induced ischemia and lactate production (seen in 36%) in a group of 14 patients. In another study, one of 2 patients with lactate production showed ST segment depression in response to pacing vs 4 out of 14 with no lactate production [34]. The character and frequency of chest pain in response to pacing stress were similar in patients with and without cardiac lactate production in most of the studies. Thus it seems that cardiac ischemia in the form of myocardial lactate release is inconclusively related to electrocardiographic signs of ischemia and to the occurrence of chest pain. Even in the study by Arbogast and Bourassa [28] that prompted Kemp to coin the term syndrome X, the authors reported a discrepancy between preserved left ventricular function and electrocardiographic and metabolic signs of cardiac ischemia.

Newer studies of cardiac metabolism in syndrome X

The use of lactate production as a single marker of the metabolic changes occurring in the myocardium is a specific but, to some extent insensitive, marker of ischemia as mentioned before. In 2 recent studies, cardiac exchange of additional compounds of the glycolytic pathway and that of lipids was examined in response to pacing stress [38,39]. Both studies included consecutive patients with normal coronary arteries and exercise-induced angina pectoris and ST segment depression (syndrome X). Bøtker *et al.* [39] sub-divided patients into 2 groups: 1) those with "microvascular" and 2) patients with "non-microvascular angina" according to whether patients had reduced (<2.5) or normal (≥2.5) coronary flow reserve as assessed by intracoronary Doppler guidewire technique or positron emission tomography (in response to dipyridamol infusion). In their study Camici *et al.* [38] performed incremental pacing up to a maximal heart rate whereas Bøtker *et al.* [39] aimed for a constant pace-rate of 150 beats/min for a maximum of 10 min.

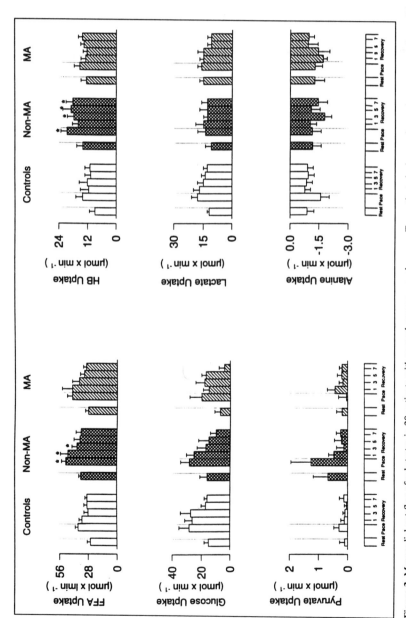

Figure 3. Myocardial net flux of substrates in 28 patients with normal coronary angiograms. Ten patients had normal exercise stress tests (controls) and 18 had positive stress tests. Patients were classified as "microvascular" (MA, n=8) or "non-microvascular angina" (non-MA, n=10) according to their coronary artery flow reserves. Positive and negative values correspond to cardiac uptake or release of substrates, respectively. Data are mean ± SEM. FFA = free fatty acids, HB = beta-hydroxybutyrate; *p<0.05 vs controls. With permission from Am J Cardiol, ref. 39.

Both studies included control groups of patients with "atypical" chest pain and both normal coronary angiograms and exercise stress tests. All syndrome X patients in these studies developed chest pain and ST segment depression in response to pacing although a higher heart rate was achieved with incremental pacing (157±16) than with constant pacing (145±5). No cardiac lactate release was observed in any patients or controls in both studies. Camici et al. [38] found identical uptake of total carbohydrates in both syndrome X and controls, but carbohydrate oxidation increased during maximal pacing only in controls. Syndrome X patients showed a greater cardiac uptake of FFA and a preference for lipid oxidation compared to controls. Cardiac pyruvate extraction was consistently lower in syndrome X than in controls and changed to a net release during and post-pacing in the former group. Syndrome X patients showed cardiac alanine uptake throughout the study whereas alanine release was seen only in controls. Myocardial energy expenditure and oxygen consumption were similar in the 2 groups at baseline but were lower in patients with syndrome X during pacing. The authors [38] concluded that the myocardial metabolic changes in syndrome X were opposite to those seen in conditions characterized by myocardial ischemia and that myocardial energy expenditure was lower in patients than controls at maximal rate-pressure product levels.

Bøtker et al. [39] on the other hand, found no differences in resting cardiac uptake of FFA, glucose, lactate, pyruvate, alanine, beta-hydroxybutyrate, citrate or oxygen when "microvascular" and "non-microvascular" groups and controls were compared (Figure 3). Cardiac uptake of FFA and beta-hydroxybutyrate were increased during pacing in "non-microvascular disease" patients compared to controls. As patients with "non-microvascular disease" had higher circulating levels of these "fuels" than controls, the observed increase in metabolite uptake is most likely to be secondary to the increased substrate availability. None of the other metabolites differed between groups during pacing and recovery. There was a continuous cardiac release of alanine and citrate as well as a small mean uptake of pyruvate in all 3 groups throughout the study period. Energy expenditure and respiratory quotients were similar in all 3 groups throughout the study. Thus, cardiac metabolism in response to pacing stress in syndrome X patients was characterized by reduced carbohydrate/FFA utilization ratio in one of the studies [38] and no differences between controls and syndrome X patients were observed in the other study, regardless of whether the patients had "microvascular disease" or not. None of these studies reported on myocardial lactate production.

The discrepancies of metabolic findings between early and recent studies are puzzling. Factors of importance may include the continuous improvements in fluoroscopy so that the likelihood of overlooking stenosed or occluded vessels are minimized at present. It is also conceivable that more strict exclusion criteria were applied in recent studies. On the other hand, the early studies reported on more than 200 cardiac metabolic examinations whereas only 30 patients were investigated in the 2 recent studies.

References

1. Opie LH. Fuels: carbohydrates and lipids. In: Opie LH, ed. The heart: Physiology and metabolism. New York: Raven Press, 1991:208-46.
2. Lassers BW, Wahlqvist ML, Kaijser L, Carlsson LA. Relationship in man between plasma free fatty acids and myocardial metabolism of carbohydrate substrates. Lancet 1971; II:448-50.
3. Neely JR, Morgan HE. Relationship between carbohydrate and lipid metabolism and the energy balance of

heart muscle. Ann Rev Physiol 1974;36:413-59.

4. Opie LH. Role of carnitine in fatty acid metabolism of normal and ischemic myocardium. Am Heart J 1979;97:375-87.

5. Randle PJ, Tubbs PK. Carbohydrate and fatty acid metabolism. In: Berne R, Sperelakis N, Geiger SR, eds. Handbook of Physiology. The Cardiovascular System. Vol. I. The Heart. American Physiological Society, Bethesda, 1979:805-44.

6. Parmeggiani A, Bowman RH. Regulation of phosphofructokinase activity by citrate in normal and diabetic muscle. Biochem Biophys Res Commun 1963;12:268-73.

7. Nielsen TT, Henningsen P, Bagger JP, Thomsen PEB, Eyjolfsson K. Myocardial citrate metabolism in control subjects and patients with coronary artery disease. Scand J Clin Lab Invest 1980;40: 575-80.

8. Kerbey AL, Randle PJ, Cooper RH et al. Regulation of pyruvate dehydrogenase in rat heart. Biochem J 1976;154:327-48.

9. Vary TC, Reibel DK, Neely JR. Control of energy metabolism of heart muscle. Ann Rev Physiol 1981;43:419-30.

10. Safer B. The metabolic significance of the malate-aspartate cycle in heart. Circ Res 1975;37:527-33.

11. Taegtmeyer H, Peterson MB, Ragavan VV, Ferguson AG, Lesch M. De novo alanine synthesis in isolated oxygen deprived rabbit myocardium. J Biochem Chem 1977;252:5010-18.

12. Taegtmeyer H, Russell R. glutamate metabolism in rabbit heart: augmentation by ischemia and inhibition with acetoacetate. J Appl Cardiol 1987;2:231-49.

13. Pisarenko OI, Lepilin MG, Ivanov VE. Cardiac metabolism and performance during L-glutamic acid infusion in postoperative cardiac failure. Clin Sci 1986;70:7-12.

14. Thomassen AR, Nielsen TT, Bagger JP, Henningsen P. Myocardial exchanges of glutamate, alanine and citrate in controls and patients with coronary artery disease. Clin Sci 1983;64:33-40.

15. Thomassen AR, Nielsen TT, Bagger JP, Thuesen L. Myocardial glutamate and alanine exchanges related to carbohydrate metabolism in patients with normal and stenotic coronary arteries. Clin Physiol 1984;4:425-34.

16. Ferrannini E. The theoretical basis of indirect calorimetry: a review. Metabolism 1988;37:287-301.

17. Thomassen A, Bagger JP, Nielsen TT, Henningsen P. Altered global myocardial substrate preference at rest and during pacing in coronary artery disease with stable angina pectoris. Am J Cardiol 1988;62:686-93.

18. Kobayashi K, Neely JR. Control of maximum rates of glycolysis in rat cardiac muscle. Circ Res 1979;44:166-75.

19. Mudge GH, Mills RM, Taegtmeyer H, Gorlin R, Lesch M. Alterations of myocardial amino acid metabolism in chronic ischemic heart disease. J Clin Invest 1976;58:1185-92.

20. Knapp WH, Helus F, Ostertag H, Tillmanns H, Kubler W. Uptake and turnover of L-(N-13)-glutamate in the normal human heart and in patients with coronary artery disease. Eur J Nuc Med 1982;7:211-15.

21. Neely JR, Feuvray D. Metabolic products and myocardial ischemia. Am J Pathol 1981;102:282-91.

22. Tischler ME, Goldberg AL. Production of alanine and glutamine by atrial muscle from fed and fasted rats. Am J Physiol 1980;238: E487-93.

23. Bagger JP Nielsen TT, Henningsen P, Thomsen PEB, Eyjolfsson K. Myocardial release of citrate and lactate during atrial-pacing induced angina pectoris. Scand J Clin Lab Invest 1981;41:431-39.

24. Camici P, Araujo LI, Spinks T et al. Prolonged metabolic recovery allows late identification of ischemia in the absence of electrocardiographic and perfusion changes in patients with exertional angina. Can J Cardiol 1986;Suppl A:131-35.

25. Segal LD, Mason DT. Effect of exercise and conditioning on rat heart glycogen and glycogen synthase. J Appl Physiol 1978;44:183-89.

26. Bagger JP. Effects of antianginal drugs on myocardial energy metabolism in coronary artery disease. Pharmacol Toxicol 1990;66(Suppl IV):1-31.

27. Wiener L, P Walinsky, Kasparian H et al. Therapeutic implications of myocardial lactate metabolism in patients considered candidates for emergency myocardial revascularization. J Thor Cardiovasc Surg 1978;75:612-20.

28. Arbogast R, Bourassa MG. Myocardial function during atrial pacing in patients with angina pectoris and normal coronary angiograms. Am J Cardiol 1973;32:257-63.

29. Bagger JP, Nielsen TT, Thomassen AT. Reproducibility of coronary haemodynamics and cardiac metabolism during pacing-induced angina pectoris. Clin Physiol 1985;5:359-70.

30. Bagger JP, Nielsen TT, Henningsen P. Increased coronary sinus lactate concentration during pacing

induced angina pectoris after clinical improvement by glyceryl trinitrate. Br Heart J 1983;50:483-90.

31. Kemp HG, Vokonas PS, Cohn PF, Gorlin R. The anginal syndrome associated with normal coronary arteriograms. Am J Med 1973;54:735-742.

32. Bemiler CR, Pepine CJ, Rogers AK. Long-term observations in patients with angina and normal coronary arteriograms. Circulation 1973;47:36-43.

33. Boudoulas H, Cobb TC, Leighton RF, Wilt SM. Myocardial lactate production in patients with angina-like chest pain and angiographically normal coronary arteries and left ventricle. Am J Cardiol 1974;34:501-5.

34. Mammohansingh P, Parker JO. Angina pectoris with normal coronary arteriograms: Hemodynamic and metabolic response to atrial pacing. Am Heart J 1975;90:555-61.

35. Opherk D, Zebe H, Weihe E *et al*. Reduced coronary dilatory capacity and ultrastructural changes of the myocardium in patients with angina pectoris but normal coronary arteriograms. Circulation 1981;63:817-25.

36. Greenberg MA, Grose RM, Neuburger N, Silverman R, Strain JE, Cohen MV. Impaired coronary vasodilator responsiveness as a cause of lactate production during pacing-induced ischemia in patients with angina pectoris and normal coronary arteries. JACC 1987;9:743-51.

37. Papanicolaou MN, Califf RM, Hlatky MA *et al*. Prognostic implications of angiographically normal and insignificantly narrowed coronary arteries. Am J Cardiol 1986;58:1181-87.

38. Camici PG, Marraccini P, Lorenzoni R *et al*. Coronary hemodynamics and myocardial metabolism in patients with syndrome X: Response to pacing stress. JACC 1991;17:1461-70.

39. Bøtker HE, Sonne HS, Bagger JP, Nielsen TT. Impact of impaired coronary flow reserve and insulin resistance on myocardial energy metabolism in patients with syndrome X. Am J Cardiol 1997;79:1615-22.

Chapter 8

ENDOTHELIAL DYSFUNCTION IN CARDIAC SYNDROME X (MICROVASCULAR ANGINA)

Kensuke Egashira, Masahiro Mohri and Akira Takeshita

For many years it has been argued that the pathogenesis of chest pain in patients with angiographically normal coronary arteries or minimal coronary artery disease (syndrome X) is multifactorial [1-3]. In a considerable proportion of patients who have atypical chest pain and no ischemic ST segment changes during pain, it is unlikely that the cause of their symptoms is cardiac. However, in the subset of patients with angina-like chest pain and stress-induced ST segment depression, a cardiac cause must be considered. Cannon *et al* [3] suggested that coronary microvascular dysfunction, with evidence of myocardial ischemia, may represent one end of the spectrum and abnormal pain perception without myocardial ischemia may represent the opposite extreme of the spectrum. Patients with anginal chest pain, stress-induced ST depression and angiographically normal coronary arteries, without coronary artery spasm, are generally assumed to have myocardial ischemia due to microvascular dysfunction (these are often considered to have cardiac syndrome X). Many studies have demonstrated that a large proportion of these patients have limited coronary vasodilatory response to pharmacological stimuli and physiological stress [1,3]. Cannon *et al* [1,2] called this group of patients with limited coronary flow reserve "microvascular angina".

Pathogenesis

Maseri *et al* [3] proposed the intriguing hypothesis that patients with cardiac syndrome X have "patchilly" distributed functional (vasoconstriction or spasm) and/or structural (organic stenosis) abnormalities in prearteriolar vessels. They considered this hypothesis useful to explain the wide spectrum of clinical symptoms seen in the absence of overt myocardial ischaemia in patients with cardiac syndrome X. These authors suggested that when a large number of prearteriolar vessels is involved, the reduced coronary flow reserve will result in more obvious myocardial ischemia. The involvement of a small number of prearteriolar vessels may result in the release of adenosine from arterioles distal to the diseased prearteriolar vessels, causing chest pain in the absence of ischemia or other detectable abnormality in coronary microcirculation.

The vascular endothelium plays an important role in the homeostasis of the blood vessel wall [6-7]. It produces various substances including nitric oxide (NO), prostacyclin and hyperpolarizing factors. These substances regulate vascular structure as well as function. Hypertension, hypercholesterolemia and aging are associated with endothelial dysfunction (abnormal release of endothelium-derived substances) of the blood vessels such as large coronary arteries [8-12]. In addition, recent evidence have demonstrated that this endothelial dysfunction is not confined to the large coronary arteries but also extends into the coronary microcirculation [8-12]. The latter concept has an important physiological implication, because more than 95% of the coronary vascular resistance resides in the microcirculation. Therefore, changes in coronary blood flow in response to stress is regulated largely by the microcirculation [13,14]. These findings suggest that endothelial dysfunction of coronary microcirculation may reduce coronary blood flow supply and thus contribute to myocardial ischemia.

There is now evidence in the literature indicating that endothelial dysfunction of the coronary microcirculation is present in patients with cardiac syndrome X [15-17]. In this chapter, we will review the current knowledge on endothelial dysfunction in the coronary microcirculation in patients with cardiac syndrome X and discuss its role in the pathogenesis of symptoms and myocardial ischemia in these patients.

Endothelial dysfunction of the coronary microcirculation in patients with cardiac syndrome X

In recent years, several studies have examined endothelial function in the coronary circulation of subsets of patients with cardiac syndrome X. Although the definition of the studied patient population varies among studies, these patients have been demonstrated to have limited endothelium-dependent increases in coronary blood flow in response to intracoronary infusion of acetylcholine. Acetylcholine-induced coronary vasodilation in humans has been shown to be inhibited in part by pretreatment with N^Gnitro-L-arginine (L-NMMA), a specific inhibitor of nitric oxide synthesis [18,19], indicating that acetylcholine dilates large epicardial and resistance coronary arteries through the endothelial release of nitric oxide in humans.

We reported that endothelium-dependent vasodilation of coronary microcirculation is impaired in patients with anginal chest pain, a positive exercise-induced ST segment depression and normal coronary arteries in the absence of risk factors for coronary atherosclerosis [15]. We studied 9 selected patients and 10 control subjects with atypical chest pain. The increase in coronary blood flow in response to acetylcholine was blunted in patients whereas the response to acetylcholine in control subjects was normal. However, the increase in coronary blood flow in response to isosorbide dinitrate and papaverine was similar between the two groups. Also, vasomotor responses of large epicardial coronary arteries to acetylcholine, isosorbide dinitrate and papaverine were similar between the two groups. Intracoronary papaverine induced myocardial lactate production suggestive of ischemia in the patients but not in the controls. We considered that these findings provide evidence of endothelial dysfunction in the coronary microcirculation in selected patients with cardiac syndrome X. In a subsequent study, we observed that L-arginine (the precursor of nitric oxide synthesis) improved endothelium-dependent vasodilation of coronary microcirculation to acetylcholine in patients with cardiac syndrome X [20], suggesting that coronary microvascular endothelial dysfunction in these patients may be related to defective synthesis of nitric oxide. A preliminary study by Bellamy et al [21] showed that oral L-arginine administration for 4 weeks increased exercise tolerance and reversed endothelial dysfunction in patients with microvascular angina. These findings suggest that nitric oxide deficiency is involved in the pathophysiology of cardiac syndrome X.

Motz *et al* [16] indicated that endothelial dysfunction of the coronary microcirculation (defined as impaired coronary blood flow response to acetylcholine but not to dipyridamole) was noted in one subset of patients with cardiac syndrome X. In other groups of patients, coronary blood flow responses to acetylcholine and dipyridamole were impaired, indicating an abnormality in microvascular smooth muscle. Quyyumi *et al* [17] examined coronary blood flow response to acetylcholine and pacing in 51 patients with cardiac syndrome X. They found a significant correlation between the coronary blood flow response to acetylcholine and the response during pacing and suggested that coronary microvascular endothelial dysfunction may contribute to reduced coronary flow reserve during atrial pacing and anginal chest pain in these patients. However, the coronary blood flow response to acetylcholine in their patients varied widely; some patients exhibited normal coronary blood flow response to acetylcholine.

Taken together, endothelial dysfunction of coronary microcirculation do occur in patients with cardiac syndrome X. However, not all of these patients have endothelial dysfunction. We consider that endothelial dysfunction in the coronary microcirculation may be closely related to the pathogenesis of cardiac syndrome X, as in our experience the majority of these patients has been shown to have microvascular endothelial dysfunction.

The relationship between the pathophysiology of cardiac syndrome X and female hormone should be mentioned. The clinical observation that the incidence of (cardiac) syndrome X is higher in women [22,23], of whom most are menopausal, raise the hypothesis that estrogen deficiency contributes to the pathogenesis of syndrome X in at least a subset of patients. There is increasing evidence that menopause is associated with endothelial dysfunction in women [23] and that estrogen treatment improves endothelial dysfunction in postmenopausal women [24-26] although the underlying mechanisms are not well understood. Rosano *et al* [27] have demonstrated that estrogen treatment reduces episodes of chest pain in daily-life in patients with cardiac syndrome X and improves exercise -induced myocardial ischemia in patients with significant coronary artery disease [28].

Does endothelial dysfunction cause myocardial ischemia?

Data in the literature supports the hypothesis that endothelial dysfunction in the coronary microcirculation may limit coronary blood supply to the myocardium at rest and/or during stress. Therefore, an important question that must be addressed is whether endothelial dysfunction, that diminishes the release of relaxing factors such as nitric oxide, can cause myocardial ischemia. Quyyumi *et al* [19] reported that intracoronary infusion of L-NMMA inhibits endothelium-derived nitric oxide and thus reduces coronary blood flow response to atrial pacing in patients with normal coronary arteriograms. However, we [20] could not reproduce this effect of L-NMMA on pacing-induced increase in coronary blood flow in humans. Nevertheless, there was no evidence of myocardial ischemia by pacing after inhibition of nitric oxide synthesis in these studies [19,20].

Studies in animals suggest that coronary blood flow during pacing and metabolic stress is modulated by multiple mechanisms acting on the coronary microcirculation [13,14]. These are nitric oxide, adenosine, ATP-sensitive K^+ channels and others. Jones *et al* [29] reported that inhibition of nitric oxide synthesis with N^ω nitro-L-arginine methyl ester (L-NAME) induced vasoconstriction of small coronary arteries, however, it dilated downstream arterioles in dogs. Since L-NAME did not affect epicardial coronary arteries, the investigators concluded that dilation of arterioles compensates for vasoconstriction due to diminished nitric oxide release in the coronary microcirculation at rest. We [30] and others [31] reported that blockade of nitric oxide with L-NAME did not impair coronary blood flow response to atrial pacing or exercise in dogs. We also reported that blockade of ATP-sensitive K^+ channel with glibenclamide partly inhibits the increase in coronary blood flow during atrial pacing in dogs by 40% [32].

It is likely therefore that the redundancy of vasodilator mechanisms for regulating coronary microvascular tone during metabolic stress may compensate for diminished release of nitric oxide. Duncker *et al* [33] demonstrated that ATP-sensitive K^+ channel blockade with glibenclamide combined with adenosine receptor blockade with 8 phenyltheophilline inhibited the increase in coronary blood flow during exercise in dogs by 60%. The same investigators also found that inhibition of nitric oxide release with blockade of ATP-sensitive K^+ channels and adenosine receptors reduced the coronary blood flow response to exercise by 80%. These findings suggest that although nitric oxide contributes to the increase in coronary blood supply to the myocardium during metabolic stress, other mechanisms compensate for the loss of nitric oxide release in the normal heart.

Evidence of myocardial ischemia in cardiac syndrome X

Zeiher *et al* [34] examined the coronary blood flow response to acetylcholine in patients with no significant coronary artery disease who had reversible thallium perfusion defect in the myocardium during exercise and 14 patients with no significant coronary artery disease who had no thallium perfusion abnormality during exercise. They found that endothelium-dependent dilation of the coronary microcirculation is markedly less in patients with exercise-induced perfusion defects than in those with no perfusion abnormality. They concluded that endothelial dysfunction in the coronary microcirculation may contribute to the ischemic manifestations of cardiac syndrome X during times of increased myocardial demand.

Experimental studies suggest that endothelium regulates coronary microvascular tone and distribution of regional flow [13,14]. Galassi *et al* [35] and Geltman *et al* [36] measured regional myocardial blood flow distribution using positron emission tomography before and after intravenous dipyridamole in a small group of patients with cardiac syndrome X. They found that patients with syndrome X have an abnormal heterogeneity of regional flow both at baseline and during coronary vasodilation provoked by dipyridamole. These authors discussed that heterogeneous distribution of myocardial blood flow in these patients is possibly due to clusters of myocardial regions with relatively higher flow at baseline and relatively lower flow during dipyridamole infusion. As stated before, we [15] demonstrated that intracoronary administration of papaverine resulted in myocardial lactate production in patients with cardiac syndrome X. We reasoned in the latter study that papaverine induced heterogeneous myocardial perfusion possibly through a steal phenomenon and thus caused myocardial ischemia. Papaverine increased coronary blood flow to a similar extent in both patients and control subjects. We have observed that a large proportion of patients with cardiac syndrome X exhibit myocardial lactate production in response to papaverine administration. However, the clinical significance and the true mechanism of papaverine-induced lactate production remains to be established.

Inobe *et al* [37] investigated the role of adenosine in the pathogenesis of syndrome X. They performed thallium myocardial scintigraphy with exercise or intravenous adenosine in 26 patients with cardiac syndrome X. Perfusion abnormalities on exercise thallium scintigraphy with anginal chest pain occurred in 14 of 26 patients with syndrome X. Adenosine induced a perfusion defect in the same myocardial area where the perfusion defect was observed at exercise in 7 of the 14 patients with syndrome X. Intravenous infusion of aminophylline, an adenosine receptor blocker, suppressed the scintigraphic perfusion defect, chest pain and ST depression in patients with syndrome X with abnormal exercise scintigrams. The investigators suggested that a heterogeneous dilation of coronary microvessels to endogenous adenosine may lead to inhomogeneous distribution of flow and thus contribute to myocardial ischemia during exercise in this subset of patients with syndrome X.

Endothelial dysfunction of the coronary microcirculation in patients with cardiac syndrome X may contribute to myocardial ischemia by causing vasoconstriction (microvascular spasm). In this regard, recent reports of Hasdai *et al* [38] are interesting. These authors [38] examined the vasomotor function of the left anterior descending coronary artery in response to acetylcholine in 20 patients with chest pain and insignificant coronary artery disease. ^{99m}Tc sestamibi was injected intravenously before the infusion of the highest dose of acetylcholine and myocardial perfusion images were obtained. According to the perfusion pattern observed, three different sub-groups were identified: perfusion defect in the study region (n=6), no perfusion defects (n=7), and perfusion defects unrelated to the study region (n=7). In the two groups without perfusion defects in the study region, the infusion of acetylcholine resulted in increased coronary blood flow. However, in patients with perfusion defects in the study region, acetylcholine decreased coronary blood flow. This was associated with only modest vasoconstriction of the large epicardial coronary arteries, indicating that the decrease in coronary blood flow seen in this patient sub-group was due to microvascular hyperconstriction (spasm). Thus, the observation of Hasdai *et al* [38] suggests that coronary microvascular spasm associated with endothelial dysfunction may decrease coronary blood flow, resulting in myocardial perfusion defects suggestive of ischemia. We have also observed that intracoronary acetylcholine can provoke myocardial lactate production associated with anginal pain and ischemic ST changes in a considerable number of patients with cardiac syndrome X [39]. In this study, patients with vasospastic angina in whom significant constriction of large epicardial coronary arteries was provoked by acetylcholine infusion were excluded. Thus, our observation suggests that acetylcholine can induce coronary microvascular spasm and thus cause myocardial ischemia in a subset of patients with cardiac syndrome X.

An animal model of long-term inhibition of nitric oxide synthesis

Obviously, the clinical correlation of endothelial dysfunction in cardiac syndrome X should be assessed in the human coronary circulation in vivo. However, if a suitable animal model would be available, it would be useful to investigate the underlying mechanisms and possible treatment. We recently created an animal model of microvascular disease by chronically administering the nitric oxide synthesis inhibitor L-NAME to pigs for 2 to 4 weeks [40,41]. Coronary microvascular endothelium seems to be dysfunctional in these animals, because the increase in coronary blood flow to the endothelium-dependent vasodilator bradykinin is impaired in L-NAME-treated animals while the coronary blood flow response to endothelium-independent vasodilators, nitroglycerin and adenosine, was similar in the two groups. Also, structural changes such as medial thickening and perivascular fibrosis are evident in this model in the prearteriolar small coronary arteries (internal diameters from 100 to 300 μm) whereas these changes were less prominent in large epicardial coronary arteries (diameters greater than 500 μm) and arterioles (diameters less than 50 μm). Although the underlying mechanisms are still unknown, these findings suggest that long-term inhibition of nitric oxide synthesis causes structural changes in coronary microvessels. We examined whether microvascular response to serotonin was altered in this model and found that intracoronary serotonin increased coronary blood flow in control animals whereas it markedly decreased coronary blood flow associated with myocardial ischemia in L-NAME-treated animals. The decrease in coronary blood flow during serotonin administration was due to microvascular hyperreactivity (spasm), because the magnitude of serotonin-induced constriction of large epicardial coronary arteries was similar between the L-NAME-treated and control animals.

We further examined whether metabolic coronary vasodilation in response to pacing-induced tachycardia is altered in this model [42]. The increase in coronary blood flow in response to atrial pacing was less in the L-NAME-treated pigs than in controls. This impaired flow response to pacing was associated with increased extraction of oxygen from the coronary circulation. The pacing-induced increase in myocardial oxygen consumption was similar in the two groups. We next examined whether angiotensin II is involved in these microvascular changes, and found that treatment with an angiotensin II type 1 receptor antagonist (CS-866) prevented the altered flow response to pacing as well as the microvascular structural changes. These findings suggest that the development of microvascular structural changes is associated with the impairment of coronary blood flow response to metabolic stimuli and that angiotensin II is likely to contribute to such changes.

This animal model with long-term inhibition of nitric oxide synthesis have several important clinical implications. First, endothelial dysfunction with a deficient NO synthesis can mediate structural as well as functional microvascular disorders. Second, coronary microvascular changes are similar to those seen in patients with cardiac syndrome X [43,44] and in patients with limited coronary vasodilatory capacity due to hypertensive heart disease [45]. Third, prearteriolar location and patchilly distribution of microvascular structural changes in this animal model mimic a hypothetical model of cardiac syndrome X as proposed by Maseri et al [3]. Finally, effects of angiotensin II receptor blockade seen in our model would be relevant to the clinical study by Kaski et *al* [46] who reported that long-term angiotensin-converting enzyme inhibition reduced exercise-induced ST depression in patients with cardiac syndrome X. Thus, this animal model would be useful for the study of pathophysiological mechanisms in microvascular disorders such as those seen in patients with syndrome X.

Conclusions

It remains to be established whether endothelial dysfunction in the coronary microcirculation is the underlying mechanism of cardiac syndrome X or an associated abnormality. However, available data in the literature are consistent with the notion that endothelial dysfunction of the coronary microcirculation may contribute to the pathogenesis and/or pathophysiology of cardiac syndrome X. How could microvascular endothelial dysfunction be involved in cardiac syndrome X? It may limit coronary blood flow increase by causing 1) impaired dilation of coronary microvessels to metabolic stimuli; 2) maldistribution of regional blood flow or blood flow steal; or 3) inappropriate microvascular constriction (spasm) at rest and/or during exercise.

The vascular endothelium is known to have multiple functions [4-6]. Endothelial dysfunction may lead to the impaired release of relaxing factors, the increased release of constricting factors, and abnormal production of cell adhesion molecules, cytokines and growth factors that induce inflammatory and proliferative changes in the blood vessel wall [4-6]. Thus, whatever the cause, endothelial dysfunction of the coronary microcirculation may be associated with, currently unknown or unrecognized, abnormalities [i.e. microvascular structural changes, spasm, local renin-angiotensin system) and cause chest pain and myocardial ischemia in patients with cardiac syndrome X.

References

1. Cannon RO, Camici PG, Epstein SE. Pathophysiological dilemma of syndrome X. Circulation 1992; 85:883-892.
2. Cannon RO, Epstein SE. Microvascular angina as a cause of chest pain with angiographically normal coronary arteries. Am J Cardiol 1988; 61:1338-1343.
3. Maseri A, Crea F, Kaski JC, Crake T. Mechanism of angina pectoris in syndrome X. J Am Coll Cardiol 1991; 17:499-506.
4. Drexler H. Endothelial dysfunction: Clinical implications. Prog Cardiovasc Dis 1997; 39:287-324.
5. Griendling KK, Alexander RW. Endothelial control of the cardiovascular system: recent advances. FASEB J. 1996; 10:283-292.
6. Moncada S, Higgs A. The L-arginine-nitric oxide pathway. N. Engl. J. Med. 1993; 329:2002-2012.
7. Zeiher AM. Schachinger V. Saurbier B. Just H. Assessment of endothelial modulation of coronary vasomotor tone: insights into a fundamental functional disturbance in vascular biology of atherosclerosis. Basic Res Cardiol 1994; 89 Suppl 1:115-128.
8. Egashira K. Suzuki S. Hirooka Y. Kai H. Sugimachi M. Imaizumi T. Takeshita A. Impaired endothelium-dependent vasodilation of large epicardial and resistance coronary arteries in patients with essential hypertension. Different responses to acetylcholine and substance P. Hypertension 1995; 25:201-206.
9. Egashira K. Hirooka Y. Kai H. Sugimachi M. Suzuki S. Inou T. Takeshita A. Reduction in serum cholesterol with pravastatin improves endothelium-dependent coronary vasomotion in patients with hypercholesterolemia. Circulation. 1994; 89:2519-2524.
10. Egashira K. Inou T. Hirooka Y. Kai H. Sugimachi M. Suzuki S. Kuga T. Urabe Y. Takeshita A. Effects of age on endothelium-dependent vasodilation of resistance coronary artery by acetylcholine in humans. Circulation 1993; 88:77-81.

98

11. Egashira K. Inou T. Hirooka Y. Yamada A. Maruoka Y. Kai H. Sugimachi M. Suzuki S. Takeshita A. Impaired coronary blood flow response to acetylcholine in patients with coronary risk factors and proximal atherosclerotic lesions. J Clin Invest 1993; 91:29-37.

12. Zeiher AM. Drexler H. Saurbier B. Just H. Endothelium-mediated coronary blood flow modulation in humans. Effects of age, atherosclerosis, hypercholesterolemia, and hypertension. J Clin Invest 1993; 2:652-62.

13. Marcus ML. Chilian WM. Kanatsuka H. Dellsperger KC. Eastham CL. Lamping KG. Understanding the coronary circulation through studies at the microvascular level. Circulation 1990; 82:1-7.

14. Chilian WM. Coronary microcirculation in health and disease. Summary of an NHLBI workshop. Circulation 1997; 95:522-528.

15. Egashira K, Inou T, Hirooka Y, et al. Evidence of impaired endothelium-dependent coronary vasodilation in patients with angina pectoris and normal coronary arteriograms. N Engl J Med 1993; 328:1659-1664.

16. Motz W. Vogt M. Rabenau O. Scheler S. Luckhoff A. Strauer BE. Evidence of endothelial dysfunction in coronary resistance vessels in patients with angina pectoris and normal coronary angiograms. Am J Cardiol 1991; 68:996-1003.

17. Quyyumi AA. Cannon RO 3d. Panza JA. Diodati JG. Epstein SE. Endothelial dysfunction in patients with chest pain and normal coronary arteries. Circulation 1992; 86:1864-1871.

18. Egashira K. Katsuda Y. Mohri M. Kuga T. Tagawa T. Kubota T. Hirakawa Y. Takeshita A. Role of endothelium-derived nitric oxide in coronary vasodilatation induced by pacing tachycardia in humans. Circ Res 1996; 79:331-335.

19. Quyyumi AA. Dakak N. Andrews NP. Gilligan DM. Panza JA. Cannon RO III. Contribution of nitric oxide to metabolic coronary vasodilation in the human heart. Circulation 1995; 92(3):320-326.

20. Egashira K, Hirooka Y, Kuga T, Mohri M, Takeshita A. Effects of L-arginine supplementation on endothelium-dependent coronary vasodilation in patients with angina pectoris and normal coronary arteriograms. Circulation 1996; 94:130-134.

21. Bellamy MF, Goodfellow J, Tweddel AC, Brownlee M, Gorman ST, Ellis GR, MacCarthy PA, Lewis MJ, Henderson AH. Oral L-arginine improves exercise tolerance and flow-mediated endothelial dysfunction in microvascular angina. Circulation 1996; 94(suppl 1):I-425.

22. Rosano GM. Collins P. Kaski JC. Lindsay DC. Sarrel PM. Poole-Wilson PA . Syndrome X in women is associated with estrogen deficiency. Eur Heart J 1995; 16:610-614.

23. Taddei S. Virdis A. Ghiadoni L. Mattei P. Sudano I. Bernini G. Pinto S Salvetti A. Menopause is associated with endothelial dysfunction in women. Hypertension 1996; 28:576-582.

24. Lieberman EH. Gerhard MD. Uehata A. Walsh BW. Selwyn AP. Ganz P. Yeung AC. Creager MA . Estrogen improves endothelium-dependent, flow-mediated vasodilation in postmenopausal women. Ann Int Med 1994; 121:936-941

25. Reis SE. Gloth ST. Blumenthal RS. Resar JR. Zacur HA. Gerstenblith G. Brinker JA. Ethinyl estradiol acutely attenuates abnormal coronary vasomotor responses to acetylcholine in postmenopausal women. Circulation 1994; 89:52-60.

26. Gilligan DM. Quyyumi AA. Cannon RO III. Effects of physiological levels of estrogen on coronary vasomotor function in postmenopausal women. Circulation. 1994; 89:2545-2551.

27. Rosano GM. Peters NS. Lefroy D. Lindsay DC. Sarrel PM. Collins P. Poole-Wilson PA . 17-beta-Estradiol therapy lessens angina in postmenopausal women with syndrome X. J Am Coll Cardiol 1996; 28:1500-1505.

28. Rosano GM. Sarrel PM. Poole-Wilson PA. Collins P. Beneficial effect of estrogen on exercise-induced myocardial ischemia in women with coronary artery disease. Lancet 1993; 342(8864):133-136.

29. Jones CJ. Kuo L. Davis MJ. DeFily DV. Chilian WM. Role of nitric oxide in the coronary microvascular responses to adenosine and increased metabolic demand. Circulation 1995; 91:1807-1813.

30. Katsuda Y. Egashira K. Akatsuka Y. Narishige T. Shimokawa H. Takeshita A. Endothelium-derived nitric oxide does not modulate metabolic coronary vasodilation induced by tachycardia in dogs. J Cardiovas Pharmacol 1995; 26:437-444

31. Altman JD. Kinn J. Duncker DJ. Bache RJ. Effect of inhibition of nitric oxide formation on coronary blood flow during exercise in the dog. Cardiovas Res 1994; 28:119-124

32. Katsuda Y. Egashira K. Ueno H. Akatsuka Y. Narishige T. Arai Y. Takayanagi T. Shimokawa H. Takeshita A. Glibenclamide, a selective inhibitor of ATP-sensitive K+ channels, attenuates metabolic coronary vasodilatation induced by pacing tachycardia in dogs. Circulation 1995; 92:511-517.

33. Duncker DJ. van Zon NS. Ishibashi Y. Bache RJ. Role of K+ ATP channels and adenosine in the regulation of coronary blood flow during exercise with normal and restricted coronary blood flow. J Clin Invest 1996; 97:996-1009.
34. Zeiher AM, Krause T, Schachinger V, Minners J, Moser E. Impaired endothelium-dependent vasodilation of coronary resistance vessels is associated with exercise-induced myocardial ischemia. Circulation 1995; 91:2345-2352.
35. Galassi AR. Crea F. Araujo LI. Lammertsma AA. Pupita G. Yamamoto Y. Rechavia E. Jones T. Kaski JC. Maseri A . Comparison of regional myocardial blood flow in syndrome X and one-vessel coronary artery disease. Am J Cardiol 1993; 72:134-139.
36. Geltman EM. Henes CG. Senneff MJ. Sobel BE. Bergmann SR. Increased myocardial perfusion at rest and diminished perfusion reserve inpatients with angina and angiographically normal coronary arteries. J Am Coll Cardiol 1990; 16:586-595.
37. Inobe Y, Kugiyama K, Morita E, Kawano H, Okumura K, Tomiguchi S, Tsuji A, Kojima A, Takahashi M, Yasue H. Role of adenosine in pathogenesis of syndrome X: assessment with coronary hemodynamic measurements and thallium-201 myocardial single-photon emission computed tomography. J Am Coll Cardiol 1996; 28:890-896.
38. Hasdai D, Gibbons RJ, Holmes DR Jr, Higano ST, Lerman A. Coronary endothelial dysfunction in humans is associated with myocardial perfusion defects. Circulation 1997; 96:3390-3395.
39. Mohri M, Koyanagi M, Egashira K, Tagawa H, Ichiki T, Shimokawa H, Takeshita A. Angina pectoris caused by coronary microvascular spasm. Lancet 1998; 351:1165-1169.
40. Kadokami T. Egashira K. Kuwata K. Fukumoto Y. Kozai T. Yasutake H. Kuga T. Shimokawa H. Sueishi K. Takeshita A. Altered serotonin receptor subtypes mediate coronary microvascular hyperreactivity in pigs with chronic inhibition of nitric oxide synthesis. Circulation 1996; 94:182-189.
41. Ito A. Egashira K. Kadokami T. Fukumoto Y. Takayanagi T. Nakaike R. Kuga T. Sueishi K. Shimokawa H. Takeshita A. Chronic inhibition of endothelium-derived nitric oxide synthesis causes coronary microvascular structural changes and hyperreactivity to serotonin in pigs. Circulation 1995; 92:2636-2644.
42. Higo T, Egashira K, Yamawaki T. Metabolic coronary vasodilation in response to pacing-induced tachycardia is impaired in an animal model of coronary microvascular disease. Circulation 1997; 96(suppl 1):I-73.
43. Suzuki H. Takeyama Y. Koba S. Suwa Y. Katagiri T. Small vessel pathology and coronary hemodynamics in patients with microvascular angina. International J Cardiol 1994; 43:139-50.
44. Mosseri M. Yarom R. Gotsman MS. Hasin Y. Histologic evidence for small-vessel coronary artery disease in patients with angina pectoris and patent large coronary arteries. Circulation 1986; 74:964-72.
45. Schwartzkopff B. Motz W. Frenzel H. Vogt M. Knauer S. Strauer BE. Structural and functional alterations of the intramyocardial coronary arterioles in patients with arterial hypertension. Circulation 1993; 88:993-1003.
46. Kaski JC, Rosano G, Gavrielides S, Chen L. Effects of angiotensin-converting enzyme inhibition on exercise-induced angina and ST segment depression in patients with microvascular angina. J Am Coll Cardiol 1994; 23:652-657.

Chapter 9

ENDOTHELIN: AN IMPORTANT MEDIATOR IN THE PATHOPHYSIOLOGY OF SYNDROME X?

Ian D. Cox and Juan Carlos Kaski

Angina pectoris with normal coronary arteries is a common clinical entity with up to 30% of patients undergoing invasive assessment for anginal chest pain having normal coronary angiograms [1, 2]. The term cardiac syndrome X to describe patients with chest pain and normal coronaries was first introduced by Kemp in 1973 [3] and is now generally confined to patients with exertional angina, completely normal coronary angiograms and a positive electrocardiographic response (> 0.1 mV of ST segment depression) to exercise testing [4]. The pathophysiology of chest pain in this patient group appears to be heterogeneous and remains the subject of considerable debate [5-7]. A non-cardiac source of pain, often originating in the gastrointestinal or musculoskeletal system, may be identified by further investigation. However, around 20% of patients appear to have objective evidence of myocardial ischemia in most series, and a mechanism involving a primary cardiac abnormality remains the most likely explanation for the symptoms in this subgroup.

Evidence for ischemia in syndrome X

In addition to electrocardiographic changes, a variety of methods have supported the existence of myocardial ischemia in a subgroup of patients with chest pain and normal coronaries. Myocardial perfusion imaging techniques with radioisotopes such as thallium-201 have also indicated that transient myocardial perfusion defects are present in approximately 30% of syndrome X patients [8-10]. Reversible abnormalities of left ventricular wall function during stress have also been reported [11], although such changes have not been demonstrated in other studies [12-14]. Metabolic evidence of ischemia in the form of myocardial lactate production has been evident in some studies of patients with angina and normal coronary arteriograms [15-17]. In a study by Opherk *et al* [15], 37% of the patients with showed myocardial lactate production although lactate production was not demonstrated in any of the controls. Furthermore, Boudoulas *et al* [18] showed that ST segment depression during atrial pacing is greater in lactate producers than non-producers and an association between disorders of microvascular vasodilatory function and lactate production has also been reported [19-21]. Rosano *et al* [22] have also recently used a specially designed coronary sinus pH electrode to demonstrate significant falls in coronary sinus pH during atrial pacing in three out of thirteen (23%) patients with chest pain and normal angiograms.

Abnormalities of coronary flow reserve

In the absence of flow limiting epicardial coronary disease, coronary flow responses are determined primarily by the vasodilator function of the coronary microvascular resistance vessels *i.e.* the small intramyocardial arteries and arterioles. In 1983, Cannon *et al* [20] used a thermodilution technique to demonstrate a limitation in the coronary flow response to rapid atrial pacing in syndrome X patients. Furthermore, the administration of ergonovine magnified this abnormal response although there was no evidence of epicardial coronary spasm. Cannon *et al* [23] concluded that the observed increase in coronary vascular resistance in these patients was due to microvascular vasoconstriction in response to ergonovine and later proposed the term *microvascular angina* to describe this mechanism. Data from a number of other invasive studies have supported the existence of abnormal coronary flow responses to atrial pacing or pharmacological stimulation in patients with chest pain and normal coronaries [17, 21, 24, 25]. Camici *et al* [26] have also used positron emission tomography (PET) to assess coronary flow responses to dipyridamole in 45 normotensive patients with chest pain and normal coronaries. They demonstrated a significantly smaller increase in myocardial perfusion in patients with exercise induced ST segment depression compared to those without such changes. However, it should be noted that there was considerable overlap between the two groups in this study and only 41% of the patients with electrocardiographic evidence of ischemia had reduced flow reserve [26].

Endothelial dysfunction

The vascular endothelium produces a variety of vasoactive substances which play a key role in the regulation of vascular smooth muscle tone and consequently, arterial blood flow [27, 28]. Endothelial derived relaxing factor (EDRF) later to be associated with the free radical nitric oxide [NO] [29, 30] was the first of these mediators to be studied in detail. *In vivo* human studies have demonstrated that infusion of NG-monomethyl-L-arginine (L-NMMA), an L-arginine analogue which competitively inhibits the production of NO [31], induces arterial vasoconstriction indicating that NO plays an important role in the regulation of basal vascular tone [32]. Consequently, endothelial dysfunction might account for the presence of abnormal microvascular responses in patients with microvascular angina. The vasodilatory activity of acetylcholine [ACh] appears to depend on the integrity of the endothelial NO system (27) and arterial vasoconstriction in response to appropriate concentrations of ACh is commonly accepted as evidence of endothelial dysfunction. Studies using ACh have demonstrated evidence of both epicardial [33, 34] and microvascular [19, 33, 35, 36] endothelial dysfunction in patients with chest pain and normal coronaries. Motz *et al* [33] found a blunted vasodilator response to ACh in 8 of 23 patients with chest pain and normal coronaries studied by an argon gas chromatographic technique; the vasodilator response to dipyridamole, a non-endothelium-dependent vasodilator was normal in all cases. Egashira *et al* [35] used intracoronary Doppler measurements to demonstrate that coronary blood flow responses to ACh were significantly reduced in a group of 9 well characterized syndrome X patients (without hypertension, hypercholesterolemia or diabetes) when compared to a control group with atypical chest pain and normal exercise ECG responses. Egashira's study also suggested that endothelial microvascular dysfunction was associated with myocardial lactate production in syndrome X. Quyyumi et al [36] demonstrated abnormalities in coronary flow responses to both ACh and atrial pacing in patients with chest pain and normal coronaries. Zeiher et al [19] similarly demonstrated microvascular endothelial dysfunction during exercise and showed that this dysfunction was associated with myocardial perfusion abnormalities. Furthermore, other authors have found evidence of impaired endothelial function in the forearm vascular bed [37] suggesting that a more generalized endothelial dysfunction extending beyond the coronary circulation may be present in syndrome X.

Possible role of endothelial vasoconstrictor mediators

The term endothelial dysfunction is frequently used synonymously with the presence of abnormal vasomotor responses to ACh. However, the vagueness of the term endothelial dysfunction underlines our lack of information regarding the precise mechanisms responsible for such abnormalities. The availability of specific pharmacological tools for investigating the role of NO have helped focus attention on this mediator and a considerable body of evidence has accumulated to support an important role for NO in this context. Quyyumi et al [38] demonstrated an association between reduced resting and stimulated bioavailability of NO and the presence of coronary risk factors in patients with angiographically normal coronaries. However, it remains unclear whether a mechanism affecting production, breakdown or signal transduction of NO is responsible for the observed abnormalities [19]. It is also clear that endothelial control of vascular function is dependent on a balanced opposition between a variety of vasodilator and vasoconstrictor mediators [28]. Therefore, other endothelial-derived mediators also require investigation; in particular, physiological antagonism to vasodilatory influences by increased endothelial production of vasoconstrictor mediators may be important. Such endothelial-derived vasoconstrictor mediators include certain prostanoids (e.g. thromboxane A2 and prostaglandin H2), components of the renin-angiotensin system and the endothelins, a family of potent vasoconstrictor peptides.

The endothelins - a family of potent vasoconstrictor peptides

The endothelins (ET) exist in three isoforms, ET-1, ET-2 and ET-3 encoded by three separate genes [39]. They are expressed widely throughout the body and have a variety of biological activities [40]. ET-1 is the only isoform synthesized by endothelial cells and is also produced by vascular smooth muscle cells. It is not stored in secretory granules within endothelial cells [41] and synthesis is regulated at the level of messenger RNA (mRNA) transcription and/or translation. It is initially synthesized as pre-pro-ET-1 [203 amino acids] which is proteolytically cleaved to big-ET-1 (39 amino acids) and thence converted to the mature form of ET-1 (21 amino acids) by the action of ET-converting enzyme which is a membrane bound glycoprotein enzyme (Figure 1) [42].

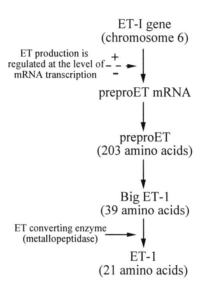

Figure 1. Synthetic pathway for endothelin -1.

As much as 75 percent of ET-1 secretion from cultured endothelial cells is directed toward the abluminal side i.e. towards the vascular smooth muscle cells [43] and in this respect ET-1 functions more as a paracrine mediator than a circulating hormone. Therefore, the measurement of circulating ET concentrations provides only an index of ET activity and may not reflect subtle differences in local ET production. A number of stimuli, including shear stress, hypoxia, thrombin, vasopressin and angiotensin II may stimulate ET-1 production. The biological activities of ET are mediated via [at least] two G-protein linked receptor subtypes - ETA and ETB. ETA receptors are present on vascular smooth muscle cells (Figure 2) and mediate a direct vasoconstriction response to ET-1 [44]. ETB receptors are expressed predominantly on endothelial cells [45] where they mediate an indirect vasodilatory action in response to ET-1 by stimulating release of NO and other endothelial-derived vasodilator mediators (e.g. prostacyclin).

ETB receptors are also present on smooth muscle cells of the aorta, pulmonary and coronary arteries [46, 47] where they mediate vasoconstriction. Intravenous infusion of ET-1 produces an initial transient vasodilation (due to endothelial ETB receptors) followed by a profound and long-lasting vasoconstriction. Haynes and Webb [48] have also demonstrated that infusion of BQ123, an ETA receptor antagonist into the forearm vascular bed causes progressive vasodilation. This suggests that endogenous production of ET-1 contributes to basal regulation of vascular tone. ET-1 also causes stimulation of vascular smooth muscle cell proliferative and synthetic functions [49].

Although the exact physiological role of ET-1 remains uncertain, an increasing body of evidence suggests that it may have pathophysiological significance in a number of disease states, particularly hypertension and heart failure. Clinical studies have also demonstrated that ET-1 levels are elevated in patients with acute coronary syndromes [50] and may also be implicated in the abnormal vasoconstrictor responses seen in such patients [51]. Recently, Krüger et al [52] have demonstrated that coronary sinus ET levels increase after short-lasting myocardial ischemia induced by atrial pacing in patients with coronary artery disease. Elevated ET-1 levels have also been observed in patients with coronary vasospasm [53, 54]. However, there is evidence to suggest that ET-1 mediated coronary vasoconstrictor effect occurs predominantly at the microvascular level [55], possibly due to the differential distribution of endothelin receptor subtypes within the coronary vasculature [56]. These findings have led to speculation that increased ET activity may be responsible for the observed coronary flow abnormalities observed in microvascular angina.

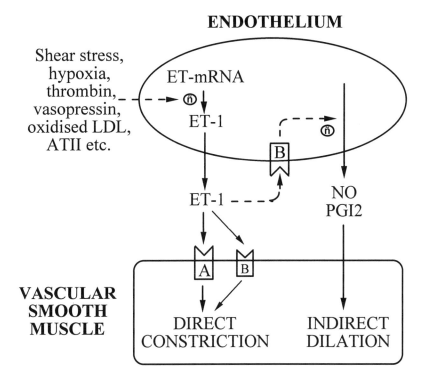

Figure 2. The vasomotor effects of endothelial-derived ET-1 are mediated via two G-protein linked receptors - **ETA** and **ETB**. They include: i) a direct vasoconstrictor effect mediated via ETA receptors which are expressed abundantly on vascular smooth muscle and too a lesser extent via ETB receptors in some vessels; and ii) an indirect vasodilator effect mediated via ETB receptors which are mainly located on endothelial cells where ET-1 binding stimulates release of vasodilator metabolites including nitric oxide (**NO**) and prostacyclin (**PGI2**).

Elevated serum endothelin levels in syndrome X

In a recent study by our group [57], plasma ET levels were measured in peripheral venous blood in 40 patients [30 women; mean age 56±8 years] with angina and normal coronary arteriograms and 21 healthy controls (17 women; mean age 53±7 years). Patients with systemic hypertension, left ventricular hypertrophy, or coronary spasm were excluded. The mean ET-1 concentration was higher in patients (3.84 ± 1.25 pg/ml) than in controls (2.88 ± 0.71 pg/ml; $p < 0.0001$). Furthermore, the time to onset of chest pain during exercise was significantly shorter in the patients with "high" ET levels (defined as > control mean + 1SD) compared to those with "low" ET-1 concentrations (n = 23). Further subgroup analysis in a larger series of patients with chest pain and normal coronary angiograms [58] has indicated that the highest plasma ET levels were observed in patients with left bundle branch block (LBBB) or previous myocardial infarction (Figure 3).

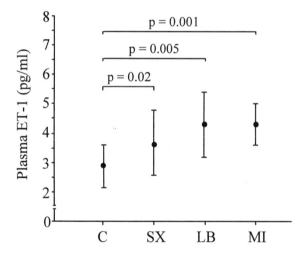

Figure 3. Analysis of plasma ET levels (mean ± SD) in different syndrome X subgroups (see text). ET levels were significantly higher in the syndrome X patients (**SX**) than controls (**C**); this difference was most pronounced in those with left bundle branch block (**LB**) or previous myocardial infarction (**MI**).

These findings raise intriguing questions about the possible pathophysiological significance of ET in syndrome X. Opherk *et al* [59] have demonstrated that LBBB identifies a subgroup of syndrome X patients at increased risk of developing impaired left ventricular contractile function during follow-up. It has also been observed that syndrome X patients with LBBB exhibit abnormal lactate metabolism during pacing stress [60]. On the basis of these observations, it has been proposed that the LBBB subgroup of syndrome X may represent a form of dilated cardiomyopathy associated with microvascular ischemia. Work in an animal model has supported the hypothesis that microvascular spasm can play a significant role in the development of myocardial injury and subsequent ventricular failure [61]. In light of our findings, one can postulate a pathophysiological model in which high plasma ET levels in syndrome X patients may contribute to the genesis of microvascular myocardial ischemia which in severe cases may lead to conduction abnormalities and progressive left ventricular dysfunction. Recent work by our group has also suggested that amongst syndrome X patients who undergo repeat angiography due to unstable symptoms, patients with LBBB are more likely to develop angiographic disease progression than those without LBBB [62]

The relationship between ET and previous myocardial infarction in patients with chest pain and normal angiograms is also of interest. As stated above, high titres of plasma ET-1 have been reported in acute myocardial infarction and unstable angina [51] and this probably reflects local ET release by the myocardial endothelium during acute coronary ischemia. We [63] have observed that an initial episode of myocardial infarction may represent the presenting symptom in some patients who subsequently develop chronic angina and are diagnosed as having syndrome X. This sequence of events suggests that the ischemic insult of myocardial infarction may lead to chronic impairment of coronary microvascular reserve even where the patency of the epicardial vessel is fully restored [63, 64]. The observed elevation of ET levels in such patients may represent an important factor in the pathophysiology of such microvascular dysfunction.

Endothelin and subangiographic atheroma in syndrome X

As already stated, *in vitro* and *in vivo* evidence has demonstrated that ET-1 can stimulate vascular smooth muscle cell proliferative and synthetic functions and that these effects can be attenuated by specific ET antagonists [49]. This suggests that ET may play an important role in atherogenesis as well as vasomotor dysfunction in patients with coronary disease. This suggestion is supported by our finding that serum ET levels correlate with the angiographic severity of coronary atherosclerotic disease [65]. Immunohistochemical techniques have also shown that ET-1 is localized to macrophage-rich areas and areas of neovascularization within atherosclerotic tissue [66-68] indicating a possible link between ET and the inflammatory mechanisms which appear to play a central role in atherogenesis. Elevated ET levels are also associated with adverse prognostic implications in patients with acute coronary syndromes [50] suggesting an association with plaque activity in the longer term.

Considerable atherosclerotic deposits may accumulate in the coronary vessel wall before lumenal stenosis is evident at angiography due to the mechanism of adaptive arterial remodeling [69]. Given that most patients diagnosed with syndrome X are middle aged or elderly and have one or more conventional coronary risk factors, it is not surprising that recent studies using intracoronary ultrasound imaging have demonstrated the presence of significant subangiographic atheroma in such patients [70, 71]. Due to lack of similar data in age matched controls, it is also difficult to determine whether the extent of such changes are any greater than might be anticipated in such a group. Nevertheless, Wiedermann *et al* [70] observed that abnormal epicardial vasomotor responses to exercise stress were associated with subangiographic atheroma in their patient group. However, in a similar study in which we also utilized

Doppler measurements of coronary flow, we were unable to establish a clear correlation between subangiographic atheroma and either epicardial or microvascular endothelium dependent responses [72]. In light of these findings, any possible relationship between elevated ET levels, endothelial dysfunction and subangiographic coronary atheroma in syndrome X remains speculative at this stage.

Coronary endothelin levels and flow responses during pacing stress

Quyyumi *et al* [36] have previously demonstrated abnormalities in coronary flow responses to both acetylcholine and atrial pacing in a group of patients with chest pain and normal coronary arteriograms. They further demonstrated that there was a strong correlation between the flow responses observed with the two stimuli and concluded that microvascular endothelial dysfunction may contribute to the reduced vasodilator reserve with atrial pacing and anginal chest pain in these patients [36]. In a recent study, we have used a thermodilution pacing catheter to investigate the relationship between plasma ET concentrations and the coronary vasomotor responses during rapid atrial pacing in a group of 19 patients with chest pain and normal coronary arteriograms (mean age 53 ± 9 years; 14 females). Exercise electrocardiography was positive (eECG+) in 10 patients and negative (eECG-) in 9 patients. Patients with epicardial coronary spasm, hypertension and left ventricular dysfunction were excluded. In each patient, the percentage fall in coronary vascular resistance (%d.CVR) following 10 minutes of rapid atrial pacing was determined. Plasma ET concentrations in simultaneously drawn arterial and coronary sinus samples were measured by radioimmunoassay. Consistent with previous studies [58], the baseline arterial ET concentration was significantly higher in the eECG+ than the eECG- group (2.24 ± 0.56 pg/ml versus 1.40 ± 0.40 pg/ml respectively; p = 0.003). The %d.CVR was significantly lower in the positive exercise ECG group than the negative exercise ECG group (27 [22-29]% versus 34 [29-45]% - median [interquartile range]; p = 0.02). However, a similar trend was evident in women compared to men in the study group (27 [23-31]% versus 34 [29-45]; p = 0.07). Multivariate regression analysis indicated that eECG positivity and age were not independent predictors of %d.CVR (p > 0.6) but that both female sex (p = 0.03) and baseline arterial ET concentration (p = 0.02) were independently predictive of %d.CVR (R-squared = 0.44, overall p = 0.02). This analysis predicts that women with high ET levels would have the lowest %d.CVR during pacing and lends further support to the hypothesis that increased ET activity represents an important aspect of microvascular endothelial dysfunction in patients with chest pain and normal coronary arteriograms. These data are also consistent with recently reported data [73] indicating an inverse correlation (R = -0.59; p < 0.05) between scintigraphically determined myocardial perfusion reserve and plasma ET levels in 32 asymptomatic patients with cardiovascular risk factors. Our results regarding the importance of gender are also intriguing important given that most series of patients with chest pain and normal coronary arteriograms have been dominated by post- and perimenopausal women [74, 75]. The hypothesis that estrogen deficiency is associated with coronary endothelial dysfunction and abnormal vasomotor control in such women has been supported by evidence from a variety of studies [75, 76]. However, serum estradiol concentrations did not correlate with either plasma ET concentration or %d.CVR in the female patients in our study; therefore, this sole factor cannot explain the observed differences.

Endothelin and peripheral vascular responses in syndrome X

As mentioned earlier, it has been suggested that the endothelial dysfunction present in some patients with syndrome X may extend beyond the coronary to involve other peripheral vascular beds [37]. However, little data exist on the relationship between ET and peripheral vascular responses in syndrome X. Preliminary work has been published by Newby *et al* [78] who performed forearm venous occlusion plethysmography on a group of 10 syndrome X patients and healthy age matched controls. They failed to demonstrate any difference in flow responses to local arterial infusion of ACh, substance P or L-NMMA suggesting that no significant differences existed in respect to NO mediated responses. However, once again, plasma ET-1 concentrations tended to be higher in the syndrome X compared to the control group (4.9 vs 4.0 pg/ml; p = 0.1). The vasoconstriction induced by arterial infusion of ET-1 at 5 pmol/min was less in the syndrome X group than the controls (21 ± 4% vs 36 ± 3%). The authors speculated that this reduced sensitivity to exogenous ET-1 in the syndrome X group may reflect the higher baseline ET-1 levels and/or alterations in receptor expression.

Endothelin and pain perception in syndrome X

In addition to their vasoactive properties, the endothelins possess other biological activities including possible algogenic effects according to preliminary data from animal studies [79]. Data from a number of studies have also indicated that syndrome X may be associated with abnormalities of both cardiac [80, 81] and somatic [82] pain perception. This raises the possibility that elevated ET levels in patients with syndrome X [57, 58] may also be associated with previously observed pain perception abnormalities. In a recent a case control study [83], we compared somatic pain perception and serum ET levels in syndrome X patients and age-matched healthy controls. Somatic pain perception was determined in the forearm during submaximal effort tourniquet and cold immersion tests. As in previous studies [82], pain threshold to both ischemic and cold stimulation of the forearm was significantly lower in syndrome X patients compared to controls. Intriguingly, we also observed a strong negative correlation (R = 0.82; p = 0.004) between ischemic pain threshold and ET levels. The findings of this small study must be interpreted with caution; however, it is attractive to speculate that a mediator possessing both vasoactive and algogenic properties might provide a link between the observed abnormalities of both microvascular function and pain perception in syndrome X. Pursuing this line, it is also possible that elevated ET levels might contribute to both the evolution of an ischemic stimulus and its "amplification" through an algogenic mechanism. Further work, possibly employing specific ET antagonists, is required to investigate the contribution of elevated ET levels to abnormalities of both somatic and visceral nociception in syndrome X patients.

Treatment implications

Patients with syndrome X frequently remain symptomatic during clinical follow-up and may be subject to recurrent hospital admissions and repeat investigations. Therefore, effective management of this condition remains a major challenge in current cardiological practice. Future progress in the treatment of this puzzling condition must be guided by advances in our understanding of the underlying pathophysiology. As outlined above, the evidence is accumulating to support future therapeutic trials of endothelin antagonists and/or endothelin converting enzyme inhibitors in syndrome X. In view of the heterogeneity of syndrome X patients, it would be important that such trials were targeted at appropriate patient subsets who might be identified by elevated serum ET levels, LBBB and/or previous myocardial infarction [58]. However, at present therapeutic application of such agents in syndrome X remains a distant prospect.

Conclusions

The endothelins are a family of potent vasoconstrictor peptides which appear to play an important role in the normal regulation of vascular tone. Evidence form a number of studies have shown that serum ET-1 levels are elevated in patients with syndrome X. Although serum levels can only be an index of local endothelial ET-1 production which occurs mainly in the ablumenal direction, it seems possible that elevated ET-1 production may contribute significantly to microvascular dysfunction in syndrome X. In addition, ET may have algogenic properties which amplify the nociceptive impact of any ischemic stimulus.

Acknowledgements

Dr. Cox is supported by a fellowship grant from the British Heart Foundation.

References

1. Proudfit WL, Shirey EK, Sones FJ. Selective cine coronary arteriography. Correlation with clinical findings in 1,000 patients. Circulation 1966;33:901-10.
2. Kemp H, Kronmal R, Vliestra R, Frye R, and the Coronary Artery Surgery Study (CASS) participants: Seven year survival of patients with normal or near normal coronary arteriograms: a CASS registry study. J Am Coll Cardiol 1986;7:479-483.
3. Kemp H. Left ventricular function in patients with the anginal syndrome and normal coronary arteriograms. Am J Cardiol 1973;32:375-376.
4. Kaski JC. Syndrome X: a heterogeneous syndrome. Historical background, clinical presentation, electrocardiographic features, and rational management. An overview. In: Angina pectoris with normal coronary arteries: Syndrome X. Ed. Kaski JC (Kluwer Academic Publishers, Massachusetts 1994) pp.-19.
5. Cannon RO, Camici PG, Epstein SE. Pathophysiological dilemma of syndrome X. Circulation 1992;85:883-892.
6. Maseri A, Crea F, Kaski JC, Crake T. Mechanisms of angina pectoris in syndrome X. J Am Coll Cardiol 1991;17:499-506.
7. Kaski JC, Elliott PM. Angina pectoris and normal coronary arteriograms: clinical presentation and hemodynamic characteristics. Am J Cardiol 1995;76: 35D-42D.

8. Kaul S, Newell J, Chesler D, Pohost G, Okada R, Boucher C. Quantitative thallium imaging findings in patients with normal coronary angiographic findings and clinically normal subjects. Am J Cardiol 1986;57:509-512.
9. Berger B, Arbaramowitz R, Park E, *et al*. Abnormal thallium-201 scans in patients with chest pain and angiographically normal coronary arteries. Am J Cardiol 1983;52:365-370.
10. Meller J, Goldsmith S, Rudin A, *et al*. Spectrum of exercise thallium-201 myocardial perfusion imaging in patients with chest pain and normal coronary angiograms. Am J Cardiol 1979;43:717-723.
11. Cannon RO, Bonow R, Bacharach S, *et al*. Left ventricular dysfunction in patients with angina pectoris, normal epicardial coronaries and abnormal vasodilator reserve. Circulation 1985;71:218-226.
12. Arbogast R, Bourassa MG. Myocardial function during atrial pacing in patients with angina pectoris and normal coronary arteriograms. Comparison with patients having significant coronary artery disease. Am J Cardiol 1973;32:257-63.
13. Nihoyannopoulos P, Kaski JC, Crake T, Maseri A. Absence of myocardial dysfunction during stress in patients with syndrome X. J Am Coll Cardiol 1991;18:1463-1470.
14. Panza J, Laurienzo J, Curiel R, *et al*. Investigation of the mechanism of chest pain in patients with angiographically normal coronary arteries using transesophageal dobutamine stress echocardiography. J Am Coll Cardiol 1997;29:293-301.
15. Opherk D, Zebe H, Weibe E, *et al*. Reduced coronary dilator capacity and ultrastructural changes of the myocardium in patients with angina pectoris but normal coronary angiograms. Circulation 1981;63:817-25.
16. Hutchison S, Poole-Wilson P, Henderson A. Angina with normal coronary arteries. QJ Med 1989;72:677-688.
17. Camici P, Marraccinni P, Lorenzoni R, *et al*. Coronary hemodynamics and myocardial metabolism in patients with syndrome X: response to pacing stress. J Am Coll Cardiol 1991;17:1461-1470.
18. Boudoulas H, Cobb T, Leighton R, Wilt S. Myocardial lactate production in patients with angina like chest pain and angiographically normal coronary arteries and left ventricle. Am J Cardiol 1974;84:501-505.
19. Zeiher AM, Krause T, Schachinger V, Minners J, Moser E. Impaired endothelium dependent vasodilation of the coronary resistance vessels is associated with exercise-induced myocardial ischemia. Circulation 1995;91:2345-52.
20. Cannon RO, Watson R, Rosing D, Epstein S. Angina caused by reduced vasodilator reserve of the small coronary arteries. J Am Coll Cardiol 1983;1:1359-73.
21. Greenberg M, Grose R, Neuberger N, Silverman R, Strain JE, Cohen MV. Impaired coronary vasodilator reserve as a cause of lactate production during pacing induced ischemia in patients with angina pectoris and normal coronaries. J Am Coll Cardiol 1987;9:743-751.
22. Rosano G, Kaski J, Arie S, *et al*. Failure to demonstrate myocardial ischemia in patients with angina and normal coronary arteries. Evaluation by continuous coronary sinus pH monitoring and lactate metabolism. Eur Heart J 1996;17:1175-1180.
23. Cannon R, Epstein S. "Microvascular angina" as a cause of chest pain with angiographically normal coronary arteries. Am J Cardiol 1988;61:1338-1343.
24. Legrand V, Hodgson JM, Bates ER, *et al*. Abnormal coronary flow reserve and abnormal radionuclide exercise test results in patients with normal coronary angiograms. J Am Coll Cardiol 1985;6:1245-53.
25. Bortone A, Hess O, Eberli FR, *et al*. Abnormal coronary vasomotion during exercise in patients with normal coronary arteries and reduced coronary flow reserve. Circulation 1989;79:516-527.
26. Camici P, Gistri R, Lorenzoni R, *et al*. Coronary reserve and exercise ECG in patients with chest pain and normal coronary angiograms. Circulation 1992;86:179-186.
27. Luscher TF, Vanhoutte PM. The endothelium: modulator of cardiovascular function. Boca Raton: CRC Press 1990.
28. Vanhoutte P. Other endothelium derived vasoactive factors. Circulation 1993;87 (Suppl V):V9-17.
29. Moncada S, Herman A, Vanhoutte P. Endothelium derived relaxing factor is identified as nitric oxide. Trends Pharmacol Sci 1986;8:365-368.
30. Palmer R, Ashton D, Moncada S. Vascular endothelial cells synthesize nitric oxide form L-arginine. Nature 1988;333:664-666.
31. Vallance P, Collier J, Moncada S. Nitric oxide synthesized from L-arginine mediates endothelium dependent dilation in human veins in vivo. Cardiovasc Res 1989;23:1053-1057.
32. Vallance P, Collier J, Moncada S. Effect of endothelial-derived nitric oxide on peripheral arteriolar tone in man. Lancet 1989;2:997-1000.

33. Motz W, Vogt M, Rabenau O, Scheler S, Luckhoff A, Strauer B. Evidence of endothelial dysfunction in coronary resistance vessels in patients with angina pectoris and normal coronary angiograms. Am J Cardiol 1991;68:996-1003.

34. Vrints C, Bult H, Hitter E, Herman A, Snoeck J. Impaired endothelium dependent cholinergic vasodilation in patients with angina and normal coronary angiograms. J Am Coll Cardiol 1992;19:21-31.

35. Egashira K, Inou T, Hirooka Y, Yamada A, Urabe Y, Takeshita A. Evidence of impaired endothelium-dependent coronary vasodilatation in patients with angina pectoris and normal coronary angiograms. N Engl J Med 1993;328:1659-64.

36. Quyyumi AA, Cannon RO, Panza JA, Diodati JG, Epstein SE. Endothelial dysfunction in patients with chest pain and normal coronary arteries. Circulation 1992;86:1864-71.

37. Sax FL, Cannon RO, Hanson C, Epstein SE. Impaired forearm vasodilator reserve in patients with microvascular angina. Evidence of a generalized disorder of vascular function? N Engl J Med 1987;317:1366-70.

38. Quyyumi AA, Dakak N, Andrews NP, Husain S, Arora S, Gilligan DM, Panza JA, Cannon RO. Nitric oxide activity in the human coronary circulation. Impact of risk factors for coronary atherosclerosis. J Clin Invest 1995;95:1747-1755.

39. Inoue A, Yanagisawa M, Kimura S et al. The human endothelin family; three structurally and pharmacologically distinct isopeptides predicted by three separate genes. Proc Natl Acad Sci 1989;86:2863-2867

40. Levin ER. Endothelins. N Engl J Med 1995;333(6):356-63.

41. Nakamura S, Naruse M, Naruse K, Demura H, Uemura H. Immunocytochemical localization of endothelin in cultured bovine endothelial cells. Histochemistry 1990;94:475-7.

42. Xu D, Emoto N, Giald A et al. ECE-1: a membrane bound metalloproteinase that catalyses the proteolytic activation of big endothelin-1. Cell 1994;78:473-485.

43. Yoshimoto S, Ishizaki Y, Sasaki T, Muroto S-I. Effect of carbon dioxide and oxygen on endothelin production by cultured porcine cerebral endothelial cells. Stroke 1991;22:378-83.

44. Arai H, Hori S, Aramori I et al. Cloning and expression of cDNA encoding an endothelin receptor. Nature 1990;348:730-2..

45. Sakurai T, Yanagishawa M, Takuwa Y et al. Cloning of a cDNA encoding a non isopeptide selective subtype of the endothelin receptor. Nature 1990;348:732-5.

46. MacLean MR, McCulloch KM, Baird M. Endothelin ETA and ETB receptor mediated vasoconstriction in rat pulmonary arteries and arterioles. J Cardiovasc Pharm 1994;23:838-45.

47. Teerlink JR, Breu V, Sprecher U et al. Potent vasoconstriction mediated by endothelin ETB receptors in canine coronary arteries. Circ Res 1994;74:105-114.

48. Haynes WG, Webb DJ. Contribution of endogenous generation of endothelin-1 to basal vascular tone. Lancet 1994;344:852-4.

49. Douglas SA, Vickery CL, Louden C, Ohlstein EH. Selective ETa receptor antagonism with BQ-123 is insufficient to inhibit angioplasty induced neointima formation in the rat. Cardiovasc Res 1995; 29:641-6.

50. Wieczorek I, Haynes WG, Webb DJ, Ludlam CA, Fox KAA. Raised plasma endothelin levels in unstable angina and non-Q wave myocardial infarction: relation to cardiovascular outcome. Br Heart J 1994; 72:436-441.

51. Bogaty P, Hackett D, Davies G, Maseri A. Vasoreactivity of the culprit lesion in unstable angina. Circulation 1994; 90:5-11.

52. Krüger D, Sheikhzadeh A, Giannitsis E, Stierle U. Cardiac release and kinetics of endothelin after severe short-lasting myocardial ischemia. J Am Coll Cardiol 1997;30:942-6.

53. Toyooka T, Aizawa T, Suzuki N et al. Increased plasma level of endothelin-1 and coronary spasm induction in patients with vasospastic angina pectoris. Circulation 1991;83:476-83.

54. Artigou JY, Salloum J, Carayon A et al. Variations in plasma endothelin concentrations during coronary spasm. Eur Heart J 1993;14:780-4.

55. Smith TP, Zhang L, Gugino SF, Russell JA, Canty JM. Differential effect of endothelin on coronary conduit and resistance arteries. Circulation 1995;92(Suppl.):I-320.

56. Dashwood MR, Timm M, Kaski JC. Regional variations in ETA/ETB binding sites in human coronary vasculature. J Cardiovasc Pharmacol 1995;26:351-4.

57. Kaski JC, Elliott PM, Salomone O, et al. Concentration of circulating plasma endothelin in patients with angina and normal coronary angiograms. Br Heart J 1995;74:620-4.

58. Kaski JC, Cox ID, Crook R, Salomone OA, Fredericks S, Hann C, Holt D. Differential plasma endothelin levels in subgroups of patients with angina and angiographically normal coronary arteries. Am Heart J (in press).

59. Opherk D, Schuler G, Wetterauer K, Manthey J, Schwartz F, Kubler W. Four year follow-up study in patients with angina and normal coronary arteriograms ("syndrome X"). Circulation 1989;80:1610-19.

60. Greemberg MA, Grose RM, Neuberger N, Silverman R, Strain JE, Cohen MV. Impaired coronary vasodilator responsiveness as a cause of lactate production during pacing-induced ischemia in patients with angina pectoris and normal coronary arteries. J Am Coll Cardiol 1987;9:743-51.

61. Sonneblick EH, Fein F, Capasso JM, Factor SM. Microvascular spasm as a cause of cardiomyopathies and the calcium channel blocking agent verapamil as potential primary therapy. Am J Cardiol 1985;55:179-84.

62. Cox ID, Schwartzman RA, Atienza F, Brown SJ, Kaski JC. Angiographic progression in patients with angina pectoris and normal or near normal coronary angiograms who are restudied due to unstable symptoms. Eur Heart J 1998;19:1027-1033.

63. Kaski JC, Rosano GM, Dickinson K, Martuscelli E, Romeo F. Syndrome X as a consequence of myocardial infarction. Am J Cardiol 1994;74:494-5.

64. Penny WJ, Tweddle AC, Martin W, Henderson AH. Microvascular angina may be a legacy of coronary thrombolysis. Eur Heart J 1990;11:1049-52.

65. Salomone A, Elliott PM, Calvino R, Holt D, Kaski JC. Plasma immunoreactive endothelin concentration correlates with severity of coronary artery disease in patients with stable angina pectoris and normal ventricular function. J Am Coll Cardiol 1996;28:4-19.

66. Zeiher A, Goebel H, Schlachinger V, Ihling C. Tissue endothelin-1 immunoreactivity in the active coronary atherosclerotic plaque: A clue to the mechanism of increased vasoreactivity of the culprit lesion in unstable angina. Circulation 1995; 91:941-947.

67. Dashwood MR, Timm M, Kaski JC. Regional variations in ETa/ETb binding sites in human coronary vasculature. J Cardiovasc Pharmacol 1995; 26:S351-4.

68. Timm M, Kaski JC, Dashwood MR. Endothelin-like immunoreactivity in atherosclerotic human coronary arteries. J Cardiovasc Pharmacol 1995; 26:S442-4.

69. Glagov S, Weisenberg E, Zarins C, Stankunavicius R, Kolettis G. Compensatory enlargement of human atherosclerotic arteries. N Engl J Med 1987;316:1371-1375.

70. Wiedermann O, Schwartz A, Apfelbaum M. Anatomic and physiologic heterogeneity in patients with syndrome X. J Am Coll Cardiol 1995;25:1310-7.

71. Nishimura RA, Lerman A, Chesebro JH, *et al.* Epicardial vasomotor responses to acetylcholine are not predicted by coronary atherosclerosis as assessed by intracoronary ultrasound. J Am Coll Cardiol 1995;26:41-9.

72. Cox ID, Clague J, Bagger JP, Ward DE, Kaski JC. Heterogeneity of endothelial responses in cardiac syndrome X cannot be explained solely by the presence of epicardial subangiographic atheroma. J Am Coll Cardiol 1997; 29 (Suppl A):156A.

73. Huelmos A, Garcia Velloso MJ, Gil MJ, Richter JA, Alegria E, Martinez-Caro D. Myocardial perfusion reserve and endothelin plasmatic levels in asymptomatic patients with cardiovascular risk factors. Eur Heart J 1997;18 (Suppl):P2408.

74. Kaski J, Crea F, Nihoyannopoulos P, Collins P, Maseri A, Poole-Wilson P. Syndrome X: clinical characteristics and left ventricular function - a long term follow-up study. J Am Coll Cardiol 1995;25:807-814.

75. Cannon RO. Microvascular angina: cardiovascular investigations regarding pathophysiology and management. Med Clin North Am 1988;75:1097-1118.

76. Sarrel P, Lindsay D, Rosano G, Poole-Wilson P. Angina and normal coronary arteries: gynecological findings. Am J Obstet Gynaecol 1992;167:467-472.

77. Sarrel P. Role of estrogen deficiency in women with syndrome X . In: Angina pectoris with normal coronary arteries: Syndrome X. Ed. Kaski JC (Kluwer Academic Publishers, Massachusetts 1994) pp.249-266.

78. Newby DE, Boon DA, Webb DJ. Abnormal endothelin-1 sensitivity with preservation of nitric oxide. J Am Coll Cardiol 1996;29:193A.

79. Raffa RB, Shupsky JJ, Martinez RP, Jacoby HI. Endothelin-1-induced nociception. Life Sci 1991;49: PL61-5.

80. Rosen SD, Uren NG, Kaski JC, Tousoulis D, Davies GJ, Camici PG. Coronary vasodilator reserve, pain perception, and sex in patients with syndrome X. Circulation 1994;90: 50-60.

81. Lagerqvist B, Sylven C, Waldenstrom A. Lower threshold for adenosine-induced chest pain in patients with angina and normal coronary angiograms. Br Heart J 1992;68: 282-5.
82. Turiel M, Galassi AR, Glazier JJ, Kaski JC, Maseri A. Pain threshold and tolerance in women with syndrome X and women with stable angina pectoris. Am J Cardiol 1987;60: 503-7.
83. Cox ID, Salomone O, Brown SJ, Hann CM, Kaski JC. Serum endothelin levels and pain perception in patients with cardiac syndrome X and healthy controls. Am J Cardiol 1997;80:637-9.

Chapter 10

ESTROGEN DEFICIENCY AND SYNDROME X

Peter Collins

Syndrome X - angina pectoris, ST-segment depression on the electrocardiogram during exercise, and normal coronary arteries is more frequent in women than in men. Female patients with syndrome X are often menopausal (either natural or surgical) and suffer from symptoms of ovarian insufficiency such as hot flushes and migraine. The high incidence of hysterectomies (4-times greater than an age matched United Kingdom population) and signs of ovarian insufficiency suggest that estrogen deficiency may trigger the onset of syndrome X in the majority of female patients with the condition. In postmenopausal patients with syndrome X, estrogen replacement therapy may reduce the frequency of the anginal chest pain.

Features of patients with syndrome X

Angina pectoris is usually caused by atheromatous coronary artery disease and occurs predominantly in males. Normal or nearly normal coronary arteries are found in approximately 20% of patients who undergo coronary angiography [1,2]. The majority of these patients are women [3-11]. The triad of angina pectoris, a positive exercise test and angiographically smooth coronary arteries is commonly referred to as syndrome X, a term first used by Kemp in 1973 [12]. The pathophysiology of the troublesome chest pain in syndrome X is poorly understood, but there are many suggested mechanisms [10,13,14]. Although syndrome X is likely to be a heterogeneous condition, reduced coronary flow reserve induced by dipyridamole has been reported in many patients with this diagnosis [10,15]. Most of the women with syndrome X are post-menopausal [16]. Indeed, estradiol-17β deficiency is associated with vasomotor instability and decreased arterial blood flow velocity in humans [17-20]. Acute administration of estradiol-17β improves myocardial ischemia in female patients with coronary artery disease [21,22]. It has also been shown to increase peripheral blood flow in postmenopausal women [23], and to improve endothelial function in estrogen depleted postmenopausal women [24]. Recent studies demonstrate a beneficial effect of chronic estrogen therapy on myocardial ischemia in postmenopausal women with coronary heart disease [25].

The clinical and gynecological features of female patients with syndrome X have been reported [26]. It has also been noted by other groups that of patients referred with chest pain, women were more likely to have normal coronary arteries and positive (ST segment depression) exercise tests. The female patients were also significantly older than men [11]. The possibility that acute [27,28] and chronic [29] administration of estrogen may be helpful in the treatment of syndrome X has also been investigated.

Estrogen deficiency and syndrome X

Clinical features of patients with syndrome X

The clinical and gynecological features of patients with syndrome X referred to two institutions have been reported. A total of 107 female patients with syndrome X were taken from a cohort of 134 consecutive patients that included 27 males [26]. All patients fulfilled strict criteria for syndrome X, namely typical exertional angina pectoris, positive exercise test and angiographically smooth coronary arteries, in the absence of coronary artery spasm, systemic hypertension, left ventricular hypertrophy or valvar heart disease.

Clinical status of patients was assessed which included the gynecological and cardiovascular history using a standardized questionnaire. The character and location of chest pain were determined. Musculoskeletal and esophageal causes of chest pain were excluded using radiological and manometric assessments in over half of the patients.

All patients had downsloping or horizontal ST segment depression on exercise testing and all patients had angiographically smooth coronary arteries.

Women included in the study were interviewed in order to obtain a complete cardiovascular and gynecological history. The menstrual history, onset of menopause, occurrence of gynecological surgery and presence of perimenopausal symptoms, with particular attention to those related to vasomotor instability, were noted. Type and dosage of hormone replacement therapy were obtained.

Thirty-seven patients were suffering hot flushes, 27 reported sleep disturbances and 22 migraine. These symptoms were frequently associated with chest pain. Eight women were on hormone replacement therapy (2 estrogen implants, 6 conjugated estrogens) when first seen but the dosage of hormones was found to be inadequate in that the plasma estradiol concentration remained low and/or the plasma FSH concentrations remained high.

Of the 63 menopausal patients 45 had a hysterectomy. Bilateral ophorectomy had been performed in 7 women. The distribution of hysterectomies for each age group is shown in Figure 1a. The mean delay between the hysterectomy and the onset of chest pain in the 43 women was 8±5.7 years (range 3 months -19 years). In the younger women (30-40 years) chest pain started sooner after hysterectomy (< 3 years compared to > 10 years, Figure 1b). These data suggest that estrogen deficiency may trigger syndrome X in susceptible women.

The average age of the menopause in the UK is 51 years [30,31]. Amongst the patient population 65% of women aged ≥51 years had already entered their menopause (mainly natural) [26]. Of interest, ≥50% of female patients under 51 years at the onset of angina were also menopausal. The high incidence of menopause among younger patients is explained by the increased incidence of hysterectomies. The incidence of hysterectomies in the population of this study (40%) is 4 times greater than that reported for a similar aged female population in the United Kingdom [32,33], and this incidence is even higher when considering women under 51 years. This seems to suggest that ovarian hormonal deficiency may trigger the onset of chest pain in female patients with syndrome X.

Age distribution at the onset of angina in 107 in women with Syndrome X

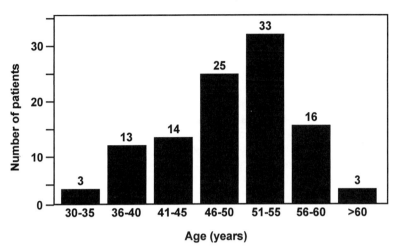

Figure 1a. Age distribution at the onset of chest pain in 107 women with syndrome X. The majority of patients were either monopausal (63) or perimenopausal (32).

Delay between hysterectomy and onset of angina women with Syndrome X

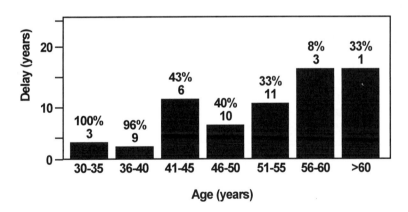

Figure 1b. Delay between hysterectomy and onset of angina in 43 women with syndrome X. The delay was shorter in younger women suggesting that abrupt changes in plasma estradiol levels may precipitate the syndrome. Digits above columns are number of patients.

Another group has reported on 160 men and women with normal coronary arteries [11]. One of the main findings was that the mean age of the 50 women was significantly greater than that of the men. Forty percent of the women and only 10% of the men had

ST segment depression on the exercise test. Of patients referred with chest pain, the women were more likely to have normal coronary arteries compared with men. The mean age of these female patients would suggest that the majority would have been menopausal.

Therapeutic role for estrogen?

Estrogen may be beneficial as a treatment in postmenopausal women with syndrome X [27,29]. Twenty-five postmenopausal patients with syndrome X completed a double-blind placebo controlled study of the effect of estradiol-17ß cutaneous patches (100 µg/24 hrs) on the frequency of chest pain and on exercise tolerance. Patients were randomized to receive either placebo or estradiol-17ß patches for eight weeks, after which patients crossed over to the other treatment. During the placebo phase, patients had a mean of 7.3 episodes of chest pain/10 days. A reduction of 3.6 episodes/10 days was observed during the estradiol-17ß phase ($p < 0.05$). No significant differences between estradiol-17ß and placebo were observed in exercise duration or in the results of other cardiological investigations.

In the treatment study there was significant reduction in the frequency of chest pain in estrogen-deficient women with syndrome X when treated with estradiol-17ß, supporting the hypothesis that estrogen deficiency may have a role in the pathogenesis of the symptoms in post-menopausal women with syndrome X [26]. Despite this beneficial effect upon chest pain there was no significant change in exercise time or in the other test results. This apparent dissociation of chest pain from exercise tolerance and ST segment changes indicates that although syndrome X is likely to be heterogeneous with multiple pathogenetic components, the chest pain in such patients may not be due to myocardial ischemia.

In a study of 15 postmenopausal women (mean age 58±6 years) with clinical syndrome X it was shown that a 24 hour treatment with 100 µg 17ß-estradiol patch improved exercise time to angina, time to 1 mm ST-segment depression and total exercise time [27]. This is an interesting result in that it is one of the few studies that have shown a beneficial effect of therapy on exercise-induced ST-segment depression in patients with syndrome X. There is a possibility that in this study the majority of the patients did have true myocardial ischemia as a cause of their chest pain, which was improved by estradiol. In a study of 15 postmenopausal women with angina and angiographically smooth coronary arteries acetylcholine-induced vasoconstriction in these patients was abolished within 24 hours by treatment with transdermal estradiol at a dose of 100 µg [28]. This would support the hypothesis that endothelial dysfunction occurs in patients with syndrome X which could be improved by estradiol.

Mechanisms of action of estrogen in syndrome X

The clinical observation that the majority of patients with syndrome X are women [3-5,12], of whom most are menopausal [26], led to the hypothesis that estrogen deficiency may play a pathophysiological role in at least a proportion of patients with syndrome X [26]. Estrogens have vasoactive properties [23,34-40], a deficiency of which is associated with vasomotor instability [18,41,42]. Estrogen replacement therapy causes normalization of the impaired peripheral skin vasodilator reserve observed in women with syndrome X [26,43]. There are a number of possible explanations for the alleviation of chest pain by 17β-estradiol observed in the present study, without invoking myocardial ischemia in the mechanism. These include relief of the prearteriolar vasoconstriction, or augmentation of adenosine-induced A_2 receptor-mediated vasodilatation by a direct action on the vascular smooth muscle cells [35,37]. The net result of either of these actions would be expected to be an increase in coronary flow with a reduced production of adenosine. Adenosine is a known algogen, excessive release of which, or sensitivity to which, is suggested as being the painful stimulus in syndrome X, resulting in exaggerated cardiac sensitivity to non-ischemic stimuli (both mechanical [44-46] and chemical, such as adenosine infusion [46]). The improvement in chest pain observed with 17β-estradiol, in the absence of improvement in cardiac testing, might, therefore, result from attenuation of adenosine production or by altering the balance or sensitivity of adenosine receptors [46,47]. Heterogeneity of adenosine receptors or sensitivity may account for regional myocardial perfusion abnormalities. Coronary vasodilatation by 17β-estradiol may also relieve myocardial ischemia in the subset of patients in whom it is manifest.

Possible analgesic mechanism of action of estrogen

The symptomatic benefits of 17β-estradiol in syndrome X may relate to an analgesic action via other, as yet poorly understood, mechanisms. Another mechanism may involve analgesic properties of estrogen. Recent animal data have shown female-male differences in pain sensitivity [48]. These differences were negated by ovariectomy and re-established after estrogen replacement. These data support the claim that estrogen has analgesic properties which may contribute to the results observed in this study. The results of a recent study by Cannon *et al* [49] suggest that imipramine, known to have visceral analgesic properties, reduces chest pain without any objective changes on formal cardiovascular testing, a response similar to that with 17β-estradiol in the present study. Alternatively, there may be central effects on psychological instability. Psychosomatic symptoms and panic disorders [50] and a general reduction in pain threshold [4] have been found to be associated with chest pain and possibly the ST segment changes in syndrome X [51]. Thus, the effects of 17β-estradiol in menopausal patients with syndrome X may be multifactorial, and may include an important improvement in the well being of patients which may increase the threshold to the perception of pain.

Endothelium-dependent effects

In postmenopausal women forearm vasodilatation induced by ACh is potentiated by the acute local administration of intravenous estradiol [52], suggesting that endothelium-dependent responses in the peripheral circulation may be modulated by steroid hormones in vivo in these women. The post-menopausal state results in an impairment in endothelial function. Estrogen increases flow-mediated vasodilation in the brachial artery of postmenopausal women [24]. There are other reports of impairment of endothelial function in syndrome X [53,54,24]), it could therefore be hypothesized that a beneficial effect of estrogen on endothelial function may be involved in the beneficial response in postmenopausal women with syndrome X. Further studies will be required to confirm this.

General conclusions

Syndrome X occurs more commonly in postmenopausal women.
These women are estrogen deficient.
Estrogen deficiency may be a trigger for the syndrome in susceptible women.
Estrogen replacement therapy in some of these women may be a useful therapy for the associated chest pain.

References

1. Phibbs B, Fleming T, Ewy GA, Butman S, Ambrose J, Gorlin R, Orme E, Mason J. Frequency of normal coronary arteriograms in three academic medical centers and one community hospital. Am J Cardiol 1988;62:472-474.
2. Likoff W, Segal BL, Kasparian H. Paradox of normal selective coronary arteriograms in patients considered to have unmistakable coronary heart disease. N Engl J Med 1967;276:1063-1066.
3. Romeo F, Gaspardone A, Ciavolella M, Gioffrè P, Reale A. Verapamil versus acebutolol for syndrome X. Am J Cardiol 1988;62:312-313.
4. Turiel M, Galassi AR, Glazier JJ, Kaski JC, Maseri A. Pain threshold and tolerance in women with syndrome X and women with stable angina pectoris. Am J Cardiol 1987;60:503-507.
5. Galassi AR, Kaski JC, Crea F, Pupita G, Gavrielides S, Tousoullis D, Maseri A. Heart rate response during exercise testing and ambulatory ECG monitoring in patients with syndrome X. Am Heart J 1991;122:458-463.
6. Pupita G, Kaski JC, Galassi AR, Vejar M, Crea F, Maseri A. Long-term variability of angina pectoris and electrocardiographic signs of ischemia in syndrome X. Am J Cardiol 1989 64:139-143.
7. Kaski JC, Crea F, Nihoyannopoulos P, Hackett D, Maseri A. Transient myocardial ischemia during daily life in patients with syndrome X. Am J Cardiol 1986;58:1242-1247.
8. Kemp HG,Jr.. Left ventricular function in patients with anginal syndrome and normal coronary arteriograms. Am J Cardiol 1973;32:375-376.
9. Cannon RO, Schenke WH, Leon MB, Rosing DR, Urqhart J, Epstein SE. Limited coronary flow reserve after dipyridamole in patients with ergonovine-induced coronary vasoconstriction. Circulation 1987;75:163-174.
10. Cannon RO, Epstein SE. "Microvascular angina" as a cause of chest pain with angiographically normal coronary arteries. Am J Cardiol 1988;61:1338-1343.
11. Foussas SG, Adamopoulou EN, Kafaltis NA, Fakiolas C, Olympios C, Pisimissis E, Siogas K, Pappas S, Cokkinos DV, Sideris D. Clinical characteristics and follow-up of patients with chest pain and normal coronary arteries. Angiology 1998;49:349-354.
12. Kemp HG,Jr., Vokonas PS, Cohn PF, Gorlin R. The anginal syndrome associated with normal coronary arteriograms. Report of a six year experience. Am J Med 1973;54:735-742.
13. Maseri A, Crea F, Kaski JC, Crake T. Mechanisms of angina pectoris in syndrome X. J Am Coll Cardiol 1991;17:499-506.
14. Rosano GMC, Lindsay DC, Poole-Wilson PA. Syndrome X: an hypothesis for cardiac pain without ischaemia. Cardiologia 1991;36:885-895.
15. Opherk D, Zebe H, Weihe E, Mall G, Dürr C, Gravert B, Mehmel HC, Schwarz F, Kübler W. Reduced coronary dilatory capacity and ultrastructural changes of the myocardium in patients with angina pectoris but normal coronary arteriograms. Circulation 1981;63:817-825.
16. Kaski JC, Rosano GMC, Collins P, Nihoyannopoulos P, Maseri A, Poole-Wilson PA. Cardiac syndrome X: clinical characteristics and left ventricular function. Long term follow-up study. J Am Coll Cardiol 1995;25:807-814.
17. Sullivan JM, Vander Zwaag R, Lemp GF, Hughes JP, Maddock V, Kroetz FW, Ramanathan KB,

Mirvis DM. Postmenopausal estrogen use and coronary atherosclerosis. Ann Intern Med 1988;108:358-363.

18. Rees MC, Barlow DH. Absence of sustained reflex vasoconstriction in women with menopausal flushes. Hum Reprod 1988;3:823-825.

19. Kronenberg F, Cote LJ, Linkie DM, Dyrenfurth I, Downey JA. Menopausal hot flushes: thermoregulatory, cardiovascular and circulating catecholamine and LH changes. Maturitas 1984;6:31-43.

20. Ginsburg J, Hardiman P. The peripheral circulation in the menopause. In: Ginsburg J, ed. The circulation in the female, Lancashire, UK: Carnforth, 1989:99-115.

21. Rosano GMC, Sarrel PM, Poole-Wilson PA, Collins P. Beneficial effect of estrogen on exercise-induced myocardial ischaemia in women with coronary artery disease. Lancet 1993;342:133-136.

22. Alpaslan M, Shimokawa H, Kuroiwa-Matsumoto M, Harasawa Y, Takeshita A. Short-term estrogen administration ameliorates dobutamine-induced myocardial ischemia in postmenopausal women with coronary artery disease. J Am Coll Cardiol 1997;30:1466-1471.

23. Volterrani M, Rosano GMC, Coats A, Beale C, Collins P. Estrogen acutely increases peripheral blood flow in postmenopausal women. Am J Med 1995;99:119-122.

24. Lieberman EH, Gerhard MD, Uehata A, Walsh BW, Selwyn AP, Ganz P, Yeung AC, Creager MA. Estrogen improves endothelium-dependent, flow-mediated vasodilation in postmenopausal women. Ann Intern Med 1994;12:936-941.

25. Webb CM, Rosano GMC, Collins P. Estrogen improves exercise-induced myocardial ischaemia in women. Lancet 1998;351:1556-1557.

26. Rosano GMC, Collins P, Kaski JC, Lindsay DC, Sarrel PM, Poole-Wilson PA. Syndrome X in women is associated with estrogen deficiency. Eur Heart J 1995;16:610-614.

27. Albertsson PA, Emanuelsson H, Milsom I. Beneficial effect of treatment with transdermal estradiol-17-beta on exercise-induced angina and ST segment depression in syndrome X. Int J Cardiol 1996; 54: 13-20.

28. Roque M, Heras M, Roig E, Masotti M, Rigol M, Betriu A, Balasch J, Sanz G. Short-term effects of transdermal estrogen replacement therapy on coronary vascular reactivity in postmenopausal women with angina pectoris and normal results on coronary angiograms. J Am Coll Cardiol 1998;31:139-143.

29. Rosano GMC, Peters NS, Lefroy DC, Lindsay DC, Sarrel PM, Collins P, Poole-Wilson PA. 17-beta-estradiol therapy lessens angina in postmenopausal women with syndrome X. J Am Coll Cardiol 1996;28:1500-1505.

30. Stanford JL, Hartge P, Brinton LA, Hoover RN, Brookmeyer R. Factors influencing the age at natural menopause. Journal of Chronic Diseases 1987;40:995-1002.

31. Jaszmann LJB. Epidemiological Climateric Syndrome. In: Campbell S, ed. Management of the Menopause and Post Menopausal Years, University Press, 1976:11-23.

32. Coulter A, McPherson K, Vessey M. Do British women undergo too many or too few hysterectomies? Soc Sci Med 1988;27:987-994.

33. Domenighetti G, Luraschi P, Casabianca A, Gutzwiller F, Spinelli A, Pedrinis E, Repetto F. Effect of information campaign by the mass media on hysterectomy rates. Lancet 1988;2:1470-1473.

34. Collins P, Rosano GMC, Jiang C, Lindsay D, Sarrel PM, Poole-Wilson PA. Hypothesis: Cardiovascular protection by estrogen - a calcium antagonist effect? Lancet 1993;341:1264-1265.

35. Chester AH, Jiang C, Borland JA, Yacoub MH, Collins P. Estrogen relaxes human epicardial coronary arteries through non-endothelium-dependent mechanisms. Cor Art Dis 1995;6:417-422.

36. Collins P, Rosano GMC, Sarrel PM, Ulrich L, Adamopoulos S, Beale CM, McNeill J, Poole-Wilson PA. Estradiol-17β attenuates acetylcholine-induced coronary arterial constriction in women but not men with coronary heart disease. Circulation 1995;92:24-30.

37. Jiang C, Sarrel PM, Lindsay DC, Poole-Wilson PA, Collins P. Endothelium-independent relaxation of rabbit coronary artery by 17β-estradiol in vitro. Br J Pharmacol 1991;104:1033-1037.

38. Gilligan DM, Quyyumi AA, Cannon RO,III. Effects of physiological levels of estrogen on coronary vasomotor function in postmenopausal women. Circulation 1994;89:2545-2551.

39. Reis SE, Gloth ST, Blumenthal RS, Resar JR, Zacur HA, Gerstenblith G, Brinker JA. Ethinyl estradiol acutely attenuates abnormal coronary vasomotor responses to acetylcholine in postmenopausal women. Circulation 1994;89:52-60.

40. Williams JK, Adams MR, Herrington DM, Clarkson TB. Short-term administration of estrogen and

122

vascular responses of atherosclerotic coronary arteries. J Am Coll Cardiol 1992;20:452-457.

41. Magness RR, Rosenfeld CR. Local and systemic estradiol-17 beta: effects on uterine and systemic vasodilation. Am J Physiol 1989;256:E536-E542.

42. Mügge A, Riedel M, Barton M, Kuhn M, Lichten PR. Endothelium independent relaxation of human coronary arteries by 17beta-estradiol in vitro. Cardiovasc Res 1993;27:1939-1942.

43. Sarrel PM, Lindsay DC, Rosano GMC, Poole-Wilson PA. Angina and normal coronary arteries in women. Gynecologic findings. Am J Obstet Gynecol 1992;167:467-471.

44. Shapiro LM, Crake T, Poole-Wilson PA. Is altered cardiac sensation responsible for chest pain in patients with normal coronary arteries? Clinical observation during cardiac catheterisation. Br Med J 1988;296:170-171.

45. Cannon RO,III, Quyyumi AA, Schenke WH, Fananapazir L, Tucker EE, Gaughan AM, Gracely RH, Cattau EL, Epstein SE. Abnormal cardiac sensitivity in patients with chest pain and normal coronary arteries. J Am Coll Cardiol 1990;16:1359-1366.

46. Lagerqvist B, Sylven C, Waldenström A. Lower threshold for adenosine-induced chest pain in patients with angina and normal coronary arteriograms. Br Heart J 1992;68:282-285.

47. Emdin M, Picano E, Lattanzi F, L'Abbate A. Improved exercise capacity with acute aminophylline administration in patients with syndrome X. J Am Coll Cardiol 1989;14:1450-1453.

48. Mogil JS, Sternberg WF, Kest B, Marek P, Liebeskind JC. Sex differences in the antagonism of swim stress-induced analgesia: effects of gonadectomy and estrogen replacement. Pain 1993;53 (1):17-25.

49. Cannon RO,III, Quyyumi AA, Mincemoyer R, Stine AM, Gracely RH, Smith WH, Geraci MF, Black BC, Uhde TW, Waclawiw MA, Maher K, Benjamin SB. Imipramine in patients with chest pain despite normal coronary angiograms. N Engl J Med 1994;330:1411-1417.

50. Bass C, Chambers JB, Kiff P, et al. . Panic anxiety and hyperventilation in patients with chest pain: a controlled study. Q J Med 1988;260:949-959.

51. Dart AM, Davies HA, Dalal J, Ruttley M, Henderson AH. `Angina' and normal coronary arteriograms: a follow-up study. Eur Heart J 1980;1:97-100.

52. Gilligan DM, Badar DM, Panza JA, Quyyumi AA, Cannon RO,III. Acute vascular effects of estrogen in postmenopausal women. Circulation 1994;90:786-791.

53. Egashira K, Inou T, Hirooka Y, Yamada A, Urabe Y, Takeshita A. Evidence of impaired endothelium-dependent coronary vasodilatation in patients with angina pectoris and normal coronary angiograms. N Engl J Med 1993;328:1659-1664.

54. Collins P. Endothelial dysfunction in patients with angina and normal coronary arteriograms. In: Kaski JC, ed. Angina pectoris with normal coronary arteries: syndrome X, Norwell, Massachusetts: Klewer, 1994:237-247.

Chapter 11

ALTERNATIVE MECHANISMS FOR MYOCARDIAL ISCHEMIA IN SYNDROME X - NEW DIAGNOSTIC MARKERS

Filippo Crea, Antonio Buffon, Achille Gaspardone, and Gaetano Lanza

Exertional chest pain, positive exercise test responses and the presence of transient ST segment depression during Holter monitoring strongly suggest the occurrence of myocardial ischemia in syndrome X. However, carefully conducted studies have failed to show: (i) myocardial lactate production during pacing [1,2]; (ii) increases in pulmonary pressure during spontaneous episodes of transient ST segment depression [3]; (iii) abnormalities of left ventricular wall motion as assessed by two-dimensional echocardiography during dipyridamole testing [4]; (iv) decreases in coronary sinus blood oxygen saturation [5] or of pH [6] during atrial pacing; (v) regional perfusion abnormalities during positron emission tomography [7]. Yet, a sizable proportion of patients with syndrome X exhibit an alteration of coronary circulation as suggested by: (i) an abnormally small increase in coronary flow in response to dipyridamole or pacing [8,9], particularly after ergonovine administration [10]; (ii) heterogeneous myocardial perfusion both at rest and during dipyridamole infusion as assessed by positron emission tomography [11,12] and (iii) a regional reduction of thallium uptake during exercise or dipyridamole infusion [13-15].

Furthermore, patients with syndrome X seem to exhibit abnormal adrenergic activity as suggested by: (i) a higher heart rate both at rest and during daily activities [16]; (ii) abnormalities of heart rate variability [12,17]; (iii) a prolongation of QTc interval [18]; (iv) a hypercontractility of the left ventricle [19]; (v) an increase of basal coronary blood flow [11] and (vi) coronary hyperactivity to adrenergic stimuli [20]. Direct measurements of plasma levels of catecholamines and myocardial density of ß-adrenergic receptor, however, led to negative or conflicting results [20-22].

Finally, patients with syndrome X frequently present other extracardiac features such as: (i) abnormal forearm vasomotor responses [23]; (ii) disorders of esophageal motility [24]; (iii) airway hyperresponsiveness [25]; (iv) hyperinsulinemia [26,27]; (v) enhanced pain perception and increased tendency to complain [28,29].

This chapter will present recent evidence which appears to shed some new light on the conflicting results relative to the presence of myocardial ischemia and impaired sympathetic function in syndrome X. We also propose a working hypothesis, which might help explaining the complex clinical picture of syndrome X.

Evidence of myocardial ischemia

In 1991 Maseri *et al* [30] proposed that syndrome X is caused by prearteriolar dysfunction in small regions sparse within the myocardium. Prearteriolar dysfunction can lead to myocardial ischemia due to both the collapse of those prearterioles showing marked vasoconstriction or to steal mechanisms. In this setting the compensatory release of adenosine, a powerful vasodilator which is known to stimulate cardiac nerve endings, and potassium leakage to the interstitium can cause chest pain and ECG changes; even in the absence of a "convincing" demonstration of myocardial ischemia [30]. The regional impairment of myocardial contractility may be negligible under the circumstances described above, because of both the rapid wash-out of anaerobic metabolites and the compensatory hypercontractility of non ischemic myocardial areas, interposed among the small ischemic regions. Furthermore, the sensitivity of traditional metabolic markers of myocardial ischemia, such as lactate production in the coronary sinus, is likely to be less than that observed when ischemia develops in large myocardial regions due to the obstruction of large epicardial vessels.

Oxidative stress products which appear to be extremely sensitive markers of myocardial ischemia may overcome the limitations of traditional markers of ischemia in patients with syndrome X. It has been shown that reperfusion of previously ischemic myocardium causes intense oxidative stress due to the production of oxygen free radicals. Although *in vivo* measurement of oxygen free radicals is difficult, plasma levels of stable lipid peroxidation products, such as lipid hydroperoxides (LH) and conjugated dienes (CD), derived from free-radical mediated oxidation of polyunsaturated membrane and circulating lipids, are accepted indices of oxidative stress [31]. The generation of lipid peroxidation products induced by oxygen free radicals is a self-propagating process which is not limited to the reperfused myocardial regions, but it occurs also in the adjacent, normally perfused, regions [32] and is eventually switched off by free radical scavengers. Buffon *et al* [33] have demonstrated a marked and sustained increase of LH and CD in the great cardiac vein, following a single brief episode of myocardial ischemia in patients undergoing elective coronary angioplasty. The same authors also measured the transcardiac production of lipid peroxides, at baseline and in response to atrial pacing, in 15 patients with syndrome X and in 5 control patients. The latter were patients undergoing cardiac catheterization because of mitral valve disease or interatrial septal defect and who had no history of chest pain, had a negative exercise test, and normal coronary arteries and left ventricular function at angiography [34]. In this study, blood samples were collected simultaneously from aorta and coronary sinus immediately before pacing, at maximal pacing rate, and at 1, 5 and 15 minutes after the end of atrial pacing. During pacing, heart rate was increased by 10 bpm every 30 seconds, until either the appearance of significant (1 mm) ST segment depression or a pacing rate of 160 bpm in those patients who did not develop ST segment changes. The target heart rate was then maintained for 3 minutes. At baseline, patients with syndrome X and controls showed similar levels of LH and CD in aorta and in coronary sinus. In patients with syndrome X, but not in control patients, LH and CD levels were slightly but significantly higher in the coronary sinus than in the aorta, suggesting persistent transcardiac production of lipid peroxides.

All patients with syndrome X developed significant ST segment depression and 14 of them complained also of typical chest pain. Conversely, none of the control patients developed pain or ECG changes. At peak heart rate, LH and CD levels were similar to those at baseline in both syndrome X and control patients. In the recovery phase, however, LH and CD in syndrome X patients exhibited a threefold increase in coronary sinus at 1 and 5 minutes, with elevated values still persisting at 15 minutes. In control patients, LH and CD levels remained unchanged in the coronary sinus throughout the study (Figure 1). This sustained oxidative stress observed in syndrome X immediately following atrial pacing is similar to that observed following coronary angioplasty [33] and strongly suggests the presence of transient myocardial ischemia. Of note, the increased transcardiac production of indices of oxidative stress observed in syndrome X even at baseline can, in turn, impair endothelial function, increase arteriolar vessel wall thickness (by stimulating smooth muscle cell proliferation), and affect myocardial cell homeostasis (membrane molecular transport, intracellular calcium-homeostasis) [35].

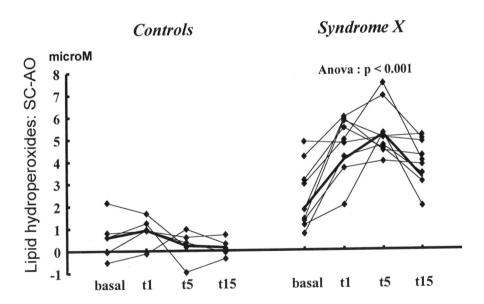

Figure 1. Cardiac production of lipid hydroperoxides in controls (left panel) and in patients with syndrome X (right panel) assessed by obtaining paired blood samples from coronary sinus (CS) and aorta (Ao) during baseline and following atrial pacing. No detectable cardiac production of lipid hydroperoxides was detectable in controls. Conversely, patients with syndrome X exhibited baseline production of lipid hydroperoxides and a further sustained increase at 1, 5 and 15 minutes after the beginning of atrial pacing.

Evidence of sympathetic dysfunction

Cardiac sympathetic function has been widely investigated in syndrome X but the results of the studies have been rather controversial. A direct assessment of cardiac adrenergic nerve function can be obtained by measuring cardiac uptake of ^{123}I-metaiodobenzylguanidine (MIBG) [36], a guanethidine analog which shares the same uptake/retention mechanisms as noradrenaline at sympathetic nerve endings [37,38].

Lanza *et al* [39] performed cardiac MIBG scintigraphy in 12 patients with syndrome X and in 10 age and sex-matched normal volunteers. Planar and SPECT scintigraphic images of the chest were obtained 0.5, 1, 2, 3, and 18 hours after the injection. Global uptake of MIBG by the heart was assessed using the heart/mediastinum ratio. To evaluate regional tracer uptake, the left ventricle was divided into 24 anatomical segments on transverse cardiac tomographic images. Semiquantitative MIBG uptake for each segment was obtained by a threshold method based on an 8 level color scale, each level corresponding to 12.5% of the maximal pixel value. Segments were scored from 0 (normal tracer uptake) to 3 (severe defect uptake). A global MIBG uptake defect score was obtained as the sum of all segmental scores for each patient. The reproducibility of MIBG results was assessed in 7 syndrome X patients at a mean follow-up of 5 months. SPECT [201]thallium stress-redistribution study was performed in 11 syndrome X patients 1 week after MIBG scintigraphy (bicycle exercise test in 10 patients, dipyridamole test in 1). Twenty-four-hour catecholamines urinary excretion was measured in 8 syndrome X patients and 7 controls.

At 3 hours, the optimal timing for the assessment of adrenergic cardiac function by MIBG uptake [36], cardiac MIBG scintigraphy appeared normal in all but 1 control subject, who showed a mild regional inferior defect. Conversely, 9 syndrome X patients (75%, $p<0.01$) showed abnormalities in cardiac MIBG uptake. On planar images cardiac MIBG uptake was totally absent in 4 patients and almost totally absent in 1. Four other patients showed inhomogeneous cardiac tracer uptake, with obvious regional defects.

The heart/mediastinum ratio, a reliable index of global cardiac MIBG uptake, was significantly lower (1.70±0.6 vs 2.2±0.3, P=0.03), and cardiac MIBG uptake defect score strongly higher (36.7±31 vs 4.0±2.5, p=0.003, Figure 2) in syndrome X patients compared to controls. Conversely, lung and salivary gland uptake of MIBG were normal and similar in patients and controls (Figure 2). There was no difference in 24-hour urinary catecholamine excretion between the 2 groups, thus suggesting that the abnormal adrenergic function in syndrome X patients was not generalized but confined to the heart.

Reversible perfusion defects on thallium stress scintigraphy were found in 5 of 11 syndrome X patients (45%). All patients with thallium defects had abnormal MIBG scintigrams, while all 3 patients with normal MIBG scintigraphy also had normal thallium images. Overall, MIBG alterations appeared much more striking and extensive than thallium defects. Of the 6 patients with normal thallium scintigraphy, one had no MIBG uptake, 2 had regional MIBG defects, and 3 had normal MIBG studies. Finally, in the 7 syndrome X patients who underwent a follow-up MIBG study, cardiac MIBG results showed a very high reproducibility (r=0.99, p<0.0001 for MIBG score).

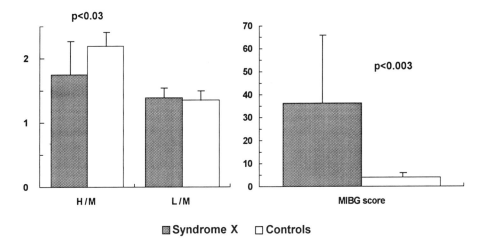

Figure 2. Heart/mediastinum ratio (H/M) and lung/medistinum ratio (L/M) of MIBG uptake (left panel) and cardiac MIBG uptake score (right panel) after 3 hours from MIBG injection in 12 patients with syndrome X and in 10 healthy control subjects.

In summary, obvious global and/or regional abnormalities in cardiac MIBG scintigraphy were observed in 75% of patients with syndrome X, with cardiac MIBG uptake being totally or almost totally absent in about 40% of patients. These findings indicate the presence of an abnormal function of efferent cardiac sympathetic nerve endings and support the cardiac origin of chest pain in these patients. The abnormalities of adrenergic activity seemed predominantly localized in the heart in our patients, as there were no differences between patients and controls in lung and salivary gland MIBG uptake and in urinary catecholamine excretion.

The lack of detectable abnormalities in cardiac MIBG scan in 25% of patients may be due to the fact that the impairment of adrenergic nerve function is a mere consequence of the primary cause(s) of the syndrome, and occurs in most, but not all, patients; alternatively, it may indicate that the mechanisms responsible for syndrome X are not necessarily the same in all patients, even when they are selected according to strict inclusion criteria.

While it is unlikely that cardiac MIBG defects reflect sympathetic denervation [40-44] in our patients, MIBG abnormalities may have different functional mechanisms, including an increased cardiac spillover of noradrenaline [45,46], which antagonizes the uptake of MIBG at nerve terminals. The increased noradrenaline spillover could help explaining several findings previously reported in these patients, including enhanced cardiac adrenergic drive [16,17,20,22], reduction of coronary flow reserve [8-10] and increased heterogeneity of myocardial perfusion [11,12]. Accordingly, reversible myocardial defects on stress thallium scintigraphy were shown in about two thirds of the patients exhibiting abnormal MIBG uptake, but in none of those with normal MIBG scan. Alternatively, MIBG alterations may be consequent to a primary microvascular dysfunction, resulting in an impairment of either uptake-1 function or of storage system [47-49].

Cell membrane dysfunction in syndrome X

Interestingly, in about one third of patients with non-insulin dependent diabetes mellitus, hyperinsulinemia is associated to an enhanced activity of the red blood cell sodium/lithium countertransport [50], which reflects the activity of the Na+-H+ exchange [51]. The latter plays a pivotal role in intracellular pH and calcium homeostasis [52]. As stimulated hyperinsulinemia is frequently found in patients with syndrome X, Gaspardone *et al* [53] investigated Na+-H+ exchange in 15 patients with syndrome X by measuring Na+-Li+ countertransport. They found that in these patients the activity of the Na+-H+ exchanger in red blood cells was about two-fold higher than that observed in an age and sex-matched control population. Of note, 14 of the 15 patients with syndrome X (93%) presented Na+-Li+ countertransport values higher than the mean + 2 standard deviations of the control group (Figure 3). These findings have been confirmed independently by Koren *et al* [54] who assessed the Na+-H+ exchange using a different methodology.

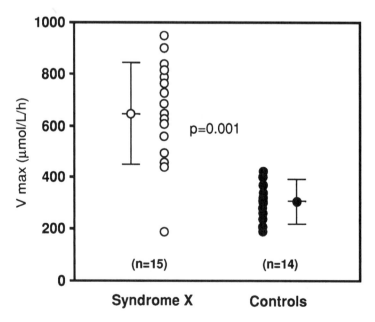

Figure 3. Activity of Na+-Li+ contertransport, an accepted marker of in vivo Na+-H+ exchange, in peripheral blood red cells of controls and patients with syndrome X. The activity of Na+-Li+ contertransport was markedly enhanced in the vast majority of patients with syndrome X.

In the same subjects, in addition to Na+-Li+ countertransport, Gaspardone *et al* assessed the activity of red blood cell Na+-K+ ATPase pump. The latter was found to be significantly reduced in patients with syndrome X compared to that measured in controls [55]. A depressed activity of the Na+-K+ ATPase pump enhances the susceptibility of microcirculation to endogenous vasoconstrictors [56].

An alteration of membrane ionic pumps as a major cause of syndrome X: a working hypothesis

The recent report by Buffon *et al* [34] of an increased release of lipid peroxidation products in the coronary sinus during atrial pacing in syndrome X, comparable to that observed following balloon occlusion in the setting of coronary angioplasty [33], seems to support that angina and ST segment changes in syndrome X are due to microvascular dysfunction resulting in myocardial ischemia. The suggested higher sensitivity of this new markers of ischemia may be related to an "explosive" generation of lipid peroxidation products following ischemia-reperfusion.

Pathogenesis of Cardiac Syndrome X

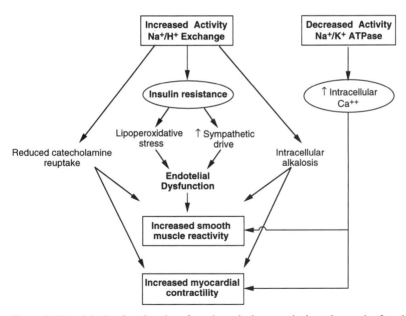

Figure 4. Potential role of an alteration of membrane ionic pumps in the pathogenesis of syndrome X. See text for explanations.

What causes microvascular dysfunction in syndrome X? The demonstration of an enhanced activity of the Na+-H+ exchange by Gaspardone *et al* [53] provides a clue to link the many and apparently different dowels of this intriguing syndrome (Figure 4).

Smooth muscle dysfunction, hyperinsulinemia and the predominance of sympathetic activity observed in patients with syndrome X may all be explained by an enhanced Na+-H+ exchange. Indeed, enhanced Na+-H+ exchange results in intracellular alkalinization and increased intracellular free calcium concentration [57]. These changes can increase coronary microvascular tone [8-10,20,21] and enhance the susceptibility of coronary microvessels to vasoconstrictor agents [9,10,20,21]. The frequent occurrence of myocardial hypercontractility [19], reduced forearm vasodilator reserve [23], abnormal esophageal motility [24] and airway hyperactivity [25] in patients with syndrome X may be due to the ubiquitous presence of this membrane ion exchanger, which is expressed in cardiac and smooth muscle cells. It is also worth noting that an enhancement of Na+-H+ exchange, throughout its effects on intracellular calcium concentration, has been indicated as a functional abnormality involved in the pathogenesis of insulin resistance and hyperinsulinemia [58]. The latter, in turn, can further enhance coronary microvascular dysfunction through an alteration of endothelial function [59] and the release of norepinephrine within the myocardium due to direct activation of perivascular sympathetic nerves [60,61]. Interestingly, the massive reduction of myocardial MIBG uptake observed in syndrome X can also be due to an increase of intracellular sodium concentration, mediated by an enhanced activity of Na+-H+ exchange, which causes a reduction of type I cathecholamine re-uptake with consequent increase of extracellular cathecholamine concentration [62]. Furthermore, the recent evidence by Gaspardone *et al* [55] of a reduced activity of Na+-K+ ATPase pump in syndrome X might help explaining another intriguing feature of the syndrome: the high prevalence of regional defects in myocardial thallium uptake [13,14,15,39], while positron emission tomography fails to detect large regions of myocardial hypoperfusion during metabolic coronary vasodilation [7,11,12]. Indeed, rather than by myocardial hypoperfusion, regional defects in myocardial thallium uptake might often be caused by an increased efflux of potassium from myocardial cells, as thallium and potassium share a similar transmembrane kinetic. Furthermore, the reduced activity of Na+-K+ ATPase pump might contribute to make smooth muscle cells more reactive to constrictor stimuli and enhance myocardial contractility (digoxin-like effect).

It must be noted, however, that the working hypothesis that an enhanced activity of the sodium-hydrogen exchange plays a key etiologic role in syndrome X fails to explain an important feature of syndrome X, the increased sensitivity to pain and the tendency to complain [28,29]. It is currently under investigation, however, whether an enhanced activity of the Na+-H+ exchange is associated to an increased sensitivity to pain. Alternatively, the latter might represent a mere unmasking feature which brings patients to medical attention and its presence may be due, therefore, to a selection bias. The working hypothesis that an enhanced activity of the Na+-H+ exchange plays a key etiologic role in syndrome X also fails to explain why MIBG uptake seems to be limited to the myocardium. It is possible that this is due to underestimation of MIBG uptake in organs different from the heart or, again, to a selection bias due to the fact that patients with predominantly myocardial sympathetic abnormalities are more likely to seek medical attention.

In conclusion, the most recent evidence suggests that patients with syndrome X do develop myocardial ischemia associated to microvascular angina. An alteration of ionic fluxes through cell membranes, in particular an enhanced activity of the sodium/hydrogen exchange, might be primarily involved in the pathogenesis of this puzzling syndrome either through a direct effect or by activating the sympathetic system. Endothelial dysfunction is another possible mechanism. The findings described in this chapter provide new grounds on which to base future research. The mechanisms described may not be limited to patients with syndrome X but they could also operate in patients with obstructive atherosclerosis in whom microvascular dysfunction may contribute to the genesis of myocardial ischemia and angina.

References

1. Arbogast R, Bourassa MG. Myocardial function during atrial pacing in patients with angina pectoris and normal coronary arteriograms. Comparison with patients having significant coronary artery disease. Am J Cardiol 1973;32:257-263.
2. Camici PG, Marracini P, Michelassi C, et al. Coronary hemodynamics and myocardial metabolism in patients with Syndrome X. J Am Coll Cardiol 1991; 17:1461-70.
3. Levy RD, Shapiro LM, Wright C, Mockus L, Fox KM Diurnal variation in left ventricular function: a study of patients with myocardial ischaemia, syndrome X, and of normal controls. Br Heart J 1987; 57:148-53.
4. Picano E, Lattanzi F, Masini M, Distante A, L'Abbate A. usefulness of a high-dose dipyridamole-echocardiography test for diagnosis of syndrome X. Am J Cardiol 1987; 60;508-12
5. Crake T, Canepa-Anson R, Shapiro LM, Poole-Wilson PA. Continuos recording of coronary sinus saturation during atrial pacing in patients with and without coronary artery disease or with syndrome X. Br Heart J 1987;57:67-72.
6. Rosano GMC, Kaski JC, Arie S, et al. Failure to demonstrate myocardial ischaemia in patients with angina and normal coronary arteries. Evaluation by continuous coronary sinus pH monitoring and lactate metabolism. Eur Heart J 1996;17:1175-80.
7. Rosen SD, Uren NG, Kaski JC, Tousoulis D, Davies GJ, Camici PG. Coronary vasodilator reserve, pain perception, and sex in patients with syndrome X. Circulation 1994;90:50-60.
8. Cannon RO III, Watson RM, Rosing DR, Epstein SE. Angina caused by reduced vasodilator reserve of the small coronary arteries. J Am Coll Cardiol 1983;1:1359-73.
9. Opherk d, Weihe E, Mall G, et al. Reduced coronary dilatory capacity and ultrastructural changes of the myocardium in patients with angina pectoris but normal coronary arteriograms. Circulation 1981;63:817-5.
10. Cannon RO, Schenke WH, Leon MB, Rosing DR, Urqhart J, Epstein SE. Limited coronary flow reserve after dipyridamole in patients with ergonovine-induced coronary vasoconstriction. Circulation 1987;75:163-74.
11. Galassi AR, Crea F, Araujo LI, et al. Comparison of regional myocardial blood flow in syndrome X and one-vessel coronary artery disease. Am J Cardiol 1993;72:134-139.
12. Meeder JG, Blanksma PK, Crijns HGJM, et al. Mechanisms of angina pectoris in syndrome X assessed by myocardial perfusion dynamics and heart rate variability. Eur Heart J 1995;16:1571-7.
13. Kaul S, Newell JB, Chesler DA, Pohost GM, Okada RD, Boucher CA: Quantitative thallium imaging findings in patients with normal coronary angiographic findings and in clinically normal subjects. Am J Cardiol 1986; 57:509-12.
14. Tweddel AC, Martin W, Hutton I: Thallium scan in syndrome X. Br Heart J 1992; 68:48-50.
15. Korhola O, Valle M, Frick MH, Wiljasalo M, RiihimäK E: Regional myocardial perfusion abnormalities on xenon-133 imaging in patients with angina pectoris and normal coronary arteries. Am J Cardiol 1977; 39:355-9.
16. Galassi AR, Kaski JC, Crea F, et al. Heart rate response during exercise testing and ambulatory ECG monitoring in patients with syndrome X. Am Heart J 1991;122:458-463.
17. Rosano GMC, Ponikowski P, Adamopoulos S, Collins P, Poole-Wilson PA, Coats AJS, Kaski JC. Abnormal autonomic control of the cardiovascular system in syndrome X. Am J Cardiol 1994;73:1174-9.
18. Rosen SD, Dritsas A, Bourdillon PJ, Camici PG. Analysis of the electrocardiographic QT interval in patients with syndrome X. Am J Cardiol 1994; 971-2.

19. Tousoulis D, Crake T, Lefroy DC, Galassi AR, Maseri-A. Left ventricular hypercontractility and ST segment depression in patients with syndrome X.

20. Montorsi P, Fabblocchi F, Loaldi A, et al. Coronary adrenergic hyperreactivity in patients with syndrome X and abnormal electrocardiogram at rest. Am J Cardiol 1991; 68:1698-1703.

21. Chauhan A, Mullins PA, Petch MC, Schofield PM. Effect of hyperventilation and mental stress on coronary blood flow in syndrome X. Br Heart J 1993;69:516-524.

22. Rosen SD, Boyd H, Rhodes CG, Kaski JC, Camici PG. Myocardial beta-adrenoceptor density and plasma catecholamines in syndrome X. Am J Cardiol 1996;78:37-42.

23. Sax FL, Cannon RO, Hanson C, Epstein SE. Impaired forearm vasodilator reserve in patients with microvascular angina. Evidence of a generalised disorder of vascular function? N Engl J Med 1987;317:1366-1370.

24. Cannon RO, Cattau EL, Yakshe PN, Maher K, Schenke WH, Benjamin SB, Epstein SE. Coronary flow reserve, esophageal motility, and chest pain in patients with angiographically normal coronary arteries. Am J Med 1990;88:217-222.

25. Cannon RO, Cattau EL, Yakshe PN, Maher K, Schenke WH, Benjamin SB, Epstein SE. Coronary flow reserve, esophageal motility, and chest pain in patients with angiographically normal coronary arteries. Am J Med 1990;88:217-222.

26. Dean JD, Jones CJH, Hutchison SJ, Peters JR, Henderson AH. Hyperinsulinaemia and microvascular angina ("syndrome X"). Lancet 1991;337:456-457.

27. Bøtker HE, Moller N, Ovesen P, Mengel A, Schmitz O, Orskov H, Bagger JP. Insulin resistance in microvascular angina (syndrome X). Lancet 1993;342:136-140.

28. Cannon RO, Quyyumi AA, Schenke WH, et al. Abnormal cardiac sensitivity in patients with chest pain and normal coronary arteries. J Am Coll Cardiol 1990;16:1359-1366.

29. Pasceri V, Lanza GA, Buffon A, Montenero AS, Crea F, Maseri A. Role of abnormal pain sensitivity and behavioral factors in determining chest pain in syndrome X. J Am Coll Cardiol 1998;31:62-66.

30. Maseri A, Crea F, Kaski JC, Crake T. Mechanism of Angina Pectoris in Syndrome X. J Am Coll Cardiol 1991;17:499-506.

31. Gutteridge JMC, Halliwell B. The measurement and mechanism of lipid peroxidation in biological systems. TIBS 1990; 15:129-135.

32. Saran M, Bors W. Radical reaction in vivo - an overview. Radiation and Environmental Biophisics 1990; 29:249-262.

33. Buffon A, Santini SA, Rigattieri S, Ramazzotti V, Summaria F, Mordente A, Liuzzo G, Biasucci LM, Crea F, Maseri A. Myocardial lipid peroxidation caused by successful coronary angioplasty. Circulation 1997; 96(Suppl.I):756.

34. Buffon A, Santini SA, Rigattieri S, Ramazzotti V, Summaria F, Mordente A, Liuzzo G, Biasucci LM, Crea F, Maseri A. Transient intracardiac lipid peroxidation induced by atrial pacing in syndrome X: a definitive demonstration of an ischemic mechanism?. Circulation 1997; 96(Suppl.I):761.

35. Kim Myung-Suk, Akera T. O_2 free radicals: cause of ischemia-reperfusion injury to cardiac Na^+-K^+-ATPase. Am J Physiol 1987; 252:H252-H257.

36. Wafelman AR, Hoefnagel CA, Maes RAA, Beijnen JH. Radioiodinated metaiodobenzylguanidine: a review of its biodistribution and pharmacokinetics, drug interactions and dosimetry. Eur J Nucl Med 1994;21:545-559.

37. Sisson JC, Shapiro B, Meyers L, Mallette S, Mangner TJ, Wieland TM, Glowniak JV, Sherman P, Beierwaltes WH. Metaiodobenzylguanidine to map scintigraphically the adrenergic nervous system in man. J Nucl Med 1987;28:1625-36.

38. Wieland TM, Brown LE, Rogers L, Worthington KC, Wu J, Clinthorne NH, Otto CA, Swanson DP, Baierwaltes WH. Myocardial imaging with a radioiodinated norepinephrine storage analog. J Nucl Med 1981;22:22-31.

39. Lanza GA, Giordano AG, Pristipino C, et al. Abnormal cardiac adrenergic nerve function in patients with syndrome X detected by [123I]metaiodobenzylguanidine myocardial scintigraphy. Circulation 1997;96:821-6.

40. Wieland TM, Brown LE, Rogers L, Worthington KC, Wu J, Clinthorne NH, Otto CA, Swanson DP, Baierwaltes WH. Myocardial imaging with a radioiodinated norepinephrine storage analog. J Nucl Med 1981;22:22-31.

41. Dae MW, Herre JM, O'Connell JW, Botvinick EH, Newman D, Munoz L. Scintigraphic assessment of sympathetic innervation after transmural versus nontransmural myocardial infarction. J Am Coll Cardiol 1991;17:1416-23.

42. Tomoda H, Yoshioka K, Shiina Y, Tagawa R, Ide M, Suzuki Y. Regional sympathetic denervation detected by iodine 123 metaiodobenzylguanidine in non-Q-wave myocardial infarction and unstable angina. Am Heart J 1994;128:452-8.

43. Hartikainen J, Kuikka J, Mantysaari M, Lansimies E, Pyorala K. Sympathetic reinnervation after acute myocardial infarction. Am J Cardiol 1996;77:5-9.

44. De Marco T, Dae M, Yuen-Gree MSF, Kumar S, Sudhir K, Keith F, Amidon TM, Rifkin C, Klinski C, Lau D, Botvinick EH, Chatterjee K. Iodine-123 metaiodobenzylguanidine scintigraphic assessment of the transplanted human heart: evidence for late reinnervation. J Am Coll Cardiol 1995;25:927-31.

45. Nakajo M, Shimabukuro K, Yoshimura H, Yonekura R, Nakabeppu Y, Tanoue P, Shinohara S. Iodine-131 metaiodobenzylguanidine intra- and extravascular accumulation in the rat heart. J Nucl Med 1986;27:84-89.

46. Imamura Y, Ando H, Mitsuoka W, Egashira S, Masaki H, Ashihara T, Fukuyama T. Iodine-123 metaiodobenzylguanidine images reflect intense myocardial adrenergic nervous acitivity in congestive heart failure independent of underlying cause. J Am Coll Cardiol 1995;26:1594-9.

47. Tsutsui H, Ando S, Fukai T, Kuroiwa M, Egashira K, Sasaki M, Kuwabara Y, Koyanagi S, Takeshita A. Detection of angina-provoking coronary stenosis by resting iodine 123 metaiodobenzylguanidine scintigraphy in patients with unstable angina pectoris. Am Heart J 1995;129:708-15.

48. Nakata T, Nagao K, Tsuchihashi K, Hashimoto A, Tanaka S, Iimura O. Regional cardiac sympathetic nerve dysfunction and the duagnostic efficacy of metaiodobenzylguanidine in stable coronary artery disease. Am J Cardiol 1996;78:292-7.

49. Takano H, Nakamura T, Satou T, Umetani K, Watanabe A, Ishihara T, Mochizuchi S, Kimura H, Honma H, Ikeda Y, Koizumi K, Arbab AS, Tamura K. Regional myocardial sympathetic dysinnervation in patients with coronary vasospasm. Am J Cardiol 1995;75:324-29.

50. Canessa M. Erythrocyte sodium-lithium countertransport: another link between essential hypertension and diabetes. Curr Opin Nephrol Hypertens 1994;3(5):511-517.

51. Kahn AM, Allen JC, Cragoe EG Jr, Shelat H. Sodium-lithium exchange and sodium-proton exchange are mediated by the same transport system in sarcolemmal vescicles from bovine superior mesenteric artery. Circ Res 1989;65:818-828.

52. Rosskopf D, Dusing R, Siffert W. Membrane sodium-proton exchange and primary hypertension. Hypertension 1993;21:607-617.

53. Gaspardone A, Ferri C, Crea F, et al. Enhanced activity of sodium-lithium countertransport in patients with cardiac syndrome X: a potential link between cardiac and metabolic syndrome X. J Am Coll Cardiol (in press).

54. Koren W, Koldanov R, Peleg E, Rabinowitz B, Rosenthal T. Enhanced red cell sodium-hydrogen exchange in microvascular angina. Eur Heart J . 1997;18:1296-1299.

55. Gaspardone A, Ferri C, Crea F, et al. Red blood cell Na^+/K^+ ATPase and $Na^+/K^+/2Cl^-$ countertransport activity in patients with syndrome X (Abstr). Eur Heart J (in press).

56. Blaustein MP. Sodium ions, calcium ions, blood pressure regulation and hypertension: a reassessment and a hypothesis. Am J Physiol 1977;232:C165-C173.

57. Rosskopf D, Dusing R, Siffert W. Membrane sodium-proton exchange and primary hypertension. Hypertension 1993;21:607-617.

58. Aviv A. The role of Ca^{2+} protein kinase C, and the Na^+-H^+ antiport in the development of hypertension and insulin resistance. J Am Soc Nephrol . 1992;3(5):1049-1063.

59. Egashira K, Inou T, Hirooka Y, Yamada A, Urabe Y, Takeshita A. Evidence of impaired endothelim-dependent coronary vasodilation in patients with angina pectoris and normal coronary angiograms. N Engl J Med 1993;328:1659-1664.

60. Anderson EA, Hoffman RP, Balon TW, Sinkey CA, Mark AL. Hyperinsulinemia produces both sympathetic neural activation and vasodilation in normal humans. J Clin Invest 1991;87:2246-2252.

61. Camici PG, Marraccini P, Gistri R, Salvadori PA, Sorace O, L'Abbate A. Adrenergically mediated coronary vasoconstriction in patients with syndrome X. Cardiovasc Drugs Ther 1994;8:221-226.

62. Ungerer M, Chlistalla A, Karoglan M, Richardt G. Regulation of cardiac uptake 1 by intra- and extraneural norepinephrine, and by transmembranous sodium gradient. Circulation 1996;94:I-128.

Chapter 12

INCREASED PLASMA MEMBRANE ION-LEAKAGE: A NEW HYPOTHESIS FOR CHEST PAIN AND NORMAL CORONARY ARTERIOGRAMS

Anders Waldenström and Gunnar Ronquist

Approximately 10-15% of all patients in the US who are subjected to coronary angiography because of anginal chest pain do not show any obvious coronary artery disease. Approximately 15% of these patients have 201-thallium myocardial perfusion defects [1,2]. Despite the normal coronary angiogram most physicians still consider the patients symptoms being due to insufficient myocardial blood perfusion. This is not surprising given the fact that symptoms in this syndrome clearly suggest the presence of myocardial ischemia. Among these are: angina pectoris like chest pains, transient ECG changes suggestive of myocardial ischemia, and myocardial perfusion defects as assessed by 201-thallium scintigraphy. Interestingly, a sizeable proportion of patients with chest pain and normal coronary arteriograms have unexplained fatigue.

In patients with myocardial ischemia these findings are often explained by an imbalance in the production and break down of ATP (Figure 1). This imbalance induces accumulation of adenosine which is known to be one of the main mediators of pain in angina pectoris, [3-7].

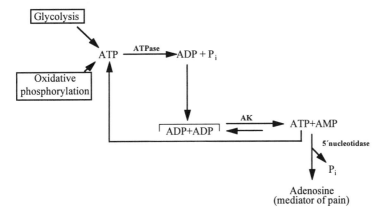

Figure 1: Metabolic coupling between increased ATPase activity and increased adenylate kinase (AK) activity in myocytes of patients with syndrome X. It is proposed that the activity of 5'nucleotidase is increased in order to drive the adenylate kinase reaction to the right leading to formation of more adenosine.

In the presence of deficient production of ATP, due to lack of electron acceptors (O_2), insufficient function of the sarcolemmal Na^+/K^+ ATPase can be observed. Under normal circumstances, this ATPase guarantees the maintenance of the electrochemical potential across the sarcolemma. Hence, in ATP deficient states (such as ischemia) the ion gradient dissipates resulting in passive potassium ion translocation to the extracellular space. This is the explanation for both the typical ST-segment changes during ischemia and the so called perfusion defects seen on 201-thallium scintigraphy. When an increase in myocardial adenosine occurs, the accumulation of extracellular potassium may induce the above mentioned ion shifts which are characteristic for ischemic heart disease and can be also observed in patients with syndrome X.

Clinical findings

In 1991 we studied twenty consecutive patients with angina pectoris, normal coronary angiography and abnormal exercise 201- thallium scans (SPECT). We carried out a number of provocative tests to explore the reasons for the anginal pain and ECG-changes [8] observed in these patients. The intra-coronary infusion of dipyridamole induced an increase of $\leq$ 200% in coronary sinus blood flow in 45% of the patients (group A) and > 200% in the remainder (group B) [8]. All patients but one developed severe chest pain during dipyridamole infusion. Despite this, myocardial lactate consumption did not change significantly and none of the patients showed ischemic ECG changes.

To assess endothelial function, intracoronary acetylcholine was infused in increasing concentrations. No ischemic ECG changes or focal changes of vessel diameter ($\geq$30%) were observed at the coronary angiography during the acetylcholine infusion. In 3 patients however, a diffuse vasoconstriction of the LAD was seen but this was not associated with perfusion defects as assessed by the 201-thallium scintigraphs. Only one patient had moderate chest pain at the highest dose of acetylcholine which continued for approximately 10 minutes. There were no signs of ischemic ECG changes during pain. Acetylcholine did not induce myocardial perfusion defects in any of the 3 patients who showed diffuse LAD vasoconstriction (30-60 %). Cold pressor testing did not cause signs of ischemia. At pacing to maximum heart rate, pain was similar in the two groups (Borg, 10-graded analogue scale). There were no differences between groups concerning ST segment changes.

Continuous 24-hour pH monitoring in the distal esophagus did not show differences in the incidence of gastroesophageal reflux or symptom index (SI%) among patients with chest pain and normal coronary arteries compared to ischemic heart disease patients who were used as a reference group. Approximately 50% of the patients with normal coronary arteriograms had chest pain during hyperventilation and ergonovine testing. Chest pain, however, was not associated with ischemic ECG changes.

The protocol used for myocardial perfusion scintigraphy and isotope angiography was as follows: At peak exercise, 201-thallium was injected into an antecubital vein 5 to 10 min after single photon emission computerized tomography (SPECT) data acquisition was started. No differences were observed in group A and group B concerning the occurrence of perfusion defects. All patients had normal left ventricular ejection fraction at rest. After exercise, the left ventricular ejection fraction was lower in group A. This study, in a limited number of patients, did not provide an explanation for the occurrence of symptoms in this patient group. Perhaps the only positive finding was that at least some patients with chest pain and normal arteriograms (group A) have a decreased coronary reserve. Patients of group A also showed chest pain at a lower pacing rate than patients of group B. In patients with dipyridamole-induced chest pains we could not find ECG signs of ischemia or lactate production. Thus our study failed to demonstrate a mechanism which could explain the chest pain of these patients. Moreover, our study also showed no definite patterns of response, thus suggesting that patients with chest pain and normal arteriograms represent a heterogeneous population. This has been recently discussed by other authors supporting the notion that multiple etiologies are likely to be responsible for the syndrome [9,10]. This led us to hypothesize that metabolic factors may be the pathogenic mechanism in at least some of the syndrome X patients. We performed another study where endomyocardial and skeletal muscle biopsies were taken from a series of patients with syndrome X. This study showed some remarkable findings (Figures 2, 3): 1) a marked decrease in ATP and increase in both ADP and AMP levels in both myocardial and skeletal muscle biopsies, and 2) increased lactate concentrations in cardiac muscle biopsies.

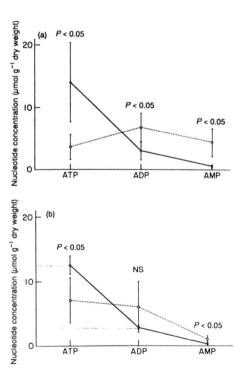

Figure 2. (a) Adenine nucleotide content (μmol g^{-1} dry weight) in endomyocardial biopsies from patients (------) and control papillary muscle (———). Note the low ATP values and inverse ATP/ADP ratio in patients. (b) Adenine nucleotide content (μmol g^{-1} dry weight) in skeletal muscle from patients (------) and controls (———). Mean values ± SD are shown. (By permission of J Internal Medicine).

138

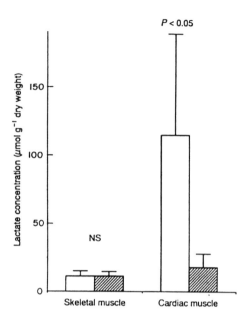

Figure 3. Skeletal and cardiac muscle content of lactate (μmol g $^{-1}$ dry weight) in patients (open bars) and controls (hatched bars). Mean values ± SD are shown. (By permission of J Internal Medicine).

The biopsy data in this study indicates the occurrence of an abnormal adenine nucleotide turnover with, possible inhibition of adenylate kinase activity *in vivo* due to elevated AMP levels. The high myocardial lactate content, as opposed to the near normal values in skeletal muscle in these patients (although the skeletal muscle biopsies showed a decrease in EC) may be explained by the fact that the skeletal muscle was truly at rest at the time of biopsy which was obviously not the case for the heart. The increased lactate levels may reflect enhanced potassium ion pumping by the Na^+/K^+ ATPase using preferentially compartmentalized ATP as substrate [11]. Hence this ATPase is fuelled by compartmentalized ATP derived from anaerobic glycolysis resulting in lactate as an end product. In a series of papers [3-7], we have shown that adenosine is an important link between ischemia and pain. This is consistent with the fact that ATP is broken down during ischemia forming *inter alia* adenosine. A decrease in ATP content represents a dangerous condition and cells may sense it and trigger the "alarm" which in this case may be represented by chest pain.

Deficient ATP production versus excessive ATP consumption in syndrome X

The present hypothesis is based on our observation of critically low ATP levels in skeletal and myocardial biopsies (low energy charge, EC)

$$EC = \frac{ATP + \frac{1}{2} ADP}{ATP + ADP + AMP} \approx 0.90$$

The most energy-demanding reactions in muscle cells are: 1) contraction and 2) ion pump activity. Because ATP levels and EC are low at rest in skeletal muscle in syndrome X patients and EC is high even during excessive muscle activity in normals, it is unlikely that a defect in the contractile system is responsible for the constantly low ATP and EC values observed in heart and skeletal muscle in patients with syndrome X. More likely, there is an excessive energy consumption due to increased ion pumping. This might be brought about by a short cut in the metabolic coupling between ATP hydrolysis and osmotic work. The critical ingredient of this hypothesis is that a leakage of potassium ions from the intra- to the extra-cellular space will activate the Na^+/K^+ ATPase in order to maintain the electrochemical gradient across the plasma membrane. This is done at the expense of an excessive breakdown of ATP which is produced by compartmentalized glycolysis involving glycolytic enzymes associated with the plasma membrane. The increased energy demand in the myocytes may result in excessive adenosine production which in turn may induce pain.

Leakage of ions can be brought about by different mechanisms one of which is incorporation of ionophores to the plasma membrane. Ionophores are organic molecules many of them derived from bacteria and viruses. Ionophores can be incorporated into biological membranes where they form ion specific channels. A common pathogen for myocarditis, the Coxsackie B3 virus, has ionophoric properties and could be the reason why patients with myocarditis have positive thallium scans.

Figure 4 illustrates the ion leakage hypothesis which may explain the occurrence of symptoms and ECG changes in patients with chest pain and normal coronary arteriograms. The following may represent a potential mechanism whereby potassium leakage through plasma membranes trigger a series of phenomena leading to "syndrome X".

1. The Na^+/K^+ ATPase pump "short cuts" and works at excessive speed because of an increase in potassium leakage along the gradient. We postulate that this is due to the "integration" of an ionophore to the plasma membrane or an ionophore-like effect.

2. There is excessive consumption of ATP and an imbalance between ATP production and consumption.

3. A decrease of ATP levels will result with an increase in ADP and AMP levels. An inverse relation between ATP and ADP will develop together with low energy charge of the cell (Figure 2). This explanation is supported by findings from muscle biopsy data and NMR spectroscopy data obtained in our patients with syndrome X [12, 13].

4. An increased adenylate kinase activity has been observed in syndrome X patients and may indicate high ATP turnover. This increased turnover mirrors the cellular "ambition" to achieve a high EC (Figure 1).

5. Increased ATP breakdown in the ATPase reaction, coupled to the adenylate kinase reaction, leads to an accumulation of AMP which, in turn, will be converted to adenosine by the 5' nucleotidase reaction in order to achieve a shift in the equilibrium reaction of adenylate kinase in favor of ATP formation. The increase in adenosine could explain the angina pectoris-like pain observed in syndrome X patients. The absence of skeletal muscle pain in spite of low ATP values and low energy charge in syndrome X patients may be caused by the low level of 5' nucleotidase in this tissue where AMP is instead converted to IMP by AMP-deaminase.

6. The present hypothesis permits also an alternative explanation to the so called

perfusion defects seen with 201-thallium scintigraphy in syndrome X. Thallium can be regarded as a potassium equivalent which distributes in the extracellular space in relation to the potassium concentration. During ischemia the Na^+/K^+ ATPase activity is inhibited because of lack of substrate. This leads to an increase of potassium ion concentration in the extracellular space. The distribution of thallium in this compartment will diminish resulting in a "cold spot" on scintigraphy. Our interpretation in syndrome X is that the primary non-ischemic leakage of intracellular potassium ions induced by an ionophore or ionophore like substance, leads to a SPECT image suggestive of ischemia but not caused by reduced perfusion.

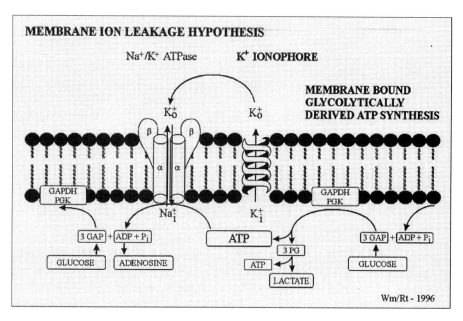

Figure 4. Schematic illustration of the plasma membrane. The Na^+/K^+ ATPase (with alfa and beta subunits) pumps potassium ions into the cell concomitantly with the extrusion of sodium ions in a stoichiometric relationship of 2 K^+ in, 3 Na^+ out per ATP. This means that not only ion gradients are created but also an electrochemical gradient develops (with the negative) charge inside the cell. The split products of the ATPase reaction, $ADP+ P_i$ will, in a process tightly bound to the plasma membrane, produce ATP by the action of membrane bound enzymes and substrates. A potassium ionophore is integrated into the membrane causing leakage of potassium ions along the gradient as indicated. The more intense the potassium leakage the faster the ion pumping required by the Na^+/K^+ ATPase in order to keep physiological ion gradients. This in turn leads to increased demands for ATP synthesis, which may explain the increased production of adenosine and lactate in this situation.

We have not been able to measure the content of adenosine in the myocardium or skeletal muscle of these patients because of its very short half life. However, we have shown that adenosine given into a coronary artery causes typical chest pain. Dipyridamole, which acts by blocking re-uptake of adenosine and thus increasing adenosine tissue levels, can also cause chest pain in syndrome X. Syndrome X patients are more "sensitive" to dipyridamole or adenosine than patients with ischemic heart disease who in turn, are more sensitive than normal controls. We believe that this is due to the presence of tissue adenosine at levels close to the threshold level for the induction of pain [7, 8].

In our own experiments, incubation of erythrocytes with different ionophores resulted in a pattern of ATP, ADP and AMP of the same type as found in syndrome X patients, [14, 15, 16]. Prolonged periods of experimentally induced ischemia in rat hearts do not induce the same nucleotide pattern. Perfusion of isolated rat hearts with a potassium ionophore induced a similar pattern of adenine nucleotides as well as an increase in lactate concentration, as observed in syndrome X patients [17]. In a Coxsackie B3 model of myocarditis in mice we have also shown a similar decrease in energy charge [18].

The applicability of our new paradigm to other disease states

Having worked with this problem over many years we have reasons to believe that there is a strong connection between syndrome X and the chronic fatigue syndrome. There are also reasons to believe that the disturbed calcium homeostasis observed in essential hypertension may be due to an increased leakage of calcium across the plasma membrane [19]. Another explanation for ion leakage across the plasma membrane may be found in the molecular structure of the membrane *per se*, i.e. the cholesterol/phospholipid relation in the membrane may determine whether the membrane is "tightly or loosely woven" allowing more or less ion leakage. We have found that the amyloid protein and its degradation products in Alzheimer's disease can function as calcium ionophores, and lead to changes in intracellular energy homeostasis. It could be speculated that this may be a pathophysiological mechanism in this disease [20, 21]. It thus seems that other diseases and not only syndrome X may be caused by a leakage of specific ions across the plasma membrane due to either incorporation of specific "false" ion channels (ionophores) or to alterations in the architecture of the plasma membrane leading to its destabilization.

Conclusion

Although there is no proof that syndrome X is caused by an excessive ion leakage across the plasma membrane, there is definitely no proof either that syndrome X is caused by myocardial ischemia. Syndrome X is clearly heterogeneous [10] and data in favor of either the ischemic hypotheses or our potassium hypothesis can only be taken as circumstantial evidence. In a situation where an objective decrease in perfusion cannot be documented other mechanisms should be postulated.

Acknowledgements

This study has been supported by grants from Medical Research Council 9X 9940 07C, Swedish Heart Lung Foundation, King Gustaf V and Queen Viktoria Foundation and Torsten and Ragnar Söderberg Foundation.

142

References

1. Kemp HG: Left ventricular function in patients with the anginal syndrome and normal coronary angiograms. Am J Cardiol 1973; 32:375-376.
2. Hutchison SJ, Poole-Wilson PA, Henderson AH: Angina with Normal Coronary Arteries: A review. Quart J Med 1988;72, No 268, pp.677-688.
3. Lagerqvist B, Sylvén Ch, Hedenström H & Waldenström A: Intravenous adenosine but not its first metabolite inosine provokes chest pain in healthy volunteers. J Cardiovasc Pharmacol 1990;16:173-176.
4. Lagerqvist B, Sylvén C, Helmius G & Waldenström A: Effects of exogenous adenosine in a patient with transplanted heart. Evidence for adenosine as a messenger in angina. Upsala J Med Sci 1990;95:137-145.
5. Lagerqvist B, Sylvén C, Beerman B, Helmius G, Waldenström A. Intracoronary adenosine causes angina pectoris like pain - an inquiry into the nature of visceral pain. Cardiovasc Res 1990; 24:609-13.
6. Lagerqvist B, Sylvén C, Theodorsen E, Kaijser L, Helmius G, Waldenström A. Adenosine-induced chest pains - a comparison between intracoronary bolus injection and steady-state infusion. Cardiovasc Res 1992; 26:810-14.
7. Lagerqvist B, Sylvén C, Waldenström A. Lower threshold for adenosine-induced chest pain in patients with angina and normal coronary angiograms. Br Heart J 1992; 68:282-285.
8. Lagerqvist B, Bylund H, Götell P, Mannting F, Sandhagen B, Waldenström A. Coronary artery vaso-regulation and left ventricular function in patients with angina pectoris-like pain and normal coronary angiograms. J Int Med 1991; 230:55-65.
9. Masahiro M, Masamichi K, Kensuke E, Hirofumi T, Toshihiro I, Hiroaki S, Akira T. Angina pectoris caused by coronary microvascular spasm. Lancet 1998; 351:1144-45.
10. Kaski J C. Chest pain and normal coronary arteriograms: role of "microvascular spasm". The Lancet 1998; 351:1165-69.
11. Weiss JN, Lamp ST. Glycolysis preferentially inhibits ATP-sensitive K^+ channels in isolated guinea pig cardiac myocytes. Science 1987; 283:67-69.
12. Waldenström A, Ronquist G & Lagerqvist B. Angina pectoirs patients with normal coronary angiograms but abnormal thallium perfusion schan exhibit low myocardial and skeletal muscle energy charge. J Int Med 1992; 231: 327-31.
13. Soussi B, Scherstén T, Waldenström A & Ronquist G. Phosphocreatine turnover and pH balance in forearm muscle of patients with syndrome X. Lancet 1993; 341: 829-830.
14. Engström I, Waldenström A & Ronquist G. Ionophore A23187 reduces energy charge by enhanced ion pumping in suspended human erythrocytes. Scand J Clin Lab Invest 1993; 53: 239-246.
15. Engström I, Waldenström A & Ronquist G. Effects of the ionophore gramicidin D on energy metabolism in human erythrocytes. Scand J Clin Lab Invest 1993; 53:247-252.
16. Engström I, Waldenström A & Ronquist G. Dissipation of the calcium gradient in human erythrocytes results in increased heat production. Clin Chim Acta 1993; 219: 113-122.
17. Martinussen HJ, Waldenström A & Ronquist G. Functional and biochemical effects of a K^+-ionophore on the isolated perfused rat heart. Acta Physiol Scand 1993; 147: 221-225.
18. Waldenström A, Fohlman J, Ilbäck N-G, Ronquist G, Häggren R & Gerdin B. Coxsacke B3 myocarditis induces a decrease in energy charge and accumulation of hyaluronan in the mouse heart. Eur J Clin Invest 1993; 23: 277-282.
19. Ronquist G, Frithz G, Soussi B, Scherstén T & Waldenström A. Disturbed energy balance in skeletal muscle of patients with untreated primary hypertension. J Int Med 1995; 238: 167-174.
20. Engström I, Ronquist G, Pettersson L & Waldenström A. Alzheimer amyloid ß-peptides exhibit ionophore like properties in human erythrocytes. Eur J Clin Invest 1995; 25: 471-476.
21. Sanderson KL, Butler L, Ingram VM. 1997. Aggregates of a ß-amyloid peptide are required to induce calcium currents in neuron-like human teratocarcinoma cells: relation to Alzheimer's disease. Brain Res 744:7-14.

Chapter 13

A POSSIBLE CELL MEMBRANE DEFECT IN CHRONIC FATIGUE SYNDROME AND SYNDROME X

Walter S. Watson, Abhijit Chaudhuri,
Georgina T. McCreath and Peter O. Behan

Chronic fatigue syndrome (CFS) is a common disorder characterized by symptoms of persistent and overwhelming fatigue lasting for 6 months or more in the absence of any other illness. There are a number of other non-specific symptoms such as muscle pain, headache and post-exertional malaise. The diagnosis of CFS is based on criteria laid down by the Centers for Disease Control and Prevention (Atlanta, USA) [1], and is essentially one of exclusion of all other possible causes for fatigue.

Paroxysmal chest pain is a common symptom in patients with CFS. A number of our patients were referred to us by cardiologists as their illness initially presented as chest pain presumed to be of cardiac origin. These patients were usually investigated extensively in coronary units and were eventually considered to have cardiac syndrome X. Typically, all these patients with chest pain went on to develop CFS and had a clinical course which was otherwise indistinguishable from patients who developed CFS after a viral infection [2,3]. There are a number of similarities between CFS and syndrome X:-

1) Nuclear magnetic resonance spectroscopy studies of skeletal muscle in patients with CFS [4] and syndrome X [5] show features consistent with abnormal oxidative metabolism
2) In CFS, abnormal lactate production has been found after exercise [6]. Similarly, abnormal lactate is found in patients with cardiac syndrome X during pacing [7]
3) A recent study of cerebral SPECT (single photon emission computed tomography) scans following Tc-99m HMPAO injection in syndrome X patients [8] has revealed "perfusion" defects similar to those documented in CFS patients [9]

It thus appears possible that, at least in subsets of patients, CFS and syndrome X could share a common pathogenic mechanism.

The incidental finding of a normal coronary angiogram and abnormal thallium cardiac SPECT scan in one of our patients with CFS and chest pain prompted the investigation of another potential link between CFS and syndrome X.

Cardiac SPECT scanning is a nuclear medicine technique used to identify regions of relatively under-perfused myocardial tissue [10]. The technique is based on the fact that intravenously injected radiothallium, Tl-201, behaves similarly to potassium in that it is taken up by cells via Na-K pumps in the cell membrane [11]. As this uptake is rapid, i.e. a few minutes, early relative tissue uptake of thallium is normally taken to represent relative tissue perfusion. The distribution of Tl-201 is recorded external to the using a gamma camera to detect the X-rays emitted by the thallium radiotracer. By using tomographic acquisition and analysis protocols, the distribution of thallium within the myocardium can be presented as a 3-D mapping.

Both coronary angiography and thallium cardiac SPECT scanning are routinely used in the detection of coronary artery disease (CAD). Therefore, in the setting of CAD detection, it is paradoxical for one test to be normal while the other is abnormal. However, Waldenstrom et al [12] have shown that a significant proportion of patients with syndrome X (who had normal coronary arteries by definition) had abnormal thallium cardiac SPECT scans. It is possible that myocardial ischemia caused by microvascular dysfunction could produce thallium scan defects in subjects with patent major coronary arteries; however, there is a lack of consensus as to the role of microvascular ischemia in syndrome X [13,14]. Waldenstrom and co-workers have proposed a novel hypothesis to explain their findings. They postulated that the myocardial thallium defects observed in patients with syndrome X were due to abnormal thallium uptake into the myocardial tissue rather than a failure of delivery of thallium to the tissue. They proposed that the thallium defects were the result of "leaky" cell membranes, which caused an abnormal efflux of potassium from the cells via ionophoric channels. In both red cells [15] and the isolated perfused rat heart [16] manipulated to contain potassium-leaking cell membranes, Waldenstrom and coworkers noted a relative reduction in adenosine triphosphate (ATP). Of particular interest in relation to CFS was the similar finding in the myocardium of mice infected with Coxsackie B3 virus [17]. Crucially, reduced ATP was also found in cardiac and skeletal muscle biopsies in syndrome X patients with abnormal thallium cardiac scans [12]. Waldenstrom's group postulated that the reduction in ATP was due to the compensatory upregulation of the Na-K ion pump activity required to maintain the integrity of the "leaky" cell. In turn, this upregulation of the pump was expected to cause a relative depletion of ATP, which provides most of the pump's energy.

In the light of the above findings, we decided to investigate the incidence of abnormal cardiac SPECT scans in a group of patients with CFS.

Thallium cardiac SPECT scanning in CFS

A small group of 10 adults (8 men, 2 women) with CFS involving significant exertional dyspnea underwent stress-rest/redistribution thallium-201 cardiac SPECT scanning with dipyridamole "stress" [18]. A combination of quantitative bullseye analysis and visual examination of reconstructed short and long axis views was used to identify defects in thallium uptake in the myocardium. Defects were noted in 6 out of 8 men and 1 out of 2 women. A single defect was noted in 4 subjects while 2 defects were noted in 3 subjects. The defects were either fixed or showed partial reversibility.

Although 7 out of 10 positive scans seemed to provide fairly conclusive evidence for myocardial thallium uptake abnormalities in CFS, the specificity of this type of scan is not particularly high and false positives can occur. The sensitivity and specificity for the SPECT scanning technique used in our study have been assessed at 95% and 71%, respectively [10]. Assuming that the incidence of CAD in the "normal" adult population is 4% [19], if we had studied 10 "normal" adults, we would expect 0.4 true positives and 2.8 false positives. Using the binomial theorem, it was shown that the observed "study positive rate" of 7 out of 10 was significantly greater than the expected rate of 3.2 out of 10 for "normal" adults.

Although the "thallium positive" rate was significantly higher than for a normal population, we lacked a control group. We considered that more weight would be placed on our findings if they were confirmed by an independent laboratory with a well-established normal database. Accordingly, a second group of adult subjects (6 men, 1 woman) with CFS and a history of chest pain were assessed at the Glasgow Royal Infirmary where ECG-gated planar thallium studies were performed in conjunction with exercise tolerance testing (one subject received dipyridamole instead of exercise) [20]. Radioventriculography in the resting state was also carried out to further assess wall motion and to obtain left and right ventricular ejection fractions [21]. In this second series, 6 out of 7 thallium scans were reported as abnormal with the defect size being very small/small in 3 subjects, small/moderate in 2 subjects, and moderate/large in 1 subject. All defects showed at least partial redistribution at 3-4 hours post thallium injection, while wall motion was preserved at all defect sites. LVEF values in the range 30-39% were reported as good in 4 subjects with the remaining 3 in the normal range i.e. >40%. RVEF values in the range 21-29% were reported as moderate in 4 subjects, all with slightly dilated RVs, while the remaining 3 were reported as good (2 subjects) and normal (1 subject). Resting ECG was normal in 6 out of 7 patients, while LVH and <1 mm ST depression was noted in 1 patient. No significant ECG change was noted on exercise in any of the patients. One patient with a small/moderate defect on thallium scanning subsequently had a normal coronary angiogram.

Therefore, two small but independent studies have shown that myocardial thallium defects are common in patients with CFS with the incidence of abnormal scans being significantly greater than that expected from an unselected adult population. These results are at odds with the findings of Lerner et al [22] who have recently reported normal cardiac SPECT scans in a series of 67 consecutive CFS subjects. Given the relatively poor specificity of cardiac SPECT scanning as discussed above, the statistical chance of obtaining 67 consecutive normal scans even in a normal population must be exceedingly small. Only further independent studies will cast light on this disparity.

Resting energy expenditure

An indirect way of assessing the validity of Waldenstrom's hypothesis was to measure resting energy expenditure in subjects with CFS. Resting energy expenditure (REE) is the energy expended by the fasted, awake subject in the resting state [23]. REE can be easily measured by indirect calorimetry where oxygen utilization and carbon dioxide production are measured. Approximately 30% of REE is normally utilized to maintain the sodium-potassium concentration gradients across the cell membrane [24], therefore, an upregulation of the Na-K pump should increase REE.

REE has been measured by indirect calorimetry in 11 female subjects with CFS and 11 healthy female controls. There was no significant difference in height, weight or age between the two groups. REE varies with the fat-free mass (FFM) of the body [25].

When REE was divided by FFM assessed by bioelectrical impedance measurements [26], there was no significant difference between the groups; this has also been shown in syndrome X [27]. However, there is a theoretically better predictor for REE than FFM and that is body cell mass as measured by total body potassium (TBK) [28]. The reason for this is that FFM includes the relatively variable extracellular fluid which contributes little to the REE while potassium is almost entirely intra-cellular and is a direct measure of the body cell mass. Body cell mass has been defined by Moore and colleagues as "the oxygen-exchanging, potassium-rich, glucose-oxidizing, work-performing tissue" [29]. TBK can be measured non-invasively because a tiny fraction of "normal" potassium is present as the long-lived radioisotope, K-40, which emits high-energy gamma rays. These rays can be detected external to the body using a whole body counter [30]. In this way, TBK can be measured to within few percent accuracy. Therefore, in addition to the REE and bioelectrical impedance measurements, TBK was measured in all 22 subjects in the study. The improved ability of TBK to predict REE was illustrated by the fact that, for the control group, the proportion of the variation of REE explained by TBK was 78%, while for FFM it was only 41%.

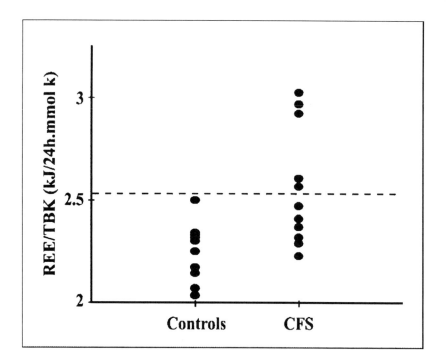

Figure 1. Resting energy expenditure expressed relative to total body potassium (the upper limit of the normal range is shown as a horizontal dashed line)

Figure 1 shows the results obtained when REE was divided by TBK for each individual subject. The ratio, REE / TBK, was significantly higher (p<0.01) for the CFS group compared to the control group (mean ± standard deviation: 2.56 ± 0.29 v 2.25 ± 0.14 expressed in units of kJ/24h.mmol K). The upper limit of normal for REE / TBK expressed as mean plus two standard deviations for the control group data is also seen on the figure indicating that 5 out of 11 of the CFS group had values above the normal range. This suggests that there was increased energy expenditure in approximately 50% of the CFS subjects, although we cannot be certain that this was due to an upregulation of the Na-K pump.

Discussion

The apparent "perfusion defects" seen in the thallium cardiac scans in CFS are unlikely to be explained by occlusive coronary vessel disease. Given the similarity between the in-vivo kinetics of thallium and potassium, a defect in cellular metabolism, as proposed for syndrome X, which allows cardiac myocytes to lose potassium to excess, provides a possible explanation for these defects [31]. Additionally, an abnormally high extracellular potassium (or an abnormally high intracellular sodium) should cause an upregulation of the cell membrane Na-K ATPase activity which in turn should increase REE.

In the present studies, cardiac thallium SPECT scans have been shown to be abnormal in the majority of patients with CFS, while REE, relative to total body potassium, was increased in about 50% of patients. These findings are not, of course, proof that a metabolic defect links CFS and syndrome X. Not all CFS subjects had abnormal cardiac scans or increased metabolic rates. Similarly, cardiac thallium scans are not abnormal in all patients with syndrome X. If there is a common link between CFS and syndrome X, it is likely that it is only present in a subset of subjects in both syndromes. This is not unreasonable given that the relatively non-specific diagnostic criteria for both syndrome X and CFS are unlikely to define pure "single pathology" groups [13,32].

Acknowledgements

We would like to thank Dr J Robinson for his help with the SGH cardiac study. In addition, we are indebted to Prof J McKillop and Dr W Martin for performing the second series of thallium scans and to Dr D C McMillan for the REE measurements. Finally, we are grateful for the assistance of the technical staff of the SGH Nuclear Medicine Department.

References

1. Fukada K, Straus SE, Hickie I, and Sharpe MC. The chronic fatigue syndrome: a comprehensive approach to its definition and study. Ann Intern Med 1994;121:953-9.
2. Behan PO and Bakheit AMO. Clinical spectrum of postviral fatigue syndrome. Br Med Bull 1991;47:793-808.
3. Behan PO and Behan WMH. Postviral fatigue syndrome. CRC Crit Rev Neurobiol 1988;4(2):157-78.
4. McCully KK, Natelson BH, Iotti S, Sisto SA, and Leigh JS. Reduced oxidative muscle metabolism in chronic fatigue syndrome. Muscle Nerve 1996;19:621-5.
5. Soussi B, Schersten T, Waldenstrom A, and Ronquist G. Phosphocreatine turnover and pH balance in forearm muscle of patients with syndrome X. Lancet 1993;341:829-30.

148

6.   Lane RJM, Burgess AP, Flint J, Riccio M, and Archard LC. Exercise responses and psychiatric disorder in chronic fatigue syndrome. Br Med J 1995;311:544-5.

7.   Boudoulas H, Tyson CC, Leighton RF, and Wilt SM. Myocardial lactate production in patients with angina-like chest pain and angiographically normal coronary arteries and left ventricle. Am J Cardiol 1974;34:501-5.

8.   Weidmann B, Jansen WC, Bock A, Assheur J, and Tauchert MO. Technetium-99m-HMPAO brain SPECT in patients with syndrome X. Am J Cardiol 1997;79:959-61.

9.   Patterson J, Aitchinson F, Wyper DJ, Hadley DM, Majeed T, and Behan PO. SPECT brain imaging in chronic fatigue syndrome. J Immunol Immunopharmacol 1995;XV:53-8.

10.   DePasquale EE, Nody AC, DePuey EG, Garcia EV, Pilcher G, Bredlau C, Roubin G, Gober A, Gruentzig A, D'Amato P et al. Quantitative rotational thallium-201 tomography for identifying and localizing coronary artery disease. Circulation 1988;77(2):316-27.

11.   Carlin RD and Jan K. Mechanism of Thallium Extraction in Pump Perfused Canine Hearts. J Nucl Med 1985;26:165-9.

12.   Waldenstrom A, Ronquist G, and Lagerqvist B. Angina pectoris patients with normal coronary angiograms but abnormal thallium perfusion scan exhibit low myocardial and skeletal muscle energy charge. J Intern Med 1992;231:327-31.

13.   Cannon III RO, Camici PG, and Epstein SE. Pathological dilemma of syndrome X. Circulation 1992;85:883-92.

14.   Rosano GM, Kaski JC, Arie S, Pereira WI, Horta P, Collins P, Pileggi F, and Poole-Wilson PA. Failure to demonstrate myocardial ischaemia in patients with angina and normal coronary arteries. Evaluation by continuous coronary sinus pH monitoring and lactate metabolism. Eur Heart J 1996;17(8):1175-80.

15.   Engstrom I, Waldenstrom A, and Ronquist G. Ionophore A23187 reduces energy charge by enhanced ion pumping in suspended human erythrocytes. Scand J Clin Lab Invest 1993;53:239-46.

16.   Martinussen HJ, Waldenstrom A, and Ronquist G. Functional and biochemical effects of a K+-ionophore on the isolated perfused rat heart. Acta Physiol Scand 1993;147:221-5.

17.   Waldenstrom A, Fohlman J, Ilback NG, Ronquist G, Hallgren R, and Gerdin B. Coxsackie B3 myocarditis induces a decrease in energy charge and accumulation of hyaluronan in the mouse heart. Eur J Clin Invest 1993;23:277-82.

18.   Watson WS, McCreath GT, Chaudhuri A, and Behan PO. Possible cell membrane transport defect in chronic fatigue syndrome? J Chron Fatigue 1997;3(3):1-13.

19.   Diamond GA and Forrester JS. Analysis of probability as an aid in the clinical diagnosis of coronary-artery disease. NEJM 1979;300:1350-8.

20.   Tweddel AC, Martin W, and Hutton I. Thallium scans in syndrome X. Br Heart J 1992;68(1):48-50.

21.   Arrighi JA, Dilsizian V. Harbert JC, Eckelman WC, Nuemann RD, editors.Nuclear Medicine: Diagnosis and Therapy. New York: Thieme; 1996; Chapter 23, Radionuclide angiography in coronary and noncoronary heart disease: Technical background and clinical applications. p. 501-31.

22.   Lerner AM, Goldstein J, Chang CH, Zervos M, Fitzgerald JT, Dworkin HJ, Lawrie-Hoppen C, Korotkin SM, Brodsky M, and O'Neill W. Cardiac involvement in patients with chronic fatigue syndrome as documented with Holter and biopsy data in Birmingham, Michigan, 1991-1993. Infect Dis Clin Pract 1997;6(5):327-33.

23.   McClave SA, Snider HL. Use of indirect calorimetry in clinical nutrition. Nutr Clin Pract 1992;7:207-21.

24.   Ackerman MJ and Clapham DE. Ion channels-Basic science and clinical disease. NEJM 1997;336(22):1575-86.

25.   Nelson KM, Weinsier RL, Long CL, Schutz Y. Prediction of resting energy expenditure from fat-free mass and fat mass. Am J Clin Nutr 1992;56(5):848-56.

26.   Hannan WJ, Cowen SJ, Plester CE, Fearon KCH, and deBeau A. Comparison of bio-impedance spectroscopy and multi-frequency bio-impedance analysis for the assessment of extracellular and total body water in surgical patients. Clin Sci 1995;89:651-8.

27.   Botker HE, Moller N, Ovesen P, Mengel A, Schmitz O, Orskov H, Bagger JP. Insulin resistance in microvascular angina (syndrome X). Lancet 1993;342(8864):136-40.

28.   Ferrannini E. The theoretical bases of indirect calorimetry: A review. Metabolism 1988;37(3):287-301.

29.   Moore FD; Oleson KH; McMurrey JD, et al. The body cell mass and its supporting environment. Philadelphia-London: W. B. Saunders; 1963.

30.   Watson WS. Total body potassium measurement--the effect of fallout from Chernobyl. Clin Phys

Physiol Meas 1987;8(4):337-41.

31. Chaudhuri A, Watson WS, Behan POB. Yehuda S, Mostofsky DI, editors.Chronic Fatigue Syndrome. New York: Humana Press; 1997; Chapter 6, Arguments for a role of abnormal ionophore function in chronic fatigue syndrome. p. 119-30.

32. Hickie I, Lloyd A, Hadzi-Pavlovic D, Parker G, Bird K, and Wakefield D. Can chronic fatigue be defined by distinct features? Psychol Med 1995;25(5):925-35.

Chapter 14

THE CHANGING CONCEPT OF SYNDROME X

Attilio Maseri, Gaetano Antonio Lanza and Antonino Buffon

The term "syndrome X" was coined by Harvey Kemp in his 1973 editorial comment [1] on a puzzling report of electrocardiographic (ECG) signs of myocardial ischemia induced by pacing in the absence of detectable left ventricular dysfunction in a group of patients with angina and normal coronary angiograms [2]. This term proved to be well chosen as during the last quarter of the century this syndrome continued to be the object of conflicting reports and a variety of pathogenetic hypotheses.

How could we get out of the dead alley?

In our opinion, the inability to get out of this dead alley is due to two major limiting factors: (1) the heterogeneity of patients included under the simplistic, extremely broad definition of syndrome X; (2) the inadequate sensitivity and specificity of the techniques used to study these patients [3].

As the local referral practices and the indications for coronary angiography vary widely, the spectrum of patients who are grouped together on the basis of only two descriptors (i.e., "anginal" symptoms and a normal coronary arteriogram) is extremely broad. In patients who fall into this broad category, the origin of the anginal pain could be either cardiac or non cardiac and, when cardiac, it could be either ischemic or non ischemic. Finally, when ischemic, the pain could either result from functional disorders of the epicardial or of the small coronary arteries, each of which, in turn, may be due to multiple causes.

A fundamental preliminary step to get out of the dead alley is to attempt a separation of patients currently labeled as "syndrome X", into distinct homogeneous clinical syndromes. This may be done on the basis of their clinical presentation and of the results of a standardized series of tests. In this process a number of questions should be answered and these are the following:

1. Is the painful stimulus coming from the heart?

A consistent association of anginal pain with detectable cardiac alterations, such as ST segment changes during exercise stress testing or Holter monitoring, a positive myocardial scintigraphy, or transient ST segment changes and anginal pain during dipyridamole testing, is likely to indicate a cardiac origin of the problem. However, this does not necessarily imply an ischemic origin. Conversely, the lack of an association of anginal pain with detectable cardiac abnormalities is compatible with a non cardiac origin of the painful stimuli. However, let's remember that even myocardial ischemia caused by large coronary artery obstructions may not be associated with recognizable ECG changes.

2. In patients with a detectable cardiac origin of the pain is there an ischemic cause?

In a minority of patients with evidence of a cardiac origin of their pain but with normal coronary arteriograms, angina can be caused by coronary artery spasm, i.e. the so-called "variant of the variant" form of angina [4]. This diagnosis is suggested by the history of spontaneously occurring angina, usually of short duration, with preserved effort tolerance and confirmed by the appropriate diagnostic tests. In this group of patients the cause of pain is ischemic.

In other patients, the cause may be ischemic or non ischemic. The inability to detect ventricular function abnormalities during a positive exercise or dipyridamole stress test, or to document myocardial lactate production during pacing induced anginal pain, stands against an ischemic origin of the painful stimulus. However, in patients with microvascular dysfunction, myocardial ischemia may be present but detectable only when a large myocardial segment is involved; ischemia may not cause appreciable contractile abnormalities or lactate production if it is very patchy, or if it results from an unevenly distributed coronary microvascular dysfunction. In the presence or absence of microvascular dysfunction, accumulation of algogenic substances, such as adenosine, could be sufficient to cause anginal pain and ECG abnormalities (Figure 1) [5].

Although myocardial lactate production is considered to represent a marker of myocardial ischemia, a more sensitive method, such as the assessment of lipid peroxide production during anginal pain [6,7], may allow the identification of an ischemic origin of the pain in those patients in whom ischemia is patchily distributed and therefore undetectable by currently used methods.

3. How can anginal pain be so disabling in the absence of detectable ischemic cardiac dysfunction?

Many patients with chest pain and normal coronary arteries have an enhanced pain sensitivity to somatic and visceral stimuli and, more specifically, to cardiac stimuli [8]. The cause for this enhanced pain sensitivity can be multiple and not necessarily the same in all patients. A patchily distributed, but intense and sustained, release of adenosine, probably as a compensatory response to inappropriate prearteriolar constriction, may be sufficient to cause severe and prolonged pain and ST segment changes, even in the absence of ischemia (Figure 1).

On the other hand, when inappropriate prearteriolar coronary vasoconstriction or ischemia cannot be demonstrated, the production of algogenic substances or pain nerve stimulation could be caused by non ischemic myocardial alterations [9,10].

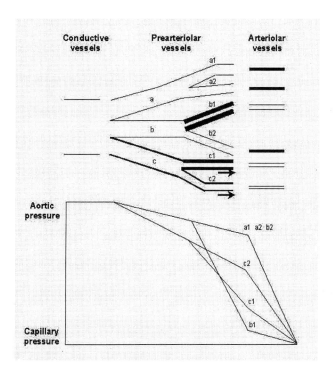

Figure 1. Model of prearteriolar constriction. Prearteriolar constriction could be patchily distributed in any myocardial layer. The regional reduction of coronary flow reserve is proportional to the severity of prearteriolar constriction and to the pressure drop at the origin of arterioles. Steal of blood flow may also occur within the same myocardial layer distal to a constricted prearteriolar branch point (c). During arteriolar dilatation and increase in flow, pressure, at the end of prearteriolar vessels, decreases further. Thus, the distending pressure at the end of the most constricted prearterioles (b1) may become lower than the critical closing pressure. Compensatory release of adenosine distal to constricted prearterioles may be sufficient to maintain blood flow, thus avoiding ischemia, but, if persistent, it may cause chest pain, by stimulating afferent receptors, particularly in patients with an enhanced pain sensitivity (Adapted from Ref. 3).

4. In patients with an ischemic origin of the pain due to microvascular alterations, what is the cause of the microvascular dysfunction?

The causes of coronary microvascular dysfunction can be several and yet produce a similar syndrome. Release of potent vasoconstrictors may represent a pathogenic mechanism. Constriction of small coronary arteries severe enough to cause massive ischemia has been observed following intracoronary administration of NPY and of endothelin in men [11] and in dogs [12], respectively. However, the cause of the microvascular dysfunction may be related not only to the potency of the stimulus but to an enhanced smooth muscle response to constrictor agents [13,14] or to some type of endothelial dysfunction [15,16]. The observation of massive defects of MIBG uptake [17] in patients with chest pain and normal coronary arteries suggests also the possibility of adrenergic dysfunction as a vasoconstrictor mechanism.

Whatever the cause of the microvascular dysfunction, available coronary dilator drugs have only weak dilator effects on small coronary prearteriolar vessels. This dilator effect may be further reduced in those prearteriolar vessels in which the increased tone exceeds the critical closing pressure, resulting in complete vessel occlusion, which in turn may prevent the local delivery of the dilator drugs (Figure 1). Structural changes of the microvessels may also play a role.

5. Amongst patients with evidence of a cardiac and/or ischemic origin of the pain, is it possible to recognize subgroups with distinct clinical syndromes?

Most patients with evidence of a cardiac origin of their pain but no evidence of coronary spasm, present with chronic, predominantly effort- and emotion-related angina. Anginal pain has a variable threshold, occurs occasionally also at rest and is often long lasting (sometimes over 30 minutes) and poorly responsive to nitroglycerin. Patients usually have a positive exercise stress test, and/or a positive Holter at very variable heart rates [18]. Their pain and exercise ECG changes are often not improved or are made worse by sublingual nitrates, in sharp contrast with findings in patients who have flow limiting coronary stenoses [19]. For these patients we have previously suggested a preliminary diagnostic approach [3] (Figure 2). Despite a history of chronic stable angina and documented transient ischemic ECG changes, the pathophysiological findings differ considerably in these patients. Indeed, they often have myocardial 201 Thallium or MIBI perfusion defects but no consistent alterations in PET studies [20,21] albeit with few exceptions [22,23]. This is a rather puzzling, still unresolved, discrepancy. Obvious ischemic abnormalities were convincingly demonstrated in a minority of cases [24], and enhanced left ventricular performance, suggesting increased sympathetic drive, was observed in others [25,26]. The majority of patients in our studies had massive deficits in MIBG uptake [17].

Another subgroup of patients can be identified who present with prolonged spontaneous episodes of severe anginal pain associated with reversible ST segment depression and/or T wave inversion, with or without elevation of cardiac enzymes. In these patients, the provocative tests for coronary spasm are negative and the ECG returns to normal in a few days. These patients however, often require re-admission to the coronary care unit due to recurrent chest pain.

The clinical presentation and features of this subgroup suggest that the underlying pathogenetic mechanisms may differ from those in the group presenting with chronic stable angina. They may also have microvascular dysfunction but the causes of the microvascular dysfunction may differ [27]. They can consist of neural stimuli (NPY and/or α-adrenergic stimulation), local production of autacoids (endothelin), and smooth muscle hyperactivity, with or without associated endothelial dysfunction. In some patients the alterations may be confined to the coronary vasculature, in others they may be part of systemic disorders, such as hypertension, metabolic syndrome X [3], or defects of membrane ionic pumps [13,14].

Additional clinical subgroups might be recognized in the future, when patients will be characterized more comprehensively on the basis of both a careful clinical history and the results of systematically applied tests.

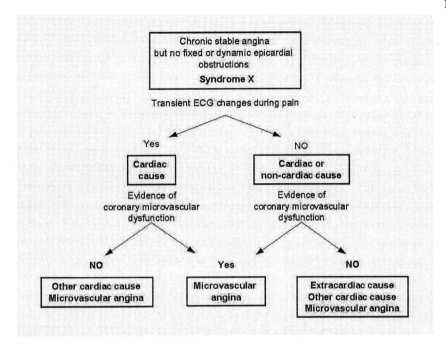

Figure 2. Diagnostic work out for patients with chronic stable angina, but without fixed or dynamic flow-limiting stenosis. The association of transient ECG changes with anginal pain indicates a cardiac origin of pain, but the absence of such changes cannot exclude a cardiac origin because of the low sensitivity of the ECG. Patients with evidence of coronary microvascular dysfunction can be diagnosed as having microvascular angina even in the absence of detectable signs of ischemia. When neither microvascular dysfunction nor ischemia can be demonstrated, they cannot be excluded because of the low sensitivity of the available techniques for detecting patchily distributed ischemia and perfusion abnormalities (Adapted by Ref. 3).

Summary

Kemp's statement in 1973, that some observations in syndrome X, "like the clues in the first half of Agatha Christie novels, may not be readily understandable, but we can be certain they are important" still stands [1]. It is sometimes difficult to distinguish relevant from confounding findings; thus, in each clinically homogeneous subgroup of patients any proposed working hypothesis must account for the salient common clinical features, for the most prevalent findings of pathophysiologic studies, and must also be compatible with the conflicting results of previous reports.

The most salient clinical features of syndrome X are represented by the following:

1. the common report of a prolonged duration of pain with no detectable cardiac ischemic manifestations;
2. the very variable anginal threshold and the common persistence of pain for several minutes after interruption of effort;

3. the poor and variable response to sublingual nitrates and the adverse effect of nitrates on the effort stress test;
4. the good long-term prognosis;
5. the often unjustified anxiety about prognosis.

The most salient pathophysiologic findings are as follows:

1. the induction of angina and ST-segment depression by dipyridamole;
2. the presence of episodes of ST-segment depression (with or without pain) not preceded by an increase in heart rate during Holter monitoring, and, conversely the absence of ST segment depression during tachycardia in the same recordings;
3. the presence of (not only thallium or potassium analogs, but also of MIBI) myocardial scintigraphic perfusion defects;
4. the discrepancy between anginal pain, ST-segment depression and detectable signs of myocardial ischemia;
5. the enhanced perception of pain.

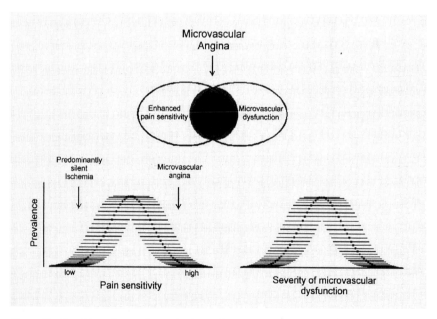

Figure 3. Possible pathogenetic mechanisms of syndrome X. The syndrome results from a variable combination of two components: an increased sensitivity to painful stimuli associated with coronary microvascular dysfunction (indicated by recurring ST-segment depression), both of which have a bell-shaped prevalence in the population. Furthermore, within individuals, either component may vary in time (indicated by the horizontal lines). In patients with a markedly enhanced sensitivity to pain, even a minimal microvascular dysfunction can cause angina. Conversely, some patients with severe microvascular dysfunction (indicated by recurring ST-segment depression) may not have chest pain and therefore will not seek medical attention. In these patients, signs of microvascular dysfunction and of myocardial ischemia will be apparent only if and when they reach the detection threshold imposed by the sensitivity of currently used diagnostic techniques. (Adapted from Ref. 3).

A patchily distributed myocardial dysfunction with a variable degree of confluence, associated with a variable increase of pain perception (3), may explain all these findings, independently of the actual causes (Figure 3). However, this working hypothesis, though plausible, does not imply that other postulated causes could also play a role in-so-far-as they account for all the relevant clinical findings listed above.

The efforts to find a single, common pathogenetic mechanisms for all patients presenting with angina and a normal coronary angiogram will continue to be unproductive and to originate conflicting reports. Only selective studies on homogenous subgroups of patients, with well defined clinical syndromes and consistent results of systematic tests, will allow the identification of specific pathogenetic and etiological mechanisms corresponding to well defined disease entities, all currently classified under the broad label of "syndrome X".

References

1. Kemp HG, Jr. Left ventricular function in patients with anginal syndrome and normal coronary arteriograms. Am J Cardiol 1973;32:375-376.
2. Arbogast R, Bourassa MG. Myocardial function during atrial pacing in patients with angina pectoris and normal coronary arteriograms. Comparison with patients having significant coronary artery disease. Am J Cardiol 1973;32:257-263.
3. Maseri A. Ischemic Heart Disease. A rational basis for clinical practice and clinical research. Churchill Livingstone Ed., 1995; pp. 507-532.
4. Cheng TO, Bashour T, Kelser G, et al.: Variant angina of Prinzmetal with normal coronary arteriograms. A variant of the variant. Circulation 1973;47:476-81.
5. Maseri A, Crea F, Kaski JC, Crake T. Mechanisms of angina pectoris in syndrome X. J Am Coll Cardiol 1991;17:499-506.
6. Buffon A, Santini S, Liuzzo G, et al. Increased lipoperoxidative stress may cause endothelial dysfunction in syndrome X. J Am Coll Cardiol 1996;29(Suppl. A):264A.
7. Buffon A, Santini SA, Rigattieri S, et al. Transient intracardiac lipid peroxidation induced by atrial pacing in syndrome X: a definitive demonstration of an ischemic mechanism? Circulation 1997;96:I-270.
8. Pasceri V, Lanza GA, Buffon A, Montenero AS, Crea F, Maseri A. Role of abnormal pain sensitivity and behavioral factors in determining chest pain in syndrome X. J Am Coll Cardiol 1998;31:62-66.
9. Poole-Wilson PA. Potassium and the heart. Clinics in endocrinology & metabolism 1984;13:249-268.
10. Waldenström A, Ronquist G, Lagerqvist B. Angina pectoris patients with normal coronary angiograms but abnormal thallium perfusion scan exhibit low myocardial and skeletal muscle energy charge. J Intern Med 1992;231:327-31.
11. Clarke JG Davies GJ, Kerwin R, et al. Coronary artery infusion of neuropeptide Y in patients with angina pectoris. Lancet 1977;i:1057-59.
12. Larkin SW, Clarke JG, Keogh BE, et al. Intracoronary endothelin induces myocardial ischemia by small vessel constriction in the dog. Am J Cardiol 1989;64:956-58.
13. Koren W, Koldanov R, Peleg E, Rabinowitz B, Rosenthal T. Enhanced red cell sodium-hydrogen exchange in microvascular angina. Eur Heart J 1997;18:1296-1299.
14. Gaspardone A, Ferri C, Crea F, et al. Stimulated hyperinsulinemia in patients with microvascular angina is associated with enhanced red blood cell Na+-Li+ countertransport. Eur Heart J 1997;18(Abstr Suppl):157.
15. Motz W, Vogt M, Rabenau O, Scheler S, Lockhoff A, Strauer S. Evidence of endothelial dysfunction in coronary resistance vessels in patients with angina pectoris and normal coronary angiograms. Am J Cardiol 1991;68:996-1003.
16. Egashira K, Inou T, Hirooka Y, Yamada A, Urabe Y, Takeshita A. Evidence of impaired endothelium-dependent coronary vasodilation in patients with angina pectoris and normal coronary angiograms. N Engl J Med 1993;328:1659-64.

17. Lanza GA, Giordano AG, Pristipino C, at al. Abnormal cardiac adrenergic nerve function in patients with syndrome X detected by [123I]metaiodobenzylguanidinw myocardial scintigraphy. Circulation 1997;96:821-6.

18. Lanza GA, Manzoli A, Pasceri V, *et al.* Ischemic-like ST-segment changes during Holter monitoring in patients with angina pectoris and normal coronary arteries but negative exercise testing. Am J Cardiol 1997;79:1-6.

19. Lanza GA, Manzoli A, Bia E, Crea F, Maseri A. Acute effects of nitrates on exercise testing in patients with syndrome X. Clinical and pathophysiological implications. Circulation 1994:90:2695-2700.

20. Camici PG, Gistri R, Lorenzoni R, *et al.*. Coronary reserve and exercise ECG in patients with chest pain and normal coronary angiograms. Circulation 1992;86:179-186.

21. Rosen SD, Uren NG, Kaski JC, Tousoulis D, Davies GJ, Camici PG. Coronary vasodilator reserve, pain perception, and sex in patients with syndrome X. Circulation 1994;90:50-60.

22. Galassi AR, Crea F, Araujo LI, *et al.* Comparison of regional myocardial blood flow in syndrome X and one-vessel coronary artery disease. Am J Cardiol 1993;72:134-139.

23. Meeder JG, Blanksma PK, Crijns HGJM, *et al.* Mechanisms of angina pectoris in syndrome X assessed by myocardial perfusion dynamics and heart rate variability. Eur Heart J 1995;16:1571-7.

24. Crake T, Canepa-Anson R, Shapiro L, Poole-Wilson PA. Continuous recording of coronary sinus oxygen saturation during atrial pacing in patients with coronary artery disease or with syndrome X. Br Heart J 1988;59:31-38.

25. Camici PG, Marraccini P, Lorenzoni R, Buzzigoli G, Pecori N, Perissinotto A, Ferrannini E, L'Abbate A, Marzilli M. Coronary hemodynamics and myocardial metabolism in patients with syndrome X: response to pacing stress. J Am Coll Cardiol 1991;17:1461-1470.

26. Tousoulis D, Crake T, Lefroy D, *et al.* Left ventricular hypercontractility and ST segment depression in patients with syndrome X. J Am Coll Cardiol 1993;22:1607.

27. Strauer BE. The significance of coronary reserve in clinical heart disease. J Am Coll Cardiol 1990;15:775.

Chapter 15

ASSESSMENT OF CORONARY BLOOD FLOW RESERVE - TECHNIQUES AND LIMITATIONS

Antonio L'Abbate

Coronary blood flow reserve

Coronary blood flow reserve can be defined as the amount by which coronary blood flow increases in response to maximal arteriolar dilation induced by physical or pharmacological stimulation. Thus, the term *coronary reserve* can also be used to indicate the amount of arteriolar tone superimposed on minimal (anatomical) resistance. Finally, as heart work is strictly dependent on coronary flow, coronary reserve can also be equated to *cardiac work reserve*. In fact, coronary arteriolar tone accurately adapts blood supply to moment by moment changes in myocardial energy demand. It is generally thought that arteriolar tone restricts blood flow to the minimal level compatible with tissue demand, as documented by the broad arteriovenous oxygen extraction characteristic of the coronary circulation.

In the clinical setting, the assessment of coronary reserve is mainly applied to the functional evaluation of coronary stenosis as in the absence of collateral circulation, the additional resistance caused by a stenosis is compensated by a parallel amount of arteriolar vasodilation. The "residual" arteriolar tone and the increment in cardiac work which occur before myocardial ischemia develops are inversely related to the severity of the obstruction.

Assessment of coronary reserve is also applied to other pathophysiological conditions not necessarily associated with coronary atherosclerosis, such as systemic hypertension, aortic valve disease, hypertrophic cardiomyopathy, dilated cardiomyopathy, syndrome X and others. In the absence of coronary stenosis, the genesis of ischemia is attributed - by exclusion - to a reduction of coronary reserve due to microvascular impairment of tissue perfusion. However the nature and mechanisms of such an impairment may vary and frequently remain speculative. Structural as well as functional alterations in the coronary microvasculature may cause, as a final effect, an increase in coronary resistance, which in turn may be responsible for myocardial ischemia, even in the absence of coronary stenosis.

On the basis of the above definition of coronary reserve, its assessment requires the measurement of maximal coronary flow increment, relative to baseline.

Coronary reserve is commonly expressed as the ratio between maximal myocardial blood flow, measured after abolition of arteriolar tone, and resting flow. Using this ratio, rather than absolute values of resting and maximal flows, allows one to disregard the mass of perfused tissue and makes it easier to compare results in different patients, based on "relative" individual changes. This approach is pertinent when coronary flow is assessed by methods that do not allow accurate and specific measurements of flow (i.e. flow per gram of myocardium). Using the "ratio" approach, however, one cannot tell whether coronary reserve is reduced because of an increased resting flow or because of a reduced maximal flow, or both. This limitation can be overcome only by measuring blood flow per unit mass. In this instance, both resting and maximal flow values can be easily compared with normal values.

An additional problem in the assessment of coronary reserve is caused by the transmural inhomogeneity of flow, which results from differences in vascularity, metabolism and tissue pressure in the outer and inner layers of the left ventricular wall. At present, technical limitations exist to measure transmural differences in myocardial blood flow, which preclude the assessment of abnormal coronary reserve limited to the subendocardial layer.

Moreover, even when standardized (class and dose) exogenous vasodilators or physical stimuli are used there is no guarantee that attainment of maximal vasodilation will be achieved in every patient.

Techniques for measuring coronary blood flow

The clinical assessment of coronary blood flow and of its alterations is still a difficult task, in spite of the relatively large number of available techniques. This results from the fact that none of the available techniques is ideal. The "ideal" technique should be one that is performed non-invasively, provides regional, transmural and specific flow and, finally, allows repeated measurements in a short time interval. The main characteristics of clinically available techniques are summarized in Table 1.

Coronary sinus thermodilution

Coronary sinus thermodilution is based on the indicator-dilution principle: cold saline is infused continuously into the coronary sinus and the blood temperature measured a few centimeters downstream to the site of injection to assess the amount of blood that circulates in the vessel and therefore "dilutes" the "tracer". If this procedure is performed in the great cardiac vein rather than in proximity to the atrial outlet of the coronary sinus, it permits to calculate the amount of blood flowing from the anterior wall rather than from the entire left ventricular myocardium [1-2]. This technique allows repeated measurements of flow. Due to the lack of information about specific flow (i.e., flow per unit mass), comparison of absolute flow values in different patients is not possible with this method. However, it allows a comparison between relative changes in perfusion.

Inert gas wash-out

Inert gas wash-out analysis is also based on the indicator-dilution theory. Measurement

Table 1. Assessment of coronary blood flow

TECHNIQUES	INVASIVENESS	TOTAL FLOW quantitative ml/min	TOTAL FLOW specific ml/min/g	REGIONAL FLOW quantitative ml/min	REGIONAL FLOW specific ml/mg/g	FLOW DISTRIBUTION
Coronary sinus thermodilution	YES	YES	—	YES (GCV-LDA)	—	—
Coronary sinus sampling of diffusible tracers	YES	YES+	YES	—	—	—
Intracoronary injection of radioactive diffusible tracers. External acquisition	YES	—	YES	—	YES	—
Intravascular coronary Doppler FLOW VELOCITY *	YES	—	—	YES	—	—
Transesophageal Echo (TEE) *	SEMI-	—	—	YES (LAD)	—	—
SPECT myocardial scintigraphy	NO	—	—	—	—	YES
Positron emission tomography (PET)	NO	YES depending on number of slices	YES depending on number of slices	YES	YES	YES
Contrast echocardiography	YES/NO (1)	—	—	—	—	YES

GCV= great cardiac vein

+ = only for left coronary injection

* = flow velocity can be transformed in flow if the vascular section at the site of sampling is known

(1) = depending on the site of injection (intracoronary vs intravenous)

of myocardial blood flow can either be obtained by the analysis of tracer wash-out in the coronary sinus (obtaining the average specific flow in the left ventricle) [3] or by the analysis of the residue in each region of the left ventricle [4]. This latter approach requires the intracoronary injection of a diffusible radioactive tracer (usually Xenon-133) and the external detection of its myocardial content over time; it provides specific flow values in different regions of the left ventricular myocardium and imaging of flow distribution. This approach has major limitations under conditions of flow heterogeneity as the normoperfused region accumulates more tracer and it is therefore mathematically over represented. As a consequence, the contribution of normoperfused areas to global flow is overestimated [5]. Additionally, coronary flows higher than 2 ml/g/min cannot be accurately measured, thus hampering the accuracy of flow measurements during pharmacologic vasodilation or maximal exercise [6].

Doppler tip devices

Doppler tip devices analyze the shift in ultrasound frequency produced by the movement of red blood cells in the blood stream. The magnitude of Doppler effect is proportional to the velocity of the circulating blood, therefore the continuous determination of reflected sound frequency allows to monitor phasic and average blood flow velocity. Doppler probes can be mounted either on the tip of a 3F catheter - which can be advanced into the proximal epicardial coronary - or on the top of a guidewire which allows to overpass stenosis and reach more distal vascular segments [7]. If associated with the measurement of distal coronary pressure, this method may be able to directly quantify the coronary resistance offered by the vasculature located distally to the stenosis without the need for assumptions related to stenosis severity and local hydraulics. When ultrasonic flowmeters are employed, two important parameters should be considered. First, that the magnitude of the Doppler shift is dependent on the angle between the piezoelectric crystal and the blood column, being largest at 45 degree. Second, that to convert measurements of blood flow velocity to absolute flow, the cross-sectional area of the vessel must be known and the velocity profile must be relatively flat [8]. This limitation is of less importance when coronary reserve is evaluated as the ratio of maximal to baseline flow velocity. In this setting, epicardial vasomotion is usually blunted by vasorelaxant drugs (usually intracoronary nitrates). Using this pretreatment strategy, the measured shifts in flow velocity directly reflect changes in blood flow.

Transesophageal echocardiography

Transesophageal echocardiography (TEE) allows the semi-invasive visualization of the proximal portion of the left anterior descending coronary artery. Doppler monitoring of the blood flow velocity in this coronary segment is made possible by its favourable spatial orientation relative to the probe. Phasic as well as average velocity values can be transformed into flow values by measurement of lumen cross-section area at the site of Doppler sampling. Repeated measurements of flow in basal conditions and following vasodilating or inotropic drugs can easily be obtained. Feasibility of the technique is quite high, reaching values of around 70-90%.

Positron emission tomography

Positron emission tomography permits accurate noninvasive quantitative regional measurements of blood flow per unit volume of tissue [9]. The two most common flow tracers are ^{13}N-Ammonia [10] and ^{15}O-water [11]. The first molecule, is almost completely extracted from the myocardium. Since arterial concentration can easily be measured within the left ventricular chamber during the first pass of ammonia, myocardial blood flow can be computed using either compartmental analysis [12] or first pass approach [13]. Both methods proved to be accurate in assessing regional blood flow as compared to the gold standard method of labeled microspheres. The myocardial extraction of ammonia decreases at high flow; due to this phenomenon a correction becomes necessary when evaluating high blood flow [13]. ^{15}O-water is a freely diffusible indicator; basically, with this tracer, measurement of blood flow can be obtained by the analysis of its washout curve. Both tracers require a steady state period of at least 1-2 minute to allow reliable quantitative measurements. Because of the insufficiently high spatial resolution of this technique, no information can be obtained about transmural blood flow distribution. Two to three measurements of flow can be obtained in the same session.

Single photon perfusion scintigraphy

Single photon perfusion scintigraphy allows imaging of flow distribution within the left ventricular wall, but not quantitative measurements of flow. Thus this technique cannot be used for quantitative assessment of coronary reserve.

Contrast echocardiography

Contrast echocardiography represents a novel way of investigating myocardial perfusion distribution in man. Due to the availability of contrast agents that may cross the pulmonary barrier this approach can be totally noninvasive. At present, this technique does not allow quantitation of flow.

Flow and pressure measurements

The quantitation of coronary reserve by simply measuring maximal and baseline flow, even if normalized for myocardial mass, can not be justified on a theoretic ground, as it disregards the second dimension of coronary reserve, i.e. perfusion pressure.

This crucial problem is illustrated in Figure 1a, where the relationship between aortic pressure and coronary blood flow is shown. From this figure the bidimensionality of coronary reserve can be argued. Flow reserve does not result from a monodimensional comparison of two flow values, but rather from the area limited by the pressure-flow relations obtained in the presence and in the absence of arteriolar tone. It should be evident from Figure 1a that two flow measurements may lead to very different values of flow ratio, and thus of computed coronary reserve, depending upon the corresponding pressure. Furthermore, it should be considered that: 1) at each level of pressure the autoregulatory curve continuously moves up and down depending upon

164

the beat-by-beat myocardial metabolic demand (which in turn is directly, but not exclusively, related to aortic pressure); and 2) the slope of the relation obtained during vasodilation is significantly affected by heart rate due to its effects on diastolic time.

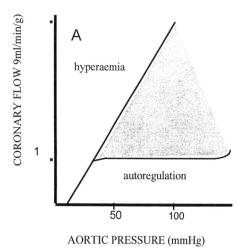

Figure 1a. Pressure-flow relations obtained in the anesthetized open-chest dog at constant myocardial oxygen consumption with intact autoregulation and following intracoronary adenosine infusion (hyperaemia). The grey area represents the coronary flow reserve, that is the amount by which coronary flow may increase for each value of pressure when arteriolar tone is abolished by adenosine.

Thus, disregarding blood pressure and heart rate while measuring coronary reserve may be a source of significant error. In order to normalize flow values (F) for the corresponding pressure (P), the ratio P/F is commonly used and quoted as coronary resistance. It should be emphasized, however, that even during maximal vasodilation, the attempt to equal P/F to coronary resistance is biased by the existence of a positive intercept of the pressure/flow curves on the pressure axis, the so-called *critical closing pressure*. In this case, resistance is equal to (P-I)/F, where *I* is the intercept value on the pressure axis. Because of this, the higher the intercept and the lower the aortic pressure corresponding to flow measurement, the more significant the deviation from a correct measurement of resistance if the P/F ratio is simply used. The estimation of *I* might come only from multiple measurements of hyperemic flow over a wide range of aortic pressures and their extrapolation to zero flow.

An alternative approach to the construction of pressure-flow curves is the use of flow and pressure values obtained in a single diastole, using Doppler catheters [14]. Unfortunately, the single beat model is strongly affected by intramyocardial capacitance [15]. In fact, capacitance forces permit flow to continue in the distal vessels at a time when flow in the proximal artery has already stopped and viceversa.

In conclusion, in contrast to animal studies, where phasic and transmural flow can be accurately measured, the assessment of coronary resistance and thus of coronary reserve in humans is far from satisfactory. This is due to the difficulty of measuring regional myocardial blood flow per unit mass of tissue and, more importantly, to the fact that potential contributions of extravascular forces and coronary capacitance are generally not taken into account. In view of these limitations, care should be taken in interpreting the relatively minor alterations in minimal resistances often observed in clinical studies.

Ways of vasodilating the coronary vascular bed

In order to assess minimal coronary resistance, several methods and agents have been proposed to "maximally" vasodilate the coronary arterial bed, i. e. transient coronary occlusion [16], papaverine [17], adenosine [18] and dipyridamole [17]. Coronary occlusion has frequently been used in dog experiments, however, several studies documented that this approach does not always induce maximal vasodilation [19]. In humans, the use of this technique is hampered by a number of ethical and methodological considerations. Obviously, the experimental occlusion of a normal coronary artery is not possible in humans. However, this procedure can be performed in stenotic segments during coronary angioplasty.

Papaverine has widely and safely been used as a coronary vasodilator in patients with coronary artery artery disease [17], syndrome X [20] and hypertension [21]. As this drug requires administration by direct intracoronary injection, it has mainly been used in conjunction with monitoring of intracoronary flow velocity. Intracoronary injection of adenosine [18] provides a similar degree of vasodilation as papaverine. However, due to the effects of adenosine on the conduction system, care must be taken not to inject this agent into a coronary artery supplying the sinus node or the atrio-ventricular node. Differently from papaverine, intravenous injection of adenosine can be used for noninvasive evaluation of maximal coronary blood flow [22].

Another agent widely employed in the clinical setting is dipyridamole. This drug has been safely used for noninvasive evaluation of maximal blood flow with a variety of methods [17, 23]. However, its use for evaluation of minimal "anatomical" resistance has not been conclusively ascertained. In fact, the adequate dose for maximal vasodilation is still a matter of controversy (0.56 mg/Kg or 0.84 mg/Kg of body weight). In addition, in a recent study, it has been demonstrated that under certain circumstances (e.g., in syndrome X patients) high dose dipyridamole submaximally vasodilates the coronary circulation [24]. It should be noted that with the injection of adenosine the coronary vasculature is exposed to high concentrations of the short acting exogenous adenosine, while with dipyridamole the vessels are exposed to progressively high concetration of endogenous adenosine.

In order to dilate the arteriolar vessels in a more physiologic way, cardiac work may be increased by atrial pacing [25], exercise [26] or by the administration of dobutamine [27]. However, in order to abolish vascular tone, it becomes essential to reach maximal cardiac work. Due to its simple acquisition, rate-pressure product is frequently used as "the" clinical index of cardiac work. However, it should be considered that it only represents a crude approximation as it does not take into account the effects of wall stress and contractility [28].

166

Pathogenetic interpretation of findings

As shown in Figure 1b, the mechanisms by which coronary reserve may be reduced can be graphically summarized as follows: 1) a decrease in coronary resistance at rest secondary to increased cardiac work and decreased arteriolar tone, as it occurs in hyperdynamic states; 2) a decrease in the slope of the hyperemic curve as it occurs with coronary stenosis of large vessels or hypertrophy of small vessels' wall or even during tachycardia because of the reduction in the diastolic perfusion time; or 3) an increase in pressure-flow intercept, denoting either increased extravascular compression or increased vascular wall tension.

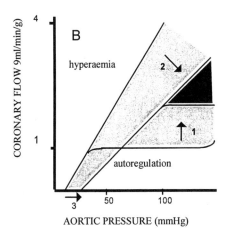

Figure 1b. Ways by which coronary reserve may be reduced: 1) increase in metabolic demand (upward shift of autoregulation curve); 2) decreased vascular section in the absence of arteriolar tone; 3) increase in the pressure value at zero flow (critical closing pressure).

Thus, in order to identify the mechanisms responsible for changes in coronary reserve, pressure-flow curves should be obtained.

In conclusion, current methods for the clinical assessment of myocardial blood flow suffer from a number of limitations and, as a consequence, several assumptions are required according to the different methods applied. Without knowledge of the closing pressure value, minimal coronary resistance will be difficult to ascertain, especially in those conditions where closing pressure is abnormally high.

Furthermore, the identification of the mechanisms responsible for impaired coronary reserve requires a great deal of information that can hardly be provided by currently available methods.

In contrast to the traditional view, it is sufficiently clear today that microvascular tone is neither exclusively located at a single level of the coronary tree such as at the arteriolar level nor is it under control of a single mechanism. It rather seems that different transversal sections (levels) of the coronary tree may modulate their tone through different mechanisms. According to this view, total coronary resistance to flow would be the result of a large number of in series and in parallel resistance values, which may change individually, or in families, in response to different mechanisms and mediators. These changes may operate in the same direction so to amplify the final result both in term of vasodilation or vasoconstriction or, conversely, in opposite direction, with a variable integrated result on flow. Our recent understanding of the controlling role of coronary endothelium in the regulation of myocardial perfusion has challenged the traditional view according to which coronary flow is mainly, if not exclusively, controlled by the metabolic modulation of arteriolar tone at the level of myocardial subunitis. However, although alterations in the endothelium-mediated control of coronary tone of large as well as small vessels has been documented in a wide number of diseases, the actual contribution of these alterations to reduced coronary reserve, as assessed by arteriolar vasodilation, remains undefined. This target could be accomplished by comparing coronary reserve measurements before and after restoration of endothelial function.

Coronary reserve in syndrome X

A reduction in coronary flow reserve, firstly reported by Opherk *et al.* [29] using the argon wash-out method, has been subsequently confirmed in a significant proportion of syndrome X patients by several investigators using different techniques such as coronary sinus thermodilution [30-33] and positron emission tomography [34-36].

Although thermodilution prevents the correct attribution of an impaired coronary reserve to increased resting flow or to decreased maximal flow, both the argon method and positron emission tomography have generally documented a reduction in maximal coronary blood flow. However, the precise site of coronary vascular abnormality downstream from the epicardial vessels, or the nature of increased vascular resistance, are still unknown. Endothelial dysfunction of the coronary microvessels [37] as well as adrenergically mediated vasoconstriction [38] have been proposed as putative mechanisms.

However originated, the increase in minimal coronary resistance is used as the strongest argument in favour of the ischemic nature of syndrome X. In fact, a reduced coronary reserve in conjunction with the presence of angina and electrocardiographic ST-T alterations closes the loop of the classical ischemic cascade. The only variation would consist in moving the cause of perfusion abnormality from epicardial to intramural coronary arteries, i.e., microvascular angina [39].

However, whether myocardial ischemia is part of syndrome X is still a matter of controversy. Several points are against this hypothesis: First, in patients with syndrome X, routine provocative tests easily reproduce angina and ST-segment depression, but not the abnormalities of ventricular wall motion usually seen in coronary artery disease. By contrast, a hypercontractile heart, both at rest and during stress, is encountered in many of the patients with syndrome X [33, 40]. Next, in a carefully selected population of patients with angina and electrocardiographic ST-segment depression during effort, angiographically normal coronary arteries, negative ergonovine tests, and no cardiac or systemic disease, we did not observe any metabolic alteration indicative of ischemia during maximal atrial pacing in spite of the presence of angina and ST-segment depression [33]. The only detected metabolic deviation from "normality" was an impaired carbohydrate oxidation, with net release of pyruvate during pacing.

Also, when patients with left bundle branch block are excluded, the prognosis of syndrome X patients appears to be not significantly different from that of the general population [41]. Finally, common anti-ischemic drug treatment is almost invariably unable to relieve symptoms in syndrome X patients.

Thus, on the basis of the above points, it can be postulated that syndrome X is characterized by the paradox of reduced coronary reserve in the absence of obvious myocardial ischemia. Such a consideration can hardly be conceived in the classic pathophysiological frame of ischemic heart disease. Theoretically, an impaired coronary reserve could be compatible with the absence of ischemia provided any of the following occurs:

1. A decrease of cardiac performance to match a lower energy supply;
2. Larger transmyocardial extraction of substrates;
3. Increased cardiac efficiency, i.e., less energy consumption for the same "external" work.

The first condition seems not to be the case in syndrome X, as left ventricular performance, both at rest and during exercise, is normal or even increased [33, 40].

The study of Camici *et al* [33] shows that during atrial pacing patients with syndrome X were able to reach rate-pressure products similar to those observed in the control group, but with a lesser increment of great vein flow, no increase in oxygen extraction and less energy expenditure.

On the basis of these results, a supernormal (highly efficient) heart rather than an ischemic heart should be postulated in patients with syndrome X.

References

1. Ganz W, Tamura K, Marcus HS, Donoso R, Yoshida S, Swan HJC. Measurement of coronary sinus blood flow by continuous thermodilution in man. Circulation 1971; 44: 181-195.
2. Pepine CJ, Mehta J, Webster WW Jr, Nichols WW. In vivo validation of a thermodilution method to determine left ventricular blood flow in patients with coronary disease. Circulation 1978; 58: 795-802.
3. Klocke FJ, Bunnel IL, Greene DG, Wittenberg SM, Visco JP. Average coronary blood flow per unit weight of left ventricle in patients with and without coronary artery disease. Circulation 1974; 50: 547-559.
4. Cannon PJ, Dell RB, Dwyer EM Jr. Measurement of regional myocardial perfusion in man with ^{133}Xenon and a scintillation camera. J Clin Invest 1972; 51: 964-977.
5. Klocke FJ. Coronary blood flow in man. Prog Cardiovasc Dis 1976; 19: 117-166.
6. Engel HJ: Assessment of regional myocardial blood flow by the precordial 133xenon clearance technique. In: The pathophysiology of myocardial perfusion, 58, W Shaper (ed), Amsterdam, Elsevier, North Holland Medical Press 1979.
7. Ofili EO, Kerten MJ, Labovitz AJ *et al*. Analysis of coronary blood flow velocity in angiographically normal and stenosed coronary arteries before and after endolumen enlargement by angioplasty. J Am Coll Cardiol 1993; 21: 308-316.
8. Hartley CJ, Cole JS. An ultrasonic pulsed Doppler system for measuring blood flow in small vessels. J Appl Physiol 1974; 37: 626-629.
9. Bergmann SR, Fox KA, Geltman EM, Sobel BE. Positron emission tomography of the heart. Prog Cardiovasc Dis 1985; 28 (Suppl 3): 165-194.
10. Schelbert HR, Phelps ME, Hoffman EJ, Huang SC, Selin CE, Kuhl DE. Regional myocardial perfusion assessed with N-13 labeled ammonia and positron emission computerized axial tomography. Am J Cardiol 1979; 43: 209-218.

11. Bergmann SR, Fox KAA, Rand AL, *et al*. Quantification of regional myocardial blood flow in vivo with H215O. Circulation 1984; 70: 724-733.

12. Hutchins GD, Schwaiger M, Rosenspire K, Krivokapich J, Schelbert H, Kuhl DE. Noninvasive quantification of regional blood flow in the human heart using N-13 ammonia and dynamic positron emission tomographic imaging. J Am Coll Cardiol 1990; 13: 1032-1042.

13. Bellina CR, Parodi O, Camici P, Salvadori PA, Taddei L, Fusani L, Guzzardi R, Klassen GA, L'Abbate A, Donato L. Simultaneous in 'vitro and in vivo validation of ^{13}N-ammonia for the assessment of regional myocardial blood flow. J Nucl Med 1990; 31: 1335-1343.

14. Mancini JGB, McGillem MJ, DeBoe SF, Gallagher KP. The diastolic hyperemic flow versus pressure relation. Circulation 1989; 80: 941-950.

15. Dole WP, Bishop VS. Influence of autoregulation and capacitance on diastolic coronary pressure-flow relationship in the dog. Circ Res 1982; 51:261-270.

16. Coffman JD, Gregg DE. Reactive hyperemia characteristics of the myocardium. Am J Physiol 199: 1143, 1960.

17. Wilson RF, White CW: Intracoronary papaverine: an ideal coronary vasodilator for studies of the coronary circulation in conscious humans. Circulation 1986; 73: 444-451.

18. Wilson RF, Wyche K, Christensen BV, Zimmer S, Laxson DD. Effects of adenosine on human coronary arterial circulation. Circulation 1990; 82: 1595-1606.

19. L'Abbate A, Camici P, Trivella MG, Pelosi G, Davies GJ, Ballestra AM, Taddei L. Time dependent response of coronary flow to prolonged adenosine infusion: doubling of peak hyperaemic flow. Cardiovasc Res 1981; 15: 282-286.

20. Chauhan A, Mullins PA, Petch MC, Schofield PM. Is coronary flow reserve in response to papaverine really normal in syndrome X? Circulation 1994; 89: 1998-2004.

21. Harrison DG, Marcus ML, Dellsperger KC, Lamping KG, Tomanek RJ. Pathophysiology of myocardial perfusion in hypertension. Circulation 1991; 83 (Suppl III): III-14-18.

22. Marzilli M, Klassen GA, Marraccini P, Camici P, Trivella MG, L'Abbate A. Coronary effects of adenosine in conscious man. Eur Heart J 1989; 10 (Suppl F): 78-81.

23. Gould KL, Schelbert HR, Phelps ME, Hoffman EJ. Noninvasive assessment of coronary stenoses with myocardial perfusion imaging during pharmacological vasodilation. V Detection of 47 percent diameter stenosis with intravenous nitrogen-13 ammonia and emission computed tomography in intact dogs. Am J Cardiol 1979; 43: 200-208.

24. Holdright DR, Lindsay DC, Clarke D, Fox K, Poole-Wilson PE. Coronary flow reserve in patients with chest pain and normal coronary arteries. Br Heart J 1993; 17: 513-519.

25. Neglia D, Parodi O., Gallopin M, Sambuceti G, Giorgetti A, Pratali L, Salvadori P, Michelassi C, Lunardi M, Pelosi G, Marzilli M, L'Abbate A. Myocardial blood flow response to pacing tachycardia and to dipyridamole infusion in patients with dilated cardiomyopathy without overt heart failure. A quantitative assessment by positron emission tomography. Circulation 1995; 92: 796-804.

26. Beller GA, Gibson RS. Sensitivity, specificity, and prognostic significance of noninvasive testing for occult or known coronary disease. Prog Cardiovasc Dis 1987; 29: 241-270.

27. Mason JR, Palac RT, Freeman ML, Virupannavar S, Loeb HS, Kaplan E, Gunnar RM. Thallium scintigraphy during dobutamine infusion: non-exercise dependent screening test foro coronary disease. Am Heart J 1984; 107: 481-485.

28. Ross J Jr, Sonnenblick EH, Kaiser GA, Frommer PL, Braunwald E. Electroaugmentation of ventricular performance and oxygen consumption by repetitive application of paired electrical stimuli. Circ Res 1965; 16: 332.

29. Opherk D, Zebe H, Weihe E, Mall G, Durr C, Gravert B, Mehmel HC, Schwarz F, Kubler W. Reduced coronary dilatory capacity and ultrastructural changes of the myocardium in patients with angina pectoris but normal coronary arteriograms. Circulation 1981; 63: 817-825.

30. Cannon RO, Watson RM, Rosing DR, Epstein SE: Angina caused by reduced vasodilator reserve of the small coronary arteries. J Am Coll Cardiol 1983; 1: 1359-1373.

31. Virtanen KS. Evidence of myocardial ischemia in patients with chest pain syndromes and normal coronary angiograms. Acta Med Scand 1984; 694 (Suppl): 58-68.

32. Bortone AS, Hess OM, Eberli FR, Nonogi H, Marolf AP, Grimm J, Krayenbuehl HP. Abnormal coronary vasomotion during exercise in patients with normal coronary arteries and reduced coronary flow reserve. Circulation 1989; 79: 516-527.

33. Camici PG, Marraccini P, Lorenzoni R, Buzzigoli G, Pecori N, Perissinotto A, Ferrannini E, L'Abbate A, Marzilli M. Coronary hemodynamics and myocardial metabolism in patients with syndrome X: response to pacing stress. J Am Coll Cardiol 1991; 17: 1461-1470.

34. Geltman EM, Henes CG, Sennett MJ, Sobel BE, Bergmann SR. Increased myocardial perfusion at rest and diminished perfusion reserve in patients with angina and angiographically normal coronary arteries. J Am Coll Cardiol 1990; 16: 586-595.

35. Galassi AR, Araujo LI, Crea F, Kaski JC, Lammertsma AA, Yamamoto Y, Rechavia E, Jones T, Maseri A. Myocardial blood flow is altered at rest and after dipyridamole in patients with Syndrome X. J Am Coll Cardiol 1991; 17: 227. (abstract)

36. Camici PG, Gistri R, Lorenzoni R, Sorace O, Michelassi C, Bongiorni MG, Salvadori PA, L'Abbate A. Coronary reserve and exercise-ECG in patients with chest pain and normal coronary angiograms. Circulation 1992; 86: 179-186.

37. Motz W, Vogt M, Rabenay O, Scheler S, Luckhoff A, Strauer BE. Evidence of endothelial dysfunction in coronary resistance vessels in patients with angina pectoris and normal coronary angiograms. Am J Cardiol 1991; 68: 996-1003.

38. Camici PG, Marraccini P, Gistri R, Lorenzoni R, Sorace O, L'Abbate A. a_1-adrenergic tone and coronary reserve in patients with Syndrome X. Circulation 1991; 84 (suppl II): II-424. (abstract)

39. Cannon RO, Epstein SE. "Microvascular angina" as a cause of chest pain with angiographically normal coronary arteries. Am J Cardiol 1988; 61: 1338-1343.

40. Picano E, Lattanzi F, Masini M, Distante A, L'Abbate A: Usefulness of high-dose dipyridamole-echocardiography test for diagnosis of Syndrome X. Am J Cardiol 1987; 60: 508-512.

41. Opherk D, Schuler G, Wetterauer K, Manthey J, Schwarz F, Kubler W. Four-year follow-up study in patients with angina pectoris and normal coronary arteriograms. Circulation 1989; 80: 1610-1616.

Chapter 16

THE ROLE OF ECHOCARDIOGRAPHY IN DIAGNOSIS AND MANAGEMENT OF CARDIAC SYNDROME X

Petros Nihoyannopoulos

The term "syndrome X", in its strict definition, includes patients with exertional chest pain usually indistinguishable from atherosclerotic coronary artery disease, a positive exercise test and completely normal coronary angiography. Left ventricular hypertrophy, coronary artery spasm, conduction defects and valvular heart disease are normally excluded from this definition [1-4]. The possible role of myocardial ischemia in the pathogenesis of syndrome X has been supported by the observation, in some patients, of coronary sinus lactate production during atrial pacing [5,6], the demonstration of abnormal left ventricular systolic function during exercise [6] and the presence of reversible defects by thallium scintigraphy [7-9]. Objective evidence of myocardial ischemia is however rarely found in patients with syndrome X. Several authors have failed to demonstrate myocardial perfusion defects or hemodynamic abnormalities in well characterised syndrome X patients [10,11].

Modern two-dimensional echocardiography not only does assess cardiac anatomy and ventricular function at rest but also during stress [12]. The use of two-dimensional echocardiography during stress has assumed such popularity in recent years in the assessment of patients with known or suspected coronary artery disease that it has, in many instances, replaced the more expensive nuclear modalities. Further, Doppler techniques, which are commonly utilised to assess valvular lesions can also be employed to assess left ventricular diastolic function, a marker which temporally precedes and outlasts the onset of transient myocardial ischemia [13].

Assessment of resting cardiac anatomy and ventricular function

In the assessment of chest pain, the hallmark of patients with syndrome X, it is important to rule out any significant macroscopic cardiac pathology e.g. valvular or myocardial disease which may be responsible for the patient's symptoms (Table 1).

Mitral valve prolapse has long been associated with chest pain [14] although the mechanism of chest pain in this condition are speculative. The diagnosis of mitral valve prolapse syndrome is based on the presence of anatomic mitral valve prolapse, usually with excessive mitral valve tissue (floppy valve) which can readily be identified by two-dimensional echocardiography and supported by the associated symptom complex. Doppler echocardiography may also detect the presence or absence of mitral regurgitation, which can add to the diagnosis.

Table 1. Cardiac conditions associated with "atypical" (non-anginal) chest pain

---

1. Mitral valve prolapse ("floppy valve")
2. Ventricular hypertrophy
3. Hypertrophic cardiomyopathy
4. Pericardial disease/effusion
5. Right ventricular pathology (overload)
6. Left ventricular dysfunction (cardiomyopathy)
7. Myocarditis
8. Infiltrative disorders (sarcoidosis, amyloidosis, hemosiderosis)

Left ventricular hypertrophy, from whatever cause, is often associated with chest pain. Echocardiography is usually employed to answer the question of whether or not a patient has ventricular hypertrophy. In this instance, it is important to remember that using echocardiography we measure left ventricular wall thickness. In general, when ventricular wall thickness exceeds 12 or 13mm, it is assumed that there is ventricular hypertrophy. Ventricular hypertrophy, however, means myocyte increase in size which can occur even though the wall thickness remains within normal limits [15]. For this reason, the electrocardiogram may have increased sensitivity over echocardiography in the diagnosis of ventricular hypertrophy [16]. Chest pain is one of the main symptoms in patients with hypertrophic cardiomyopathy and this condition therefore needs to be excluded in patients with angina and normal coronary arteriograms. An important diagnostic feature is the detection of hypertrophic cardiomyopathy in the presence of asymmetric ventricular hypertrophy.

It is important to remember that the echocardiogram may also show increased wall thickness without patients necessarily having hypertrophy. Typically, cardiac infiltration with amyloid involves the interstitial tissue among myocytes which retain a normal size. Because of interstitial infiltration however, the echocardiogram will show an increased wall thickness.

For the diagnosis of left ventricular hypertrophy, ideally one should look at the relationship of left ventricular mass to left ventricular cavity size and to the total hemodynamic load imposed on the left ventricle. These geometric patterns are defined by the *relative wall thickness ratio,* which is the thickness of the posterior wall divided by left ventricular radius in diastole. This formula has been developed to define wall stress based on the Marquee de La Place relationship which states that left ventricular wall stress (S) is directly proportional to intracavitary pressure (P) and chamber radius (R) and is inversely related to wall thickness (T): $S = P \times R / T$.

Pericardial effusion and pericardial thickening are other common causes of chest pain that mimic angina and can readily be identified using two-dimensional echocardiography. Once pericardial effusion has been noted, the presence of pericardial constriction or tamponade can also be determined using Doppler velocity variations during the respiratory cycle.

Left and right ventricular function can be ascertained with great accuracy using two-dimensional echocardiography. Right ventricular hypertrophy, dilatation or dysfunction can often cause chest pain and, of course, echocardiography has a crucial role in the correct diagnosis of these entities.

Left ventricular function, both global and regional, can be described with great accuracy using two-dimensional echocardiography. For this purpose the left ventricle is typically "divided" into 16 regions [17] which correspond to the various coronary vascular beds. This represents an easy and highly accurate method to assess ventricular function and offers the advantage that when each one of the 16 segments appears normal, there is no need to proceed to further time consuming volume calculations. A number of methods exist at present for the determination of ventricular volumes but all rely on geometric assumptions of the left ventricle which may or may not be valid in every clinical condition. Furthermore, a high level of expertise is necessary in order to provide reproducible measurements of ventricular volumes. In everyday practice however, the commonest way to assess left ventricular function in the vast majority of echocardiography laboratories is eye-balling. When LV function appears normal to the experienced observer, there is usually no further need for sophisticated calculations.

When a regional wall motion abnormality is detected at rest, the diagnosis of coronary artery disease is highly suspected. It is important to remember however that myocardial ischemia is not the only cause for resting regional myocardial dysfunction. Abnormal septal motion can also occur in several other conditions such as abnormal intracardiac conduction (bundle branch block, WPW), right ventricular volume or pressure overload, focal myocarditis and cardiac sarcoidosis. All these conditions can cause chest pain and can readily be detected by the resting echocardiogram.

Assessing left ventricular function during stress

This is now the most important role of echocardiography in patients with syndrome X. As early as 1935, Tennant and Wiggers [18] noted the loss of regional myocardial contraction occurring during coronary artery occlusion. Studies at rest, in which progressive coronary stenosis is produced in the conscious dog, have shown a linear correlation between regional wall motion and subendocardial blood flow in contrast with a poor correlation with sub-epicardial blood flow. A 20% decrease in blood flow produces a corresponding small reduction in systolic wall thickening [19]. This close coupling between the level of ischemia, as assessed by reduced regional blood flow, and regional contraction suggests in the strongest possible way that regional wall motion is a sensitive and meaningful marker of acute ischemia [20].

The use of stress testing to detect reversible left ventricular contractile dysfunction is based on the concept of myocardial oxygen supply and demand. The demand side of the equation is highly dependent upon many factors, including left ventricular pressure, volume, wall stress, heart rate and contractility. All of these parameters relate to myocardial oxygen consumption, mainly through their combined effect on left ventricular wall forces linked together by the Marquee de La Place's equation. All of these parameters will tend to increase during dynamic stress with exercise or pharmacological stress utilising inotropic stimulation (e.g. dobutamine).

Systolic myocardial thickening ceases when ischemia involves the inner half of a segment of the left ventricular wall as a result of coronary artery stenosis [21]. However, it is possible that myocardial ischemia limited to the inner 10-20% of the myocardial wall could remain undetected [19]. Similarly, a patchy distribution of

174

myocardial ischemia distal to isolated, abnormally constricted small blood vessels could also be insufficient to induce detectable wall motion abnormalities. In both these theoretical assumptions, the reduction in myocardial contraction caused by localised ischemia would also be masked by augmentation of contractile performance in normally perfused areas [22].

Reversibility of regional dysfunction: The return of myocardial function to normal after restoration of regional myocardial flow may vary. Regional wall motion abnormalities may improve or indeed completely resolve over 2 to 3 weeks after a 2 hour period of coronary occlusion in the conscious dog [23]. A number of studies have shown that post-ischemic dysfunction (or stunning) occurs after release of a 15 minute coronary occlusion and that recovery requires many hours or days [23,24]. The rate of recovery appears to be related to the extent and severity of coronary artery disease [25].

Patients with syndrome X

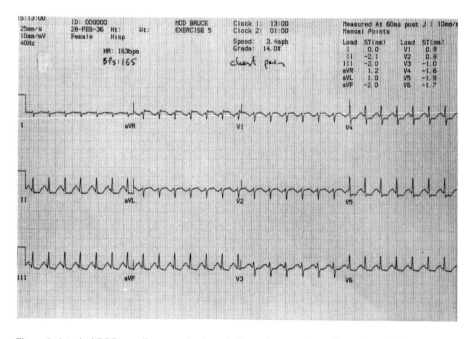

Figure 1. A typical ECG recording at maximal treadmill test from a patient with syndrome X. There is 1.7 to 2.1 mm ST depression in the inferior and lateral leads, indistinguishable from atheromatous coronary artery disease, with concomitant reproduction of patient's symptom of angina. This patient had an entirely normal left ventricular function, both at rest and immediately after exercise (see text for details).

Based on the above concepts, it may be assumed that if patients with syndrome X were to suffer from myocardial ischemia, wall motion abnormalities should occur during inotropic provocation of chest pain and/or ECG changes. To test this hypothesis, a study was conducted in our institution using exercise echocardiography as well as atrial pacing [26]. We have shown that in patients with syndrome X, left ventricular function on exertion and during atrial pacing is normal, despite the occurrence of concomitant anginal pain and ST segment depression on the ECG. Figure 1 demonstrates the ECG from a typical patient with syndrome X immediately after maximal exercise. This 62 year old female had an entirely normal echocardiogram at rest as well as after maximal stress but had a clearly ischemic looking ECG. It is noticeable that she was able to exercise for 13 minutes on the Modified Bruce protocol raising her heart rate from 92 to 163 bpm (107% of her maximal predicted for age), thus attaining a maximal work load of 8 METs. Her angina and typical ECG changes in the inferior and lateral leads were reproduced (Figure 1). The echocardiogram however was entirely normal when recorded 35 secs after cessation of the treadmill.

One of the characteristic ECG patterns in those patients with syndrome X is the rather rapid recovery of the ST-changes after cessation of exercise, usually within a minute. Figure 2 demonstrates the summary of the progressive increase in heart rate throughout the stress test, up to 163 and ST depression down to 2.1 mm. Importantly, after cessation of exercise, the ST segment depression and heart rate both returned to normal in just under one minute. It is therefore crucial for the echocardiographic images to be captured quickly after cessation of exercise. In our study [26], the first images were obtained at an average time of 20.6 secs and completed by 54.1 secs. Importantly, all images were acquired while the ECG was still abnormal.

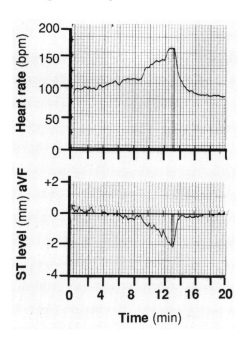

Figure 2. A characteristic pattern of progressive increase in heart rate and ST depression from the same patient as in figure 1. Notice that after cessation of exercise, the heart rate and ST depression rapidly normalise in just under a minute.

176

Quantitative assessment of systolic wall thickening is also important for the accurate assessment of left ventricular systolic function. One way is to digitise the left ventricular wall by tracing the epicardial and endocardial surface and display it in a three-dimensional representation (Figure 3). When looking at the 18 patients we studied [26], the average systolic wall thickening of all myocardial regions was increased from 47.1% to 74% during atrial pacing despite reproduction of chest pain and ECG changes and this was observed in each of the anterior, lateral, inferior and septal regions. This finding is in sharp contrast with the findings in patients with atherosclerotic coronary artery disease, who have indistinguishable symptoms and ECG changes on exercise but develop detectable wall motion abnormalities during stress.

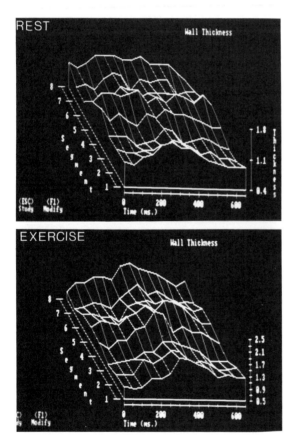

Figure 3. Digitised echocardiographic images from a patient with syndrome X at rest (top) and immediately after treadmill exercise (bottom) displaying regional wall thickening from a short axis projection. Myocardial segments are displayed in the Z axis from 1 to 8 with the anterior septum, anterior free wall, lateral, postero-lateral, posterior, infero-posterior, inferior wall and posterior septum, respectively. In the horizontal axis is displayed the timing of contraction from 0 at the onset of QRS complex and every 50 milliseconds thereafter, up to 600 milliseconds into systole. In the vertical axis (Y axis) is displayed the wall thickness in centimetres. Notice that there is a significant increase in regional wall thickness throughout systole at peak exercise compared to that at rest, particularly occurring at approximately 300 msec from the QRS complex.

Another elegant study by Panza *et al* [27] confirmed the absence of wall motion abnormalities during stress by performing transesophageal dobutamine stress echocardiography in patients with syndrome X. What was interesting from this later study was the fact that 18% of their patients with syndrome X also had reversible thallium perfusion deficits on the stress images and another 16% of patients, had a decreased ejection fraction. Importantly, these findings of the radionuclide studies were not related to the presence of ischemic-like repolarisation changes on the treadmill exercise ECG [27] nor to the patients symptoms. Whether the results of the radionuclide studies constitute a false positive result or a failure to detect ischemia during stress echocardiography remains unclear. The failure to link the reversible thallium defects to the clinical or treadmill exercise outcome however, points more towards the direction of a false positive thallium result. In any way, if myocardial ischemia is assumed to be limited and patchy [28] within the normal, 10 mm thick myocardium and surrounded by healthy muscle, as has been suggested in some patients with syndrome X, it is then questionable that it could ever be detected by SPECT in view of its poor spatial resolution which approaches 12 mm.

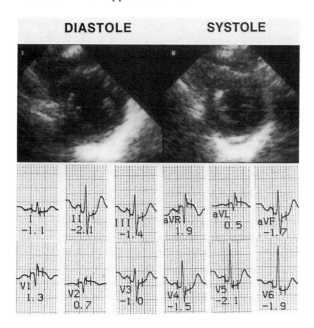

Figure 4. Parasternal short axis views in diastole (left) and systole (right) with concomitant ECG tracing at peak dobutamine stress echocardiography from a patient with syndrome X. While the ECG shows unequivocal ST depression in the inferior and lateral leads, the whole of the left ventricle contracts perfectly well with concentric systolic wall thickening throughout.

Figure 4 demonstrates one of our typical syndrome X patients during dobutamine stress. The echocardiographic images in the short axis are taken during maximum stress in diastole and systole at the same time where there were marked ischemic-like ECG changes and the patient complained of her usual chest pain. It is clearly noticeable that the whole of myocardium contracts symmetrically with concentric increase in wall thickness. It remains possible however that small, localized areas of regional ischemia surrounded by healthy myocardium are not detected with echocardiography, not because of lack of spatial resolution, which is of approximately 2 mm, but because a small localized ischemic zone might be tethered by the well contracting surrounding healthy myocardium so that any potential dysfunction would be masked. Additionally, the analysis of regional myocardial function is usually performed by averaging values from circumferencial segments located inside the 16 topographic regions following the coronary artery distribution. Although this approach represents a powerful way of assessing myocardial function, it may also 'dilute' very small, localized areas of myocardial dysfunction of a given segment.

Change in myocardial oxygen supply

Stress echocardiography has also been performed using dipyridamole infusion which, unlike exercise and dobutamine, it causes peripheral vasodilatation. The intravenous administration of dipyridamole causes arteriolar vasodilatation by preventing the cellular uptake of adenosine. Dipyridamole administration results in a small drop of systemic blood pressure and reflex tachycardia. Thus, myocardial oxygen requirements remain practically unchanged. In the presence of severe coronary stenosis, intravenous dipyridamole causes transmural "steal" due to redistribution of myocardial blood flow with a diversion of blood away from the endocardium and towards epicardial regions. Redistribution of blood may also occur within endocardial layers as a result of "luxury" perfusion of regions supplied by normal vessels. In a previous study [29] however, no wall motion abnormalities had been detected despite the reproduction of ischemic ECG changes and patients symptoms.

Assessing left ventricular diastolic function

Doppler evaluation of left ventricular inflow velocity profile has been shown to provide a clinically useful measure of left ventricular diastolic function [30]. With the patients in sinus rhythm the usual waveforms of early (E) and late (A) left ventricular diastolic filling are obtained. From these waveforms of the mitral velocity flow profile can be derived many parameters, all serving as an index of left ventricular diastolic function. The isovolumic relaxation time (IVRT) is usually obtained with pulsed doppler with the transducer slightly tilted anteriorly in order to obtain the clutter artefact of the aortic valve closure simultaneously with the early filling waveform (E wave).

The transmitral inflow profiles heavily depend on age, heart rate and patients loading conditions. A reduction in left ventricular filling pressures by intravenous nitroglycerin produces a reduction in the peak E wave and therefore a decrease in the E/A ratio [31]. It is attractive to measure transmitral diastolic indices to assess ischemia as diastolic abnormalities precede systolic events [32]. The development of ECG changes or symptoms of angina occur even later along the ischemic cascade.

Evaluation of the doppler response to dipyridamole stress was undertaken by Mazeika and colleagues [33] who examined patients with normal coronaries and in patients with significant coronary artery disease with and without inducible ischemia. Both ejection and diastolic flow indices were evaluated and when compared between groups, there was no significant difference in the doppler parameters. The only significant divergent response occurred in the ejection indices in patients with extensive ischemia. Another limiting factor in interpreting diastolic changes is the fact that the heart rate response limits interpretation of the separate mitral inflow waveforms so interpretation is mainly focused upon the systolic ejection indices. It is therefore not entirely surprising that there is little data available in the literature regarding doppler diastolic indices in patients with syndrome X.

Conclusion

Echocardiography is of pivotal importance in patients with chest pain and it should be performed early in order to exclude any resting ventricular or valvular dysfunction. If the patient complains of exertional chest pain with equivocal ECG changes, then stress echocardiography is probably the less expensive and most accurate stress test linked to an imaging modality. While a negative stress echocardiography test does not exclude minor coronary artery disease, it does rule out significant coronary disease. At present, there is no evidence that patients with syndrome X develop myocardial dysfunction, either systolic or diastolic, during chest pain episodes.

References

1. Kaski JC, Crea F, Nihoyannopoulos P, Hackett D, Maseri A. Transient myocardial ischemia during daily life in patients with syndrome X. Am J Cardiol 1986; 58: 1242-47.
2. Levy RD, Shapiro LM, Wright C, Mockus L, Fox KM. Syndrome X: the hemodynamic significance of ST segment depression. Br Heart J 1986; 56: 353-57.
3. Crake T, Canepa-Anson R, Shapiro L, Poole-Wilson PA. Continuous recording of coronary sinus oxygen saturation during atrial pacing in patients with coronary artery disease or with syndrome X. Br Heart J 1988; 59: 31-8.
4. Kemp HG. Left ventricular function in patients with anginal syndrome and normal coronary arteriograms. Am J Cardiol 1973; 32: 375-76.
5. Boudoulas H, Cobb TC, Leighton RF, Wilt CM. Myocardial lactate production in patients with angina-like chest pain and angiographically normal coronary arteries and left ventricle. Am J Cardiol 1974; 34: 501-5.
6. Cannon RO, Bonow RO, Bacharach SL, et al. Left ventricular dysfunction with angina pectoris, normal epicardial coronary arteries and abnormal vasodilator reserve. Circulation 1985; 71: 218-26.
7. Berger BC, Abramowitz R, Park CH et al. Abnormal thallium 201 scans in patients with chest pain and angiographically normal coronary arteries. Am J Cardiol 1983;52:365-70.
8. Legrand V, Hodgson J McB, Bates ER et al. Abnormal coronary flow reserve and abnormal radionuclide exercise test results in patients with normal coronary angiograms. J Am Coll Cardiol 1985; 6: 1245-53.
9. Tweddel A, Martin W, Hutton I. Thallium scans in syndrome X. Br Heart J 1992;68:48-50.
10. Green LH, Cohn PF, Holman L, Adams DF, Markis JE. Regional myocardial blood flow in patients with chest pain syndromes and normal coronary arteriograms. Br Heart J 1978; 40: 242-49.
11. Wieshammer S, Delagardelle C, Siegel HA. Haemodynamic response to exercise in patients with chest pain and normal coronary angiograms. Eur Heart J 1986; 7: 654-61.
12. Iliceto S, Galiuto L, Marangelli V, Rizzon P. Clinical use of stress echocardiography. Factors affecting diagnostic accuracy. Eur Heart J 1994;15:672-80.
13. Rokey R, Kuo LC, Zoghbi WA, Limacher MC, Quinones MA. Determination of parameters of left ventricular diastolic filling with pulsed Doppler echocardiography: comparison with cineangiography. Circulation 1985;71:543-550.

14. Boudoulas H, Wooley CF. Chest pain associated with mitral valve prolapse. Primary Cardiol 1985;11:16-25.

15. McKenna WJ, Stewart JT, Nihoyannopoulos P., McGinty F, Davies MJ. Hypertrophic cardiomyopathy without hypertrophy; two families with myocardial disarray in the absence of increased myocardial mass. Br Heart J 1990; 63: 287.

16. Ryan MP, Cleland JGF, French J, Joshi j, Choudhury L, Chojnowska L, Michalak E, Al-Mahdawi S, Nihoyannopoulos P, Oakley CM. The standard electrocardiogram as a screening test for hypertrophic cardiomyopathy. Am J Cardiol 1995;76:689-694.

17. American Society of Echocardiography Committee on Standards, Subcommittee on Quantitation of Two-dimensional Echocardiograms. Recommendations for quantitation of the left ventricle by two-dimensional echocardiography. J Am Soc Echocardiogr 1989;2:358-67.

18. Tennant R, Wiggers CJ The effect of coronary artery occlusion on myocardial contraction Am J Physiol 1935;12:351.

19. Gallagher KP, Matsuzaki M, Osakada G, Kemper S, Ross J Jr. Effect of exercise on the relationship between myocardial blood flow and systolic wall thickening in dogs with acute coronary stenosis. Circ Res 1983; 52: 716-29.

20. Leighton RF, Nelson D, Brewster P. Subtle left ventricular asynergy with completely obstructed coronary arteries. Am J Cardiol 1983; 52:693

21. Lima JAC, Becker LC, Melin JA, et al. Impaired thickening of nonischemic myocardium during acute regional ischemia in the dog. Circulation 1985; 71: 1048-59.

22. Ball RM, Bache RJ. Distribution of myocardial blood flow in the exercising dog with restricted coronary artery inflow. Circ Res 1976; 38: 60-66.

23. Theroux P, Ross J Jr, Franklin D, Kemper WS, Sasayama MS. Coronary arterial reperfusion III. Early and late effects on regional myocardial function and dimensions in conscious dogs. Am J Cardiol 1976;38:599.

24. Matsuzaki M, Gallagher KP, Kemper WS, White F, Ross J Jr. Sustained regional dysfunction produced by prolonged coronary stenosis: gradual recovery after reperfusion. Circulation 1983;68:170.

25. Tsoukas A, Ikonomidis I, Cokkinos P, Nihoyannopoulos P. Significance of persistent left ventricular dysfunction during recovery after dobutamine stress echocardiography. J Am Coll Cardiol 1997; 30: 621-6.

26. Nihoyannopoulos P, Kaski J-C, Crake T, Maseri A. Absence of myocardial dysfunction during stress in patients with syndrome X. J Am Coll Cardiol 1991, 18: 1463-70.

27. Panza JA, Laurienzo JM, Curiel RV, Unger EF, Quyyumi AA, Dilsizian V, Cannon III RO. Investigation of the mechanism of chest pain in patients with angiographically normal coronary arteries using transesophageal dobutamine stress echocardiography. J Am Coll Cardiol 1997;29:293-301.

28. Maseri A, Crea F, Kaski JC, Crake T. Mechanisms of angina pectoris in syndrome X. J Am Coll Cardiol 1991;499-506.

29. Picano E, Lattanzi F, Masini M, Distante A, L'Abbate A. Usefulness of a high dose dipyridamole-echocardiography test for diagnosis of syndrome X. Am J Cardiol 1987;60:508-512.

30. Rockey R, Kuo LC, Zoghbi WA, Limacher MC, Quinones MA. Determination of parameters of left ventricular diastolic filling with pulsed doppler echocardiography: comparison with cineangiography. Circulation 1985;71:543-550.

31. Choong CY, Herrmann HC, Weyman AE, Fifer MA. Preload dependence of doppler derived indexes of left ventricular diastolic function in humans. J Am Coll Cardiol 1987;10:800-808.

32. Labovitz AJ, Lewen MK, Kern M et al. Evaluation of left ventricular systolic and diastolic dysfunction during transient myocardial ischaemia produced by angioplasty. J Am Coll Cardiol 1987;10:748-755.

33. Mazeika PK, Nihoyannopoulos P, Joshi J, Oakley CM. Evaluation of dipyridamole-doppler echocardiography test in effort angina pectoris Am J. Cardiol 1991;68:478-84.

Chapter 17

IMAGING IN MICROVASCULAR ANGINA - WHAT'S NEW ?

Ann Tweddel

Normal or near normal coronary arteriography is a prerequisite for the diagnosis of microvascular angina. However it is often forgotten that arteriography provides merely a luminogram of the artery. This is exemplified by the demonstration of fibrous or lipid containing plaques within the artery wall using intracoronary ultrasound and Doppler, which may escape detection by contrast arteriography, particularly when located at the coronary ostium [1].

Morphological changes within the vessel wall, including calcification, may occur in 50-70% of patients thought to have arteriographically normal vessels [2]. It should also be borne in mind that the spatial limitations of contrast arteriograms do not allow demonstration of the microvasculature, which may be imaged by perfusion techniques, providing complementary information.

The earliest data demonstrating alteration of coronary vascular in the 1970's relied on measurements of coronary sinus flow [3]. These have now been largely superseded by doppler flow catheters and, most recently, doppler flow wires. Experimental studies on coronary flow reserve (CFR) suggest that in normal individuals flow reserve - or more properly velocity reserve- is 3.5 times higher than basal flow [4]. Recent data from flow wire and positron emission tomography (PET) studies suggest that normal ranges are somewhat lower - in the range of 2.7 to 2.8 [5]. These differences may be partly dependent on the measurement technique (3F Doppler tipped catheters, flow wires with spectral analysis, quantitative angiography analysis (QCA) or intra-coronary doppler for analysis of internal diameter of the vessel) or may reflect the choice of agent to produce "maximal" dilation (e.g. intra-coronary papaverine producing more intense coronary vasodilation than intra-venous dipyridamole). As with all measurements, the results require to be interpreted in the light of the limitations of the methodology.

There appears to be a uniform acceptance that a reduction in CFR is synonymous with malfunction of the microvasculature [6]. This is interesting in the light of data from Yokoyama *et al* [7] demonstrating reduced CFR in hypercholesterolemic patients without arteriographic coronary stenoses or indeed, by Uren *et al* [8] of reduced coronary vascular reserve in territories subtended by supposedly normal vessels in patients with coronary artery disease. A further interesting group of patients are those with heart transplantation, in whom abnormalities of functional imaging (reduced CFR and perfusion deficits) may precede the development of transplant arteriopathy [9,10].

Perfusion imaging

Radionuclide techniques have been used extensively to assess myocardial perfusion in patients with microvascular angina, with very variable findings. These range from no consistent abnormalities [11] to the recommendation that abnormalities on perfusion imaging should be a requirement for diagnosis.

Our own data from Xenon-133 [12] imaging suggest that, in patients with microvascular angina and without coronary artery spasm demonstrated by arteriography, when chest pain is induced by atrial pacing abnormalities occur both in myocardial distribution of flow and washout.

In reporting perfusion imaging results, various technical factors should be considered. Photon attenuation defects of the posterior myocardium, are common due primarily to low count density and of the anterior wall due to breast attenuation or overlying tissue in obese patients [13,14].

Similar consideration to technical factors should be given to flow measurements with PET. Cross-contamination of activity from the liver provides a relative increase in activity in the lateral wall. Gating the images to the electrocardiogram may increase inhomogeneity, due to partial volume effects, but changes are dependent on cardiac cycle duration and imaging technique [15]. Results of "absolute" measures of myocardial flow should therefore be interpreted with caution. The resolution of the technique does not allow for differentiation between sub-endocardial and sub-epicardial flow.

Stress induced perfusion abnormalities, using conventional thallium imaging, have been reported in patients with microvascular angina since the early 1980's [16,17]. Our own experience is that thallium perfusion abnormalities are common in patients with stress induced chest pain, suggestive of angina, with normal coronary arteriograms (98 of 100 consecutive patients). These occur throughout the myocardium, with no consistent pattern and no apparent relation between extent of defect and the presence of an electrically positive stress test [18]. This is in keeping with more recent data using single photon emission tomography (SPET), demonstrating that in patients with "strictly defined syndrome X", Thallium[201] SPET scan abnormalities are common (25/28 patients) [19].

Thallium[201] has long been criticized as a flow tracer, as it is also taken up within the myocardium in a similar manner to K^{43}, suggesting uptake within the cell. There is some recent experimental animal data confirming this, which is presumably the mechanism for demonstration of myocardial viability. The use of newer Technetium[99] perfusion agents obviates these criticisms.

We have recently completed a study where we have directly compared stress perfusion images, in patients with well documented microvascular angina obtained using Thallium[201] and Myoview (Tc[99] Tetrofosmin). Figure 1 shows an identical distribution of perfusion deficit with both agents, although deficits are more profound in the inferior surface with the technetium agent, reflecting sub-diaphragmatic attenuation in our imaging system. These results suggest that there are indeed inhomogeneities of flow distribution in these patients [20].

The demonstration of "slow flow" - or more correctly slow clearance of contrast medium at arteriography has also been related to abnormalities of perfusion imaging [21,22]. It is likely that the underlying pathophysiological mechanisms are similar, though as yet uncertain. Clearance from the myocardium is via the microvasculature and thus it is likely that this is a reflection of abnormalities either of flow or resistance, in the microcirculation.[23]

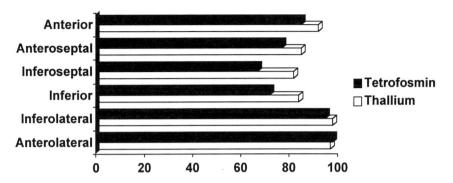

Figure 1. Myocardial perfusion imaging – Thallium vs Tetrofosmin (% reduction in counts scaled to 100% - 5 middle slices, 6 segments)

This demonstration of heterogeneity of "flow" is in keeping with recent data emerging from PET scanning, but again the literature is confusing. Galassi *et al* [24] using PET ($O^{15}CO_2$ and intravenous dipyridamole), demonstrated an increasing coefficient of variation with dipyridamole stress, similar to that seen in patients with coronary disease and significantly different from normal controls (48 ± 12, 48 ± 11 vs control 30 ± 7, p <0.01).

In patients with microvascular angina Meeder *et al* [25], using parametric PET, assessed the relationship between myocardial perfusion heterogeneity and autonomic function measured by heart rate variability. They observed a marked perfusion heterogeneity which was inversely related to autonomic tone (coefficient of variation 17 ± 3.2 vs $13.6\pm2.2\%$ in normal controls, p <0.01). The authors felt that their data supported the suggestion of increased hyper-reactivity of small vessels in this syndrome, with compensatory release of adenosine which might well be distributed in a 'patchy' fashion.

Crea *et al*, in an earlier chapter have demonstrated not only increased heterogeneity of flow in response to stress but have also reported the intriguing finding of increased resting flow in patients with microvascular angina.

Ventricular function

From the functional point of view, ventricular function at rest is not impaired and indeed may be hyperdynamic in patients with syndrome X. Earlier data [26,27] suggested that the left ventricular exercise response might be used as a diagnostic test but more recent data appear to refute these findings- with most stress technologies (stress echo and radionuclide blood pool imaging) showing no abnormality [28,29].

Our experience, using adenosine as a pharmacological stress, is that systolic function is maintained, but diastolic dysfunction is impaired, with accompanying chest pain. This may well indicate an abnormality of ventricular compliance, reflected as LV diastolic dysfunction, consequent upon subendocardial ischemia and similar to that seen in aortic stenosis (for an excellent description of this phenomenon see the editorial by Lance Gould in Circulation, [30]); or unusual handling of adenosine [31], as discussed in earlier chapters in this book.

Subendocardial ischemia

The demonstration of markers of subendocardial ischemia in the intact human present a challenge, with the limited resolution of current imaging techniques. Using SPET and PET, heterogeneous flow responses across the myocardium have been demonstrated, but with the rapidly expanding Magnetic Resonance Imaging (MRI) technology, the ability to differentiate subendocardial ischemia has become a real possibility. Using adenosine as the stressor, in patients with reduced CFR, MRI studies have shown that subendocardial flow was reduced, while epicardial flow increased [32].

The potential ability to link flow changes with metabolic changes also exists with MRI. BOLD MRI [33] uses variations of oxygen saturation of hemoglobin which result in local changes in magnetic susceptibility and consequently MRI signal - oxyhemoglobin is diamagnetic (i.e. zero) and deoxyhemoglobin is paramagnetic, with reduced T2 signal. The combination of measurement of oxygen usage in the myocardium [34,35], together with differential flow measurements within the myocardium, represent exciting possibilities for future imaging.

Summary

Heterogeneous flow responses across the myocardium in syndrome X and other conditions could be masked when techniques with limited spatial resolution are used. This may provide an explanation for the confusing literature in this regard. Imaging techniques, used appropriately, with knowledge of their strengths and limitations, can be of use as markers of flow, metabolism or function in the patient with microvascular angina and may be of inestimable value in the effort to identify the pathophysiological mechanisms that occur in this intriguing condition.

References

1. Essop AR, Scott PJ, Tweddel AC et al. The surgical implications of intraluminal coronary ultrasound. Am Heart J 1993;25:882-4.
2. Erbel R, Ge J, Bockisch A et al. Value of intra coronary ultrasound and Doppler in the differentiation of angiographically normal coronary arteries. Eur Heart J 1996; 17:880-889.
3. Kemp HG. Left ventricular function in patients with anginal syndrome and normal coronary arteriograms. Am J Cardiol 1973; 32:375-6.
4. Wilson RF, White CW. Intracoronary papaverine: an ideal coronary vasodilator for studies of the coronary circulation in conscious humans. Circulation 1986; 73:444-51.
5. McGinn AL, White CW, Wilson RF. Interstudy variability of coronary vasdilator reserve: influence of heart rate, arterial presure and ventricular preload. Circulation 1990; 81:1319-30.
6. Opherk D, Zebe H, Schuler G, Weihe E, Mall G, Kubler W. Reduced coronary reserve and abnormal exercise left ventricular reserve in patients with syndrome X. Arch Mal Coeur 1983; 76: 231-235.
7. Yokoyama I, Ohtake T, Monomura S-I et al. Reduced coronary flow reserve in hypercholesterolemic patients without overt coronary stenosis. Circulation 1996; 94:3232-3238.
8. Uren NG, Marraccini P, Gistri R, de Silva R, Camici PG. Altered coronary vasdilator reserve and metabolism in myocardium subtended by normal arteries in patients with coronary artery disease. J Am Coll Cardiol 1993; 22:650-8.
9. Kern MJ, Bach RG, Mechem CJ et al. Variations in normal coronary vasodilator reserve stratified by artery, gender, heart transplantation and coronary artery disease. JACC 1996; 28:1154-60.
10. Puskas C, Kosch M, Kerber S et al. Progressive heterogeneity of myocardial perfusion in heart transplant recipients detected by Thallium-201 myocardial SPECT. J Nucl Med 1997; 38:760-5.
11. Cannon R, Epstein SE. "Microvascular angina" as a cause of chest pain with angiographically normal coronary arteries. Am J Cardiol 1988; 61:1338 -1343.
12. Tweddel AC, Martin W. Myocardial perfusion imaging with Xenon-133. In What's New in Cardiac

Imaging? Ed EE van der Wall Kluwer Academic Publishers 1992; 41-48.

13. Elson SH, Clark WS, Williams BR. Is 'diaphragmatic ' attenuation a misnomer? Int J Card 1997; 130:161-64.

14. Prvulovich EM, Lonn AHR, Bomanji JB *et al*. Transmission scanning for attenuation correction of myocardial 201 Tl images in obese patients. Nucl Med Commun 1997; 18:207-218.

15. Bartlett ML, Bacharach SL, Voipio-Pulkki LM, Dilsizian V. Artifactual inhomogeneities in Myocardial PET and SPECT scans in normal subjects. J Nuc Med 1995: 36:188-195.

16. Canty JM, Klocke FJ. Reduced myocardial perfusion in the presence of pharmacologic vasodilator reserve. Circulation 1985;71:370-377.

17. Berger BC, Abramowitz R, Park CH *et al*. Abnormal thallium-201 scans in patients with chest pain and angiographically normal coronary arteries. Am J Cardiol 1983; 52:365-370.

18. Tweddel AC, Martin W, Hutton I. Thallium scans in Syndrome X. Br Heart J 1992; 68:48-50.

19. Kao CH, Weng SJ, Ting CT, Chen YT. Thallium 201 myocardial SPET in strictly defined Syndrome X. Nucl Med Commun 1995; 16:640-646.

20. Tweddel AC, Jones EA, Evans W *et al*. Vascular or myocardial abnormality in microvascular angina: Thallium and Technetium perfusion imaging compared. Heart 1996; 75:54.

21. Cesar LA, Ramires JA, Serrano CV *et al*. Slow coronary run-off in patients with angina pectoris: clinical significance and thallium -201 scintigraphic study. Braz J Med Biol Res 1996; 29:(5) 605-13.

22. Ciavolella M, Avella A, Bellagamba S *et al*. Angina and normal epicardial coronary arteries: radionuclide features and pathophysiological implications at long term follow- up. Cor Art Dis 1994; 5:493-99.

23. Marcus ML, Chillian WM, Kanatsuka H *et al*. Understanding the coronary circulation through studies at the microvascular level Circulation 1990; 82:1-7.

24. Galassi AR, Crea F, Araujo LI *et al*. Comparison of regional myocardial blood flow in Syndrome X and one vessel coronary disease. Am J Cardiol 1993; 72:(2) 134.

25. Meer JG, Blanksma PK, Crijns HJG. Mechanisms of angina pectoris in Syndrome X assessed by myocardial perfusion dynamics and heart rate variability. Eur Heart J 1995; 16 1571-7.

26. Cannon RO, Bonow RO, Bacharach SL *et al*. Left ventricular dysfunction in patients with angina pectoris, normal epicardiac coronary arteries and abnormal vasodilator reserve. Circulation 1985; 71:218-26.

27. Legrand V, Hodgson J, Bates E *et al*. Abnormal coronary flow reserve and abnormal radionuclide exercise test result in patients with normal coronary arteriograms. J Am Coll Cardiol 1985; 6:1245-53.

28. Panza JA, Laurienzo JM, Curiel RV *et al*. Investigation of the mechanism of chest pain in patients with angiographically normal coronary arteries using transesophageal dobutamine stress echocardiography. J Am Coll Cardiol 1997; 29:293-301.

29. Nihoyannopoulos P, Kaski JC, Crake T, Maseri A. Absence of myocardial dysfunction during stress in patients with syndrome X. J Am Coll Cardiol 1991; 18:1463-70.

30. Gould KL. Why Angina Pectoris in aortic stenosis. Circulation 1997; 95:790-2.

31. Inobe Y, Kugiyama K, Morita E *et al*. Role of adenosine in pathogenesis of syndrome X: assessment with coronary hemodynamic measurements and Thallium-201 myocardial Single -Photon Emission Computed Tomography. JACC 1996; 28:890-6 .

32. Hundley WG, Lange RA, Clarke GD *et al*. Assessment of coronary arterial flow reserve in humans with magnetic resonance imaging. Circulation 1996; 93:(8) 1502-8.

33. Wilke N, Jerosch-Herold M, Wang Y *et al*. Myocardial perfusion reserve: Assessment with multisection, quantitative first'-pass MR imaging. Radiology 1997; 204:373-384.

34. Kone BC. A 'BOLD' new approach to renal oxygen economy. Circulation 1996; 94:3067-68.

35. Li D, Dhawale P, Rubin PJ *et al*. Myocardial signal response to dipyridamole and dobutamine: demonstration of the BOLD effect using a double -echo gradient-echo sequence. Magn Res Med 1996; 36:16-20.

Chapter 18

ASSESSMENT OF QUALITY OF LIFE IN PATIENTS WITH SYNDROME X

Felipe Atienza and José A. De Velasco

When you can measure what you are speaking about
and express it in numbers, you know something about it;
but when you cannot measure it... your knowledge is
of a meagre and unsatisfactory kind.
Lord Kelvin, Lecture at the Institute of Civil Engineers, 1883.

Patients with chest pain and normal coronary angiograms have a favorable long-term prognosis regarding life expectancy, being their survival rate similar to that of the general population. The main clinical problem in these patients is not an increased risk of developing coronary events, but the presence of disabling and recurrent symptoms. Reassurance by the physician often fails to improve symptoms and these patients continue to attend outpatient clinics, are frequently admitted to CCU for unstable angina or suspected myocardial infarction, and the great majority take cardiac medications [1-4]. This makes syndrome X patients heavy "consumers" of health care resources [5,6]. Previous studies have shown that approximately 75% of patients with syndrome X remain chronically disabled with significant limitation to their daily life activities, usually due to persistent chest pain [3,7-9]. The socio-economic consequences of syndrome X are considerable as between 32% and 51% of patients remain unable to work after angiography and 45% remain or become unemployed [3,7,8]. Thus, despite the good vital prognosis patients with syndrome X seem to have an impaired quality of life.

Quality of life

The term "health-related quality of life" or "quality of life" refers to *changes in physical, functional, mental, and social health* due to the presence of a disease or condition [10]. Since health has been defined as a *"complete state of physical, mental and social well-being and not merely the absence of disease"*, the assessment of quality of life becomes crucial for a comprehensive evaluation of patients [11]. In this context, recent years have witnessed a growing interest in broadening the parameters used to evaluate patients in both clinical practice and research, beyond traditional therapeutic indicators such as prolonged survival, retardation of disease progress, and control of symptoms [12].

Quality of life assessment is particularly important in the realm of chronic disease where the impact of the disease on functional, psychological and social health to the individual requires greater attention [12]. This relatively new concept has evolved to meet the need for more comprehensive measurements of treatment outcome. It allows the assessment of the global impact of disease on the individual by including physical, psychological and social functioning measures. The notion of "quality of life" can more fully describe the health status of populations or disease groups [13,14]. Moreover, quality of life measurements are useful to suggest possible areas which may benefit from a particular form of treatment, and to evaluate the impact of this treatment. It also provides the means to assess the socio-economic impact of a particular disease and the treatment implemented. Quality of life evaluation should include sociomedical status, function in daily-life, performance of social roles, intellectual capability, emotional stability and life satisfaction. These multifaceted components, some of which reflect the patients' perception, have been collectively termed "quality of life" [15].

It is important to stress that not only acute processes but also chronic conditions are associated with adverse effects on most aspects of daily-life [16]. The clinical profile of syndrome X follows the same pattern than that seen in most chronic diseases. Long-term follow-up studies have shown that a sizeable proportion of syndrome X patients remain significantly symptomatic, the majority requiring multiple drug combinations which may in turn cause side effects, and further hospital admissions and investigations are usually needed [3-9]. Etiologic therapy is possible in just a few patients, making symptomatic treatment the cornerstone of syndrome X patients' management. On the other hand, quality of life's impairment in patients with angina pectoris due to coronary artery disease is well recognized. When compared with other chronic diseases, angina has more impact on quality of life than hypertension, diabetes and chronic obstructive airways disease, but less than heart failure or acute myocardial infarction [16]. Despite its importance, there is a paucity of data regarding the impact of syndrome X on quality of life.

The importance of subjective variables in the assessment of health status

When assessing the health status of our angina patients, we often relay on relatively objective data such as the physician's reports of symptoms, angina diaries or exercise test results. Most clinicians base their clinical judgement on these objective measures of outcome, but this laudable and essential desire of objectivity may divert us from subjective important measures. Moreover, these objective measures are not exempt of problems; e.g. exercise stress testing does not necessarily correlate with daily-life activity of patients and the NYHA classification has both high interobserver variability and low correlation with exercise testing. Moreover the Canadian Cardiovascular Society Classification may be sensitive only to fairly dramatic changes in chest pain [17-19]. More informative data on frequency, duration and severity of chest pain can be obtained by patients diary cards, but these are time consuming and rather cumbersome for the patient. Hence, while objective measures are important, they are often poor indicators of the patient's physical and emotional well-being, and hardly reflect the capacity to function in day-to-day activity [20]. To better understand the full impact of a disease on an individual's lifestyle we need more subjective measurements than those based on laboratory tests [21].

Relief of pain, decreased consumption of nitrates, or increased exercise performance are usually considered surrogates of quality of life in patients with angina pectoris. The effects of angina are not limited to just the patient perception of pain or exercise limitation. The symptom of angina affects all aspects of the patients' lives. In addition to a reduction in physical mobility, several studies have shown that patients with angina are more socially isolated, have trouble to sleep, difficulties to cope with their families and friends, and have fewer holidays and hobbies compared with those who do not have angina [16,20,22]. The administration of a quality of life questionnaire in these circumstances helps the respondent to consider many facets of life that can be affected by these symptoms and thereby yield a more thoughtful and reliable assessment compared to that provided by isolated questions or angina diaries. A key feature of quality of life questionnaires is that the patient, rather than the health care provider, rates the impairment related to each item. This is important since their perspectives can be quite different [23].

An important goal of medical therapy for patients with syndrome X should be to improve patients symptoms and function during daily activities. Numerous physiologic end points such as exercise tolerance tests have been used as surrogate measures of therapeutic benefits. However, sensitivity, specificity and predictive value of changes in physiologic measures as indices of beneficial and adverse effects of treatment on patient's life-style have not been clearly defined. Therefore, a more direct measure that comprehensively assesses the effects of treatment in the individual patient's life-style is critical for the evaluation of syndrome X. Since the agreement between objective and subjective measures is only moderate, clearly a combination of both subjective and objective variables may provide better information about the effectiveness of an intervention [20].

Need for a specific questionnaire to assess quality of life

Quality of life assessment mainly depends on the use of questionnaires. The choice of a questionnaire will obviously depend on the nature of the underlying disease, for its content must be closely related to the nature of the medical condition being treated as well as to the effects of the drug or other treatment under assessment [24]. Many generic questionnaires have been developed for the assessment of quality of life in a wide variety of health states, conditions and diseases [16,25,26]. The major limitation of such generic measures is that they may not adequately cover certain topics of particular relevance for a given disease or treatment. Generic questionnaires are most useful when conducting general surveys on health or making comparisons between disease states, but they lack specificity and sensitivity and may not detect subtle but important points relevant to a particular condition [16].

Disease-specific questionnaires focus on domains most relevant to the disease or condition under study and on characteristics of patients in whom the condition is most prevalent. These are appropriate for clinical trials in which specific therapeutic interventions are evaluated [10]. Despite the fact that syndrome X patients have angina-like chest pain, these patients differ from coronary artery disease patients in many respects. In the clinical setting, it seems that patients with normal coronary arteries may have a different quality of life and functional status than those with coronary artery stenoses. Several characteristics of syndrome X could explain this different clinical perception: e.g. the female predominance, the atypical features of chest pain and a greater proportion of painful episodes, an abnormal pain perception, the high prevalence of psychological disorders and the recurrent hospital admissions, as well as lack of specific treatments in most instances [3-9,27-29]. There are few disease-specific quality of life questionnaires for use in angina pectoris [20,30,31] and most of them do not cover the characteristic features of syndrome X.

In 1994, Cannon *et al* [32] demonstrated that the administration of imipramine improves symptoms in patients with chest pain and normal coronary angiograms. However, this paper did not assess the effects of imipramine on patients' quality of life. In a letter to the editor regarding Cannon et al's paper [32], it was suggested that measures of clinical efficacy like quality of life would be desirable before recommending the use of such treatment in practice [33]. In his reply, Cannon acknowledged the lack of an instrument for objectively assessing quality of life in this type of patient [34]. A recent study that assessed the impact of imipramine treatment on syndrome X patients' quality of life using a generic non-specific questionnaire, failed to demonstrate an improvement on quality of life despite the fact that active treatment considerably reduced the number of chest pain episodes [35]. The authors interpreted that this was due to the high incidence of side effects of treatment that negatively counterbalanced its beneficial effects on chest pain. Perhaps, the fact that in this study the investigators used a generic non-specific questionnaire was responsible for the failure to detect subtle changes not specifically assessed by the questionnaire. Hence, it would therefore seem desirable to develop and validate a disease specific questionnaire as part of the comprehensive assessment of syndrome X patients and its treatment. To meet this need, we have validated a self-administered quality of life questionnaire specific for syndrome X patients [12-15,36,37].

Quality of life questionnaire for syndrome X patients

The new questionnaire includes a comprehensive yet focused pool of 45 questions that cover the most relevant and specific domains that encompass quality of life. The questions are grouped in nine different scales or categories. A total score is obtained for every patient, where higher scores indicate worse quality of life. Thus, the total score provides a measurement of patients' overall quality of life.

In our study we found that quality of life is impaired in patients with syndrome X. The majority of them were symptomatic during the two weeks of the study: 31 (47%) required sublingual GTN to control their symptoms (16.9 ± 26.4 doses in two weeks), 24 (36%) reported worsening of symptoms, and only 2 patients were completely asymptomatic during the study period (Table 1).

When quality of life total scores were classified according to chest pain characteristics it became apparent that patients with greater symptomatic impairment, e.g. more frequent or severe angina episodes, had the highest score indicating poorer quality of life. Quality of life scores were increasingly higher in patients with more frequent attacks or more severe chest pain episodes, showing the ability of the questionnaire to discriminate groups of patients with different clinical status (Table 2).

Moreover, a significant correlation was found between total score and the number of chest pain episodes, the magnitude of pain and GTN consumption. This correlation was especially significant for the scales of chest pain, pain perception, general health and physical exertion.

Table 1. Characteristics of chest pain episodes (n = 56)

Number of episodes in 2 weeks	Frequency	(%)
<5 episodes	10	(18%)
5 – 15 episodes	31	(55%)
>15 episodes	15	(27%)
Pain level of chest pain episodes (from 0 - 10)		
<2·4	14	(25%)
2.4 - 4.7	26	(46%)
>4.7	16	(24%)

Table 2. Comparison of the ability of the questionnaire to discriminate according to attack rate and chest pain level

Attack rate/wk	<3	3-7	>7	P
Total Score	71 ± 42	84 ± 28	122 ± 24	0.004
Chest pain level	<2.5	2.5-4.7	>4.7	
Total Score	61 ± 33	96 ± 30	113 ± 25	0.0006

Mean ± SD; p = Kruskal-Wallis difference between groups

The distribution of the scores according to the Canadian Cardiovascular Society showed a similar relationship. Quality of life total scores were increasingly higher in patients who were in class II compared to those in class I, while patients in class III-IV had the lowest quality of life (Table 3). As could have been expected, these differences were particularly significant for the scales of chest pain, pain perception, physical exertion, general health and social function.

Finally, the questionnaire demonstrated to be able to detect clinically significant changes in quality of life over time. After follow-up, all quality of life profiles were significantly better for patients whose clinical status improved compared to those who remained stable or worsened. Patients who remained clinically stable during follow-up showed no changes in total scores. In patients whose symptoms worsened, total score increased and, conversely, score decreased in those patients whose symptoms improved (Table 4).

Table 3. Total scores according to the Canadian Cardiovascular Society Classification (n = 63)

	n	Mean	SD	Conf. Interval
Class I	5	36.2	13.7	19.1 to 53.2
Class II	38	87.6	28.4	78.3 to 97
Class III-IV	20	119.4	23.6	08.3 to 130.4

Kruskal-Wallis difference between groups (p <0.0001)

Table 4. Test-retest analysis for determination of reliability and responsiveness. Total scores results

	N	PRE	POST	p
Stable	37	87 ± 30	81 ± 30	ns
Worsening	24	108 ± 31	116 ± 31	0.02
Improvement	5	55 ± 37	39 ± 28	0.04

mean $\pm$ SD; p = Wilcoxon test difference

Our results indicate that quality of life, and most of its different domains are significantly affected by syndrome X. The domains which showed higher impairment in these patients were those of chest pain, pain perception, physical exertion, general health and social function. Persistent chest pain appears to be particularly important in its effects on quality of life. In our study, the severity and frequency of chest pain were the main determinants of their functional disability and quality of life impairment. The quality of life questionnaire provides a comprehensive evaluation of the domains affected by the chest pain. Therefore, this specific quality of life questionnaire for syndrome X patients seems to be a valid, sensible and reliable tool. It enables measurement of quality of life in a standardized fashion, providing a quantitative measure that allows to compare quality of life in different patients and to assess changes over time as well as the effect of therapeutic interventions.

Syndrome X treatment objectives. Role of quality of life questionnaires in the management of syndrome X patients´ in clinical practice and trials

Patients with chest pain and normal coronary angiograms are a heterogeneous population with regard to the possible underlying pathophysiological cause of their symptoms [27]. Although the cause of chest pain is thought to be multifactorial, syndrome X has adverse effects on quality of life, regardless of the etiology proposed to explain the symptoms. It is the duration of the disease, the clinical presentation with stable vs. unstable symptoms, and the severity of chest pain which determines the extent to which quality of life will be impaired [7-9]. While the underlying mechanisms to explain symptoms in patients with normal coronary angiograms are elucidated, given the excellent prognosis of these patients, the primary treatment endpoint should perhaps be the control of chest pain. This should enable them to enhance function in everyday life and achieve the highest level of well-being. Perhaps all clinical trials in syndrome X should include measures of functioning and well-being to begin to shed light on treatment effects. Moreover, accomplishing this goal may reduce health care costs because the estimated advantage of one treatment over another in cost-effectiveness can be substantially altered by adjusting the primary measure of effectiveness for quality of life [10]. However, the majority of the pharmacological trials to date have evaluated the effect of treatment mainly based on the electrocardiographic signs of ischemia during exercise or ambulatory ECG monitoring rather than on symptoms or the impact of symptoms on quality of life. The effects of treatments on quality of life should not be ignored and the inclusion of validated quality of life specific questionnaires in future studies must be encouraged. Patient self-assessment questionnaires represent a promising step in an effort to learn more about this puzzling syndrome and the efficacy of medical interventions.

The questionnaire developed by the authors is available on request.

References

1.   Kemp HG, Kronmal RA, Vlieststra RE, Frye RL. Seven year survival of patients with normal or near normal coronary arteriograms: a CASS registry study. J Am Coll Cardiol 1986;7:479-83.
2.   Opherk D, Shuler G, Wetterauer K, Manthey J, Schwarz F, Kubler W. Four-year follow-up study in patients with angina pectoris and normal coronary arteriograms ("Syndrome X"). Circulation 1989;80:1610-6.
3.   Kaski JC, Rosano GMC, Collins P, Nihoyannopoulos P, Maseri A, Poole-Wilson PA. Cardiac syndrome X: clinical characteristics and left ventricular function. Long-term follow-up study. J Am Coll Cardiol 1995;25:807-14.
4.   Lichtlen PR, Bargheer K, Wenzlaff P. Long-term prognosis of patients with angina-like chest pain and normal coronary angiographic findings. J Am Coll Cardiol 1995;25:1013-8.
5.   Cox ID, Schwartzman RA, Atienza F, Brown SJ, Kaski JC. Angiographic progression in patients with angina pectoris and normal or near normal coronary angiograms who are restudied due to unstable symptoms. Eur Heart J 1998; 19:1027-33.
6.   Keavney B, Haider YM, McCance AJ, Skehan JD. Normal coronary angiograms: financial victory from the brink of clinical defeat? Heart 1996;75:623-25.
7.   Lavey EB, Winkle RA. Continuing disability of patients with chest pain and normal coronary arteriograms. J Chron Dis 1979;32:191-6.
8.   Bass C, Wade C, Hand D, Jackson G. Patients with angina with normal or near normal coronary arteries: clinical and psychosocial state 12 months after angiography. Br Med J 1983;287:1505-8.
9.   Chauhan A, Mullins PA, Thuraisingham SI, Petch MC, Schofield PM. Clinical presentation and functional prognosis in syndrome X. Br Heart J 1993;70:346-51.
10. Testa MA, Simonson DC. Assessment of quality-of-life outcomes. N Engl J Med 1996;334:835-40.
11. Constitution of the World Health Organization. In: World Health Organization. Handbook of basic documents. 5ᵗʰ ed. Geneva: Palais des Nations, 1952:3-20.
12. Aaronson NK. Quantitative issues in health-related quality of life assessment. Health Policy 1988;10:217-30.
13. Fletcher AE, Hunt BM, Bulpitt CJ. Evaluation of quality of life in clinical trials of cardiovascular disease. J Chron Dis 1987;40:557-566.
14. Kaplan RM. Health-related quality of life in cardiovascular disease. J Cons Clin Psych 1988;56:382-

194

92.

15. Wenger NK, Mattson ME, Furberg CD, Elinson J. Assessment of quality of life in clinical trials of cardiovascular therapies. Am J Cardiol 1984;54:908-13.

16. Stewart AL, Greenfield S, Hays RD, Wells K, Rogers WH, Berry SD, Mc Glynn EA, Ware JE Jr. Functional status and well-being of patients with chronic conditions. JAMA 1989;262:907-13.

17. Goldman L, Hashimoto B, Cook EF, Loscalzo A. Comparative reproducibility and validity of systems for assessing cardiovascular functional class: advantages of a new specific scale. Circulation 1981;64:1227-1234.

18. Goldman L, Cook F, Mitchell N, Flatley M, Sherman-Cohn PF. Pitfalls in the serial assessment of cardiac functional status. J Chron Dis 1982;35:763-771.

19. CASS Principal Investigators and their associates: Coronary artery surgery study (CASS). A randomised trial of coronary artery bypass surgery. Quality of life in patients randomly assigned to treatment groups. Circulation 1983;68:951-960.

20. Wilson A, Wiklund I, Lahti T, Wahl M. A summary index for the assessment of quality of life in angina pectoris. J Clin Epidemiol 1991;44:981-8.

21. Cowley AJ. The clinical impact of coronary artery disease; are subjective measures of health status more relevant than laboratory-assessed exercise tolerance? Eur Heart J 1995;16:1461-2.

22. Skinner JS, Albers CJ, Hall RJC, Adams PC. Comparison of Nottingham Health Profile (NHP) scores with exercise duration and measures of ischaemia during treadmill exercise testing in patients with coronary artery disease. Eur Heart J 1995;6:1561-5.

23. Rector TS, Cohn JN. Assessment of patient outcome with the Minnesota Living with Heart Failure questionnaire: Reliability and validity during a randomized, doble-blind, placebo controlled trial of pimobendan. Am Heart J 1992;124:1017-1024.

24. Barnett DB. Assessment of quality of life. Am J Cardiol 1991;67:41C-44C.

25. Dupuy HJ. The Psychological General Well-Being (PGWB) Index; In: Wenger NK, Mattson ME, Furberg CF, Elinson J, Eds. Assessment of Quality of Life in Clinical Trials of Cardiovascular Therapies. New York: Le Jac; 1984:170-83.

26. Bergner M, Bobbitt RA, Carter WB, Gilson BS. The Sickness Impact Profile: development and final revision of a health status measure. Med Care 1981;19:787-805.

27. Cannon RO III, Camici PG, Epstein SE. Pathophysiological dilemma of syndrome X. Circulation 1992;85:883-92.

28. Lantiga LJ, Sprafkin RP, McCroskery JH, Baker MT, Warner RA, Hill EN. One-year psychosocial follow-up of patients with chest pain and angiographically normal coronary arteries. Am J Cardiol 1988;62:209-13.

29. Chauhan A, Mullins PA, Thuraisingham SI, Taylor G, Petch MC, Schofield PM. Abnormal cardiac pain perception in syndrome X. J Am Coll Cardiol 1994;24:329-35.

30. Velasco JA, Del Barrio V, Mestre MV, Penas C, Ridocci F. Validación de un nuevo questionario para evaluar la calidad de vida en pacientes postinfarto. Rev Esp Cardiol 1993;46:552-8.

31. Marquis P, Fayol C, Joire JE. Clinical validation of a quality of life questionnaire in angina pectoris patients. Eur Heart J 1995;16:1554-60.

32. Cannon RO III, Quyyumi AA, Mincemoyer R, Stine AM, Cracely RH, Smith WB, Geraci MF, Black BC, Uhde TW, Waclawiw MA, Maher K, Benjamin SB. Imipramine in patients with chest pain despite normal coronary angiograms. N Engl J Med 1994;330:1411-7.

33. Venes DJ. (Letter to the editor). N Engl J Med 1994;331:882.

34. Cannon RO III. (Reply). N Engl J Med 1994;331:883.

35. Cox ID, Hann CM, Kaski JC. Low dose imipramine improves chest pain but not quality of life in patients with angina and normal coronary angiograms. Eur Heart J 1998;19:250-254.

36. Kirshner B, Guyatt G. Methodological framework for assessing health indices. J Chron Dis 1985;38:27-36.

37. Mayou R, Bryant B. Quality of life in cardiovascular disease. Br Heart J 1993;69:460-6.

Chapter 19

TREATMENT OF PATIENTS WITH ANGINA AND NORMAL CORONARY ARTERIOGRAMS

Giuseppe M.C. Rosano, Gabriele Fragasso, Sergio L. Chierchia

The long term prognosis of patients with chest pain and normal coronary arteries, is good and similar to that of the general population with regard to survival and occurrence of major cardiovascular effects. However, despite the good prognosis, quality of life in syndrome X patients is often poor, as discussed by Atienza *et al* in another chapter of this book. Indeed, approximately 75% of syndrome X patients continue to report chest pain at follow-up, and in 20-30% the chest pain remains unchanged or deteriorates [1-4]. Despite reassurance, a large proportion of patients continue to see a doctor, attend casualty departments and have repeat hospitalizations and diagnostic examinations, including repeat coronary angiography [2-4]. About 50% of patients with angina and normal coronary arteriograms remain out of work as they are extremely limited in their daily activities, with relevant socio-economical implications [2,4].

Given the fact that prognosis is good in patients with angina and normal coronary arteriograms and that the limiting factor is chest pain, the primary goal regarding treatment of syndrome X appears to be the control of chest pain. Probably because chest pain in syndrome X mimics true angina pectoris, the majority of the pharmacological studies carried out in these patients have evaluated the effects of antianginal agents not only on symptoms but, principally, on electrocardiographic signs of ischemia. Drugs commonly used for treatment of coronary heart disease (i.e. β-blockers and calcium antagonists) have been tried in patients with syndrome X with controversial results.

β-blockers and calcium antagonists

ß-blockers have been tested in patients with angina and normal coronary arteriograms not only because of their anti-ischemic and anti-anginal effect but also because of their effect upon heart rate which, as discussed in chapter 17, is increased in a subset of these patients. ß-blockers are particularly effective in controlling chest pain in patients with increased sympathetic activity but they are also effective in patients with a "normal" autonomic control of the cardiovascular system. Romeo *et al* [5] observed that acebutolol improved exercise tolerance in patients with syndrome X who had signs of increased sympathetic activity during exercise, while verapamil was effective in all patients, irrespective of their sympathetic status [5]. Similar results were reported by

Montorsi *et al* [6] who suggested that ß-blockers may be effective in syndrome X patients with both inverted T waves on the resting electrocardiogram and signs of adrenergic hyperactivity following cold pressor testing. Fragasso *et al* [7] have recently shown that chronic therapy with β-blockers improves symptoms, exercise tolerance and the left ventricular filling pattern of patients with syndrome X. This effect is not dependent upon the reduction of heart rate as the i.v. infusion of atenolol decreases heart rate to a degree similar to that obtained with chronic therapy, which does not have any effect on left ventricular filling pattern. More recently, Leonardo *et al* [8] have reported a good correlation between control of anginal symptoms and normalization of increased sympathetic drive in patients with angina and normal coronary arteriograms who received chronic therapy with atenolol. Therefore, it seems plausible that ß-blockers may be effective in controlling symptoms of patients with angina and normal coronary arteriograms by reducing the abnormally increased sympathetic activity of these patients.

Calcium channel blockers are also effective for control of chest pain in patients with angina and normal coronary arteriograms. Positive effects of calcium antagonists upon coronary vasomotor tone have been reported by Cannon *et al* [9] and by Montorsi *et al* [10,11] in patients without signs of adrenergic hyperactivity. Conversely, a consistent reduction of the episodes of ST segment depression on ambulatory electrocardiographic monitoring with propranolol but not with verapamil has been reported by Bugiardini *et al* [12]. These discrepancies may be dependent upon different patient selection and pathogenetic mechanisms. The patient population studied by Montorsi *et al* [10-11] differed from that studied by Bugiardini *et al* [12] since Montorsi *et al* [10-11] excluded patients with an increased sympathetic drive, who might have benefited from ß-blockers. Therefore, despite their potential beneficial effect upon episodes of ST segment depression, calcium antagonists may not be universally useful in the treatment of patients with angina and normal coronary arteriograms.

Nitrates

Although sublingual nitrates are extremely effective to relieve chest pain caused by transient myocardial ischemia in patients with coronary artery disease they are effective in less than 50% of patients with syndrome X [3-4]. Lanza *et al* [13] have suggested that acute nitrate administration may worsen exercise-induced ST-segment depression in patients with syndrome X. More recently, Buffon *et al* [14] from the same group of investigators reported that acute nitrate administration resulted in slow contrast media run-off in the epicardial coronary arteries of patients with syndrome X. They interpreted this finding as a paradoxical microvascular response to nitrates but no pathophysiological investigation was carried out to explain the phenomenon. Despite the effect observed in these small studies, nitrates continue to be a therapeutic option in at least 40-50% of patients with syndrome X.

Recently, Pasceri *et al* [15] studied the effect of antianginal therapy with ß-blockers in patients with Syndrome X. They also compared the effects of calcium-antagonists and nitrates in 10 patients with syndrome X, in a double-blind cross-over study. After a 4 week run-in period patients were randomized to receive amlodipine 10 mg od, atenolol 100 mg od or isosorbide mononitrate 40 mg od for a period of 4 weeks. Every patient received treatment with the 3 drugs. The number of anginal episodes was significantly reduced by atenolol but not by nitrate or the calcium antagonist. Quality of life improved significantly with both atenolol and amlodipine (Table 1).

Table 1. Effect of antianginal therapy on chest pain and quality of life in patients with syndrome X

VARIABLE	Run-in	ISMN	AML	ATEN
Anginal episodes	23 ± 18	24 ± 22	21 ± 22	15 ± 13[*]
Quality of life	22 ± 16	30 ± 27	51 ± 25[*]	59 ± 29[*]
Pts improved		4	5	6
Pts worsened		3	3	0

[*]=p> 0.05 vs run-in
[†] Adapted from Pasceri *et al.* Eur Heart J 1997 (abstract) [15]
ISMN = isosorbide mononitrate; AML = amlodipine; ATEN = atenolol; Pts = patients

Thus, ß-blockers seem to be amongst the most effective standard anti-anginal therapy to control symptoms in patients with angina and normal coronary arteriograms. Although this beneficial effect may be in part due to their anti-ischemic properties, it is likely that their positive action in Syndrome X is also due to their effects on the increased sympathetic activity of these patients.

In patients in whom standard anti-anginal therapy is not effective, alternative forms of treatment have been proposed for the control of symptoms. These are based on epidemiological or pathophysiological grounds and aim to affect microvascular function and/or exert analgesic effects.

Xanthine derivatives

These drugs have both analgesic and anti-ischemic effects. In a small study Emdin *et al* [16] reported a significant improvement of exercise-induced ischemia in 12 patients with syndrome X, using i.v. aminophylline. More recently, Elliott *et al* [17] examined the efficacy of oral aminophylline in patients with syndrome X. They studied 13 patients (11 women) who were randomized to receive oral aminophylline or placebo for three weeks. All patients underwent exercise stress testing and ambulatory ECG monitoring at the end of each three week period. Ten patients completed the study. The time to angina during exercise testing was longer in patients who were treated with aminophylline than in those who received placebo (mean [SD] 632 [202] seconds *vs* 522 [264] seconds, P = 0.004). Peak exercise ST segment depression , however, did not differ significantly between patients who received aminophylline and those on placebo. Six patients taking aminophylline showed a reduction in the number of episodes of chest pain. The authors concluded that oral aminophylline has a favorable effect on exercise induced chest pain in patients with syndrome X.

Antiadrenergic agents

These drugs could decrease the vasoconstrictor tone possibly consequent to an abnormal adrenergic stimulation. Galassi *et al* [18] however, did not find any beneficial effect of prazosin and clonidine on myocardial ischemia on exercise and ambulatory electrocardiographic monitoring in 12 patients with syndrome X, while an improvement in exercise tolerance has been reported by Lorenzoni *et al* [19] using selective α_1-blockers. At present no large studies have been carried out on the effect of this class of drugs upon chest pain in patients with angina and normal coronary arteriograms.

ACE-inhibitors

Studies in patients with syndrome X have suggested that patients who have increased sympathetic drive develop systemic hypertension during follow-up. It is conceivable that local renin-angiotensin modulation of coronary tone may play a role in the pathogenesis of syndrome [20]. Enhanced coronary vasoconstrictor tone in patients with syndrome X may be due to stimulation of the renin-angiotensin system. Blockade of the renin-angiotensin system should result in attenuation of the increased resistance to coronary flow as ACE-inhibitor drugs reduce sympathetic tone and prevent the development of systemic hypertension. ACE-inhibitors have been shown to reduce sympathetic activity in several pathological conditions [21]. Based on these grounds, Kaski *et al* [22] have hypothesized that ACE-inhibitors may have a role in the treatment of patients with angina and normal coronary arteriograms. These authors tested the effect of ACE-inhibitor therapy in 10 patients with angina and normal coronary arteriograms fulfilling the definition of syndrome X. After a run-in exercise test patients entered a double blind cross-over study during which they received enalapril 10 mg od for 2 weeks and placebo od for 2 weeks. All patients had an ischemic-appearing exercise test at both baseline and after placebo whilst 4 patients had a negative exercise test after the administration of enalapril. ACE-inhibition also reduced the occurrence of effort-induced chest pain and the degree of ST segment depression during exercise (1.1±0.4 vs 1.6±0.3 mm, p<0.01; enalapril vs placebo). These effects may be dependent upon an effect on the microvasculature, but may also be related to the lower rate-pressure product obtained with enalapril compared to placebo as a consequence of the blood pressure lowering effect of the drug. Several studies have suggested that ACE-inhibitors reduce the increased sympathetic drive in patients with a variety of cardiac conditions and it is therefore conceivable that ACE-inhibitors may be effective in patients with angina and normal coronary arteriograms through this mechanism.

Imipramine

Recently, Cannon *et al* [23] studied, in a randomized double-blind study of 60 patients with angina and normal coronary arteries, the effects of the administration of imipramine (50 mg), clonidine (0.2 mg) and placebo. The rationale for this study was the possible effect of imipramine and clonidine on the transmission and/or perception of visceral pain, which is likely to be increased in most of these patients. Imipramine reduced both spontaneous episodes of pain [by 57±27%, p<0.05 vs. clonidine (-21±72%) and placebo (-29±104%)], and chest pain induced by right ventricular pacing (Figure 1). Despite these encouraging results, a recent study by, Cox *et al* [24] showed that although effective in controlling anginal symptoms, imipramine was poorly tolerated because of its side effects and did, therefore, not improve quality of life in patients with angina and normal coronary arteriograms.

% Change in episodes of CP

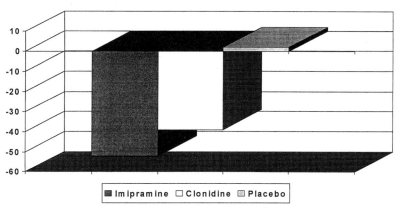

Figure 1. The effects of imipramine and clonidine on episodes of CP

Estrogens

The majority of patients with Syndrome X are women, most of whom are post-menopausal. Estrogens are vasoactive substances, and their deficiency is associated with vasomotor instability and decreased arterial flow velocity. This has led to the suggestion that estrogens may play a central role in the pathogenesis of chest pain in post-menopausal patients with Syndrome X [25-29]. This is supported by the finding that cutaneous vasodilator reserve, found to be impaired in women with Syndrome X, is normalized by estrogen replacement therapy. Rosano *et al* [30] have evaluated the effect of estrogen replacement therapy upon symptoms in female menopausal patients with syndrome X. Twenty-five post-menopausal patients with Syndrome X completed a double-blind placebo controlled study of the effects of estradiol-17ß cutaneous patches (final dose 100 µg/24 hrs) on two primary endpoints: frequency of chest pain and exercise tolerance. After a four-week period without any drugs patients were randomized to receive either placebo patches or estradiol-17ß patches for eight weeks. Subsequently patients crossed over to the other treatment. Each patient kept a daily record of chest pain, and underwent exercise testing, 48-hour ambulatory electrocardiographic monitoring and myocardial thallium[201] perfusion scan, at the end of each treatment phase. Plasma levels of estradiol-17ß were higher in the estradiol phase than during placebo (386 ± 223 vs 53 ± 51 pmol/L). In four patients plasma estradiol-17ß did not exceed 76 pmol/L during the active treatment phase, and two patients had high plasma estradiol-17ß levels (>150 pmol/L) on placebo, suggesting residual ovarian function. During the placebo phase, patients showed a mean of 7.8 episodes of chest pain/10 days (n = 25). A reduction to 3.2 episodes/10 days was observed during the estradiol 17-ß phase (p = 0.045). Of the six patients with either low estradiol-17ß levels during active treatment (n = 4) or persistent ovarian function (n = 2), only 1 patient had a reduction in chest pain with estradiol-17ß. The patients whose plasma estradiol-17ß levels increased on active treatment benefited more than those in whom plasma levels remained low (χ^2 = 4.96, p < 0.01). No significant differences were observed in exercise duration or in the results of the other cardiological tests between estradiol-17ß and placebo. The authors, therefore concluded that estrogen replacement therapy reduces the frequency of chest pain in female post-menopausal patients with Syndrome X. The patients who derived most benefit from estrogen were those who had ovarian insufficiency. The degree of improvement in the occurrence of chest pain after estrogen therapy is similar to that obtained by Cannon *et al* with imipramine [23].

Conclusions

Standard anti-anginal therapy is often ineffective in controlling symptoms in patients with angina and normal coronary arteriograms. Sublingual nitrates are used for the relief of anginal attacks and approximately 50% of patients have a good response. Amongst anti-ischemic drugs, ß-blockers and calcium channel blockers seem to be the most effective in controlling symptoms.

Since the majority of patients with angina and normal coronary arteriograms do not have myocardial ischemia, alternative forms of symptomatic treatment have been tested. Amongst these, imipramine and estrogen seem to be effective at least in a subset of patients.

Therapy in patients with angina and normal coronary arteriograms needs to be tailored according to patient characteristics. Patients with increased sympathetic drive may benefit from ß-blockers, menopausal women may have symptomatic relief of their chest pain with estrogen replacement therapy.

References

1. Romeo F, Rosano GMC, Martuscelli E, Lombardo L, Valente A: Long-term follow-up of patients initially diagnosed with syndrome X. Am J Cardiol 1993;71:669-673
2. Ockene IS, Shay MJ, Alpert JS, Weiner BH, Dalen JE: Unexplained chest pain in patients with normal coronary arteriograms: a follow-up study of functional status. N Engl J Med 1980;303:1249-1252
3. Kemp HG,Jr., Vokonas PS, Cohn PF, Gorlin R: The anginal syndrome associated with normal coronary arteriograms. Report of a six year experience. Am J Med 1973;54:735-742
4. Kaski JC, Rosano GMC, Collins,P.; Nihoyannopoulos,P.; Maseri,A.; Poole-Wilson,P.A.Cardiac syndrome X: clinical characteristics and left ventricular function. Long term follow-up study. J Am Coll Cardiol 1995; 25: 807-814
5. Romeo F, Gaspardone A, Ciavolella M, Gioffrè P, Reale A: Verapamil versus acebutolol for syndrome X. Am J Cardiol 1988;62:312-313
6. Montorsi, F. Fabbiocchi, A. Loaldi, L. Annoni, A. Polese, N. De Cesare, and M. Guazzi. Coronary adrenergic hyperrreactivity in patients with syndrome X and abnormal electrocardiogram at rest. *Am.J.Cardiol.* 68:1698-1703, 1991.
7. Fragasso G, Chierchia S, Pizzetti G, Rossetti E, Carlino M, Gerosa S, Carandente O, Fedele A, Cattaneo N: Impaired left ventricular filling dynamics in patients with angina pectoris and angiographically normal coronary arteries; effect of beta-adrenergic blockade. Heart 1997; 77: 32-39
8. Leonardo F, Fragasso G, Rosano GMC, Pagnotta P, Chierchia SL. Effect of atenolol on QT interval and dispersion in patients with syndrome X. Am J Cardiol 1997; 80: 789-90.
9. Cannon RO, Watson RM, Rosing DR, Epstein SE: Efficacy of calcium channel blocker therapy for angina pectoris resulting from small-vessel coronary artery disease and abnormal vasodilator reserve. Am J Cardiol 1985;56:242-246
10. Montorsi P, Manfredi M, Loaldi A, Fabbiocchi F, Polese A, de Cesare N, Bartorelli A, Guazzi MD: Comparison of coronary vasomotor responses to nifedipine in syndrome X and in Prinzmetal's angina pectoris. Am J Cardiol 1989;63:1198-1202

11. Montorsi P, Cozzi S, Loaldi A, Fabbiocchi F, Polese A, de Cesare N, Guazzi MD: Acute coronary vasomotor effects of nifedipine and therapeutic correlates in syndrome X. Am J Cardiol 1990;66:302-307

12. Bugiardini R, Borghi A, Biagetti L, Puddu P: Comparison of verapamil versus propranolol therapy in syndrome X. Am J Cardiol 1989;63:286-290

13. Lanza GA, Manzoli A, Bia E, et al. Deficient NO production does not play a role in syndrome X. (Abstr) Eur Heart J 1993; 14: 98

14. Buffon A, Conti E, Finocchiaro ML, Beltrame JF, Cianflone D, Crea F, Maseri A. Paradoxical effect of intracoronary nitrates on coronary blood flow in patients with syndrome X. Eur Heart J 1997; 18:169

15. Pasceri V, Colonna G, Ierardi C, Natali R, Mustilli M, Maseri A, Lanza GA. Effect of standard anti-ischemic drugs on anginal episodes in patients with syndrome X. Eur Heart J 1997; 18:629

16. Emdin M, Picano E, Lattanzi F, L'Abbate A: Improved exercise capacity with acute aminophylline administration in patients with syndrome X [see comments]. J Am Coll Cardiol 1989;14:1450-1453

17. Elliott PM, Krzyzowska-Dickinson K, Calvino R, Hann C, Kaski JC. Effect of oral aminophylline in patients with angina and normal coronary arteriograms (cardiac syndrome X). Heart 1997; 77: 523-526

18. Galassi AR, Kaski JC, Pupita G, Vejar M, Crea F, Maseri A: Lack of evidence for alpha-adrenergic receptor-mediated mechanisms in the genesis of ischemia in syndrome X. Am J Cardiol 1989;64:264-269

19. Lorenzoni R, Rosen SD, Camici PG. Effect of selective α_1 blockade on resting and hyperemic myocardial blood flow in normal humans. AM J Physiol 1996; 271: H1302-H1306.

20. Xiang JZ, Linz W, Becker H: Effects of converting enzyme inhibitors ramipril and enalapril on peptide actions and sympathetic neurotransmission in the isolated heart. Eur J Pharmacol 1984;113:215-223

21. Mancini GB, Henry GC, Macaya C, O'Neill BJ, Pucillo AL, Carere RG, Wargovich TJ, Mudra H, Lüscher TF, Klibaner MI, Haber HE, Uprichard ACG, Pepine CJ, Pitt B. Angiotensin-converting enzyme inhibition with quinapril improves endothelial vasomotor dysfunction in patients with coronary artery disease. The TREND (Trial on Reversing ENdothelial Dysfunction) study. Circulation 94:258-265, 1996.

22. Kaski JC, Rosano G, Gavrielides S, Chen L: Effects of Angiotensin-converting enzyme inhibition on exercise-induced angina and ST segment depression in patients with microvascular angina. J Am Coll Cardiol 1994;23:652-657

23. Cannon RO, Quyyumi AA, Mincemoyer R, Stine AM, Gracely RH, Smith WB, Geraci MF, Black BC, Uhde TW, Waclawiw MA, Mahrer K, Benjamin SB: Imipramine in patients with chest pain despite normal coronary angiograms. N Engl J Med 1994;330:1411-1417

24. Cox ID, Hann CM, Kaski JC. Low dose imipramine does not improve quality of life in patients with angina and normal coronary angiograms. Eur Heart J 1998;19:250-255

25. Sarrel PM, Lindsay DC, Rosano GMC, Poole-Wilson PA: Angina and normal coronary arteries in women. Gynecological findings. Am J Obstet Gynecol 1992;167:467-471

26. Williams JK, Adams MR, Klopfenstein HS: Estrogen modulates responses of atherosclerotic coronary arteries. Circulation 1990;81:1680-1687

27. Rosano GMC, Collins P, Kaski JC, Lindsay D, Sarrel PM, Poole-Wilson PA. Syndrome X is associated with oestrogen deficiency. Eur Heart J 1995; 16: 610-614

28. Rees MC, Barlow DH: Absence of sustained reflex vasoconstriction in women with menopausal flushes. Hum Reprod 1988;3:823-825

29. Rosano GMC, Sarrel PM, Poole-Wilson PA, Collins P: Beneficial effect of oestrogen on exercise-induced myocardial ischemia in women with coronary artery disease. Lancet 1993;342:133-136

30. Rosano GMC, Peters N, Lefroy D, Lindsay D, Sarrel PM, Collins P, Poole-Wilson PA. 17-beta estradiol therapy lessens angina in postmenopausal women with syndrome X. J Am Coll Cardiol 1996; 28: 1500-5

Chapter 20

MANAGEMENT STRATEGIES FOR CHEST PAIN IN PATIENTS WITH NORMAL CORONARY ANGIOGRAMS

Richard O. Cannon III

Because of the ongoing controversy regarding the etiology of symptoms in patients with chest pain despite normal coronary angiograms and ischemic-appearing ST segment depression during stress (syndrome X), we recently investigated whether these patients have confirmatory evidence of ischemia during stress [1]. Based on animal models of ischemia, we reasoned that diminished transmural contractility during stress should be a sensitive and specific marker for myocardial ischemia.

Myocardial contractile response to stress in syndrome X

Several groups have shown that dobutamine stress echocardiography accurately reveals inducible myocardial ischemia in coronary artery disease patients, and is particularly useful in patients with limited exercise capacity [2-4]. Accordingly, to determine whether patients with chest pain and normal coronary angiograms, who commonly have poor exercise tolerance, have evidence of myocardial ischemia during stress, we studied 70 patients with angina-like chest pain and normal coronary angiograms (44 women and 26 men; average age 49 years), 22 (31%) of whom had ischemic-appearing ST segment depression during treadmill exercise, thus fulfilling clinical criteria for syndrome X [1]. Eleven patients (16%) had limitation in left ventricular ejection fraction responses to exercise during radionuclide angiography and 13 (18%) had reversible perfusion defects during exercise by thallium scintigraphy, abnormalities consistent with myocardial ischemia. However, the findings of the radionuclide studies were not concordant with one another and were not related to the presence of ST segment depression during exercise testing, suggesting that all might have been "false positive" tests. The results of exercise treadmill testing and stress echocardiography from these 70 patients were compared to those of 26 normal volunteers (7 women and 19 men; average age 56 years).

We used the transesophageal route for imaging in order to maximize the number of ventricular segments visualized and the quality of images for assessment of contractility. Dobutamine infused in step-wise increments up to 40 μgm/kg/min induced chest pain in 59 patients (84%) with chest pain and normal coronary angiograms, and in none of the normal volunteers. Ischemic-appearing ST segment depression developed in 22 patients (34%) with chest pain and normal coronary angiograms, and in 2 normal volunteers (8%). Wall motion abnormalities occurred in none of the patients with chest pain and normal coronary angiograms, and in none of the normal volunteers. Further, no differences were observed in the transmural contractile response to dobutamine between patients with chest pain and normal coronary angiograms and normal volunteers (Figure 1). Indeed, within the chest pain and normal coronary angiogram group, the quantitative myocardial response to dobutamine was similar in patients with and those without ischemic-appearing ST segment depression (Figure 2). Thus, despite the frequent provocation of characteristic chest pain and in the syndrome X subset, ischemic-appearing ST segment depression, patients with chest pain and normal coronary angiograms do not demonstrate concomitant regional wall motion abnormalities and in fact show a quantitatively normal myocardial contractile response to dobutamine.

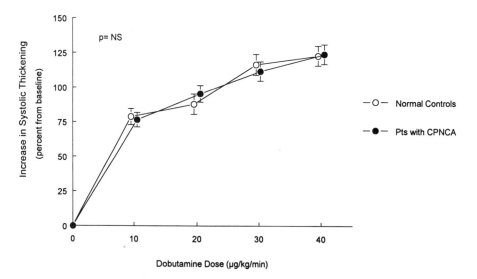

Figure 1. Comparison of the quantitative myocardial response to the infusion of incremental doses of dobutamine in normal control subjects (open circles) and in patients with chest pain and normal coronary angiograms (solid circles). The markers and error bars represent mean ± SEM. The p value corresponds to the comparison of the different responses using analysis of variance for repeated measures. Reprinted from reference 1 with permission from the American College of Cardiology.

Thus, it appears likely that the majority of patients with chest pain and normal coronary angiograms, even if selected on the basis of an ischemic-appearing electrocardiographic response to exercise associated with chest pain and labeled as having syndrome X, do not have confirmatory myocardial contractile evidence of myocardial ischemia during stress. It is possible that patchy or diffuse microvascular constriction (or absence of appropriate vasodilation) produces myocardial ischemia undetectable by currently available noninvasive or invasive techniques. However, the existence of such mild degrees of myocardial ischemia would suggest that a high rate of therapeutic success with anti-ischemic therapy should be achievable, which is contrary to the clinical experience in managing these patients.

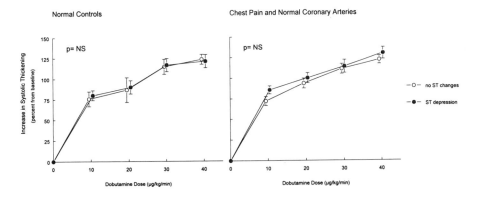

Figure 2. Comparison of the quantitative myocardial response to the infusion of incremental doses of dobutamine in subjects with (solid circles) and without (open circles) development of ST segment depression during exercise testing. Patients with chest pain and normal coronary angiograms are shown at the right, and normal control subjects are shown at the left. The markers and error bars represent mean ± SEM. Reprinted from reference 1 with permission from the American College of Cardiology.

Abnormal visceral pain sensitivity

The pain response to dobutamine stress in the absence of evidence for ischemia is consistent with our previous observation that patients with chest pain syndromes despite normal coronary angiograms have painful responses to catheter movement, contrast media injection into coronary arteries, adenosine infusion, and electrical stimulation of the right atrium and ventricle [5,6].

Whether heightened intracardiac pain sensitivity demonstrated in patients with chest pain and normal coronary angiograms represents one extreme of the normal bell curve distribution of visceral sensory function or is indicative of a true abnormality in visceral sensory function is unknown. These patients may represent the opposite end of the cardiac pain spectrum from that subgroup of patients with coronary artery disease who have "silent ischemia"; i.e., no chest pain despite myocardial ischemia. Similar observations of exaggerated visceral pain sensitivity have been made within the esophagus of patients with chest pain and normal or near-normal coronary angiograms [7], and may explain why high esophageal pressures and acid reflux, generally unrecognized by healthy subjects, cause chest pain in some patients. Additionally, exaggerated visceral pain sensitivity has been demonstrated within the rectum, sigmoid colon, and small intestines of patients with irritable bowel syndrome [8]. Thus, patients with "sensitive hearts" may represent one manifestation of chronic pain associated with heightened visceral pain sensitivity. In addition, the mechanism of exaggerated visceral pain sensitivity may be linked neurophysiologically to whatever is responsible for anxiety and panic disorders commonly noted in patients with chest pain and normal coronary angiograms [9].

The National Institutes of Health Chest Pain study

We conducted a study to categorize cardiac, gastrointestinal, psychiatric, and visceral pain sensitivity findings in a large, consecutive series of patients with chest pain and normal coronary angiograms who were referred to our institution [6]. Based on our hypothesis that patients with chest pain and normal coronary angiograms suffer from a chronic pain syndrome due to abnormal visceral pain sensitivity, we further assessed the impact of drug therapy useful in the management of chronic pain syndromes. Sixty consecutive patients (40 women and 20 men, average age 50 years) underwent baseline testing and then participated in a randomized, double-blind, placebo-controlled trial of clonidine .1 mg twice daily, imipramine 50 mg nightly with a morning placebo, or placebo twice daily (half dose for one week, full dose for 3 weeks - treatment phase), compared with an identical period of twice-daily placebo (placebo phase). Half of these patients had been hospitalized more than once because of chest pain symptoms, and 18 (30%) had undergone more than one cardiac catheterization with repeat demonstration of normal coronary arteries. The average duration of symptoms was 53 months.

Baseline testing showed that 22% of the patients had ischemic-appearing EKG responses to treadmill exercise, 17% had abnormal left ventricular functional responses to exercise (in the absence of conduction abnormalities on the electrocardiogram), 41% had esophageal dysmotility, and 63% fulfilled criteria for one or more lifetime psychiatric diagnoses (in particular, panic disorder). Eighty-seven percent had their characteristic chest pain provoked by right ventricular electrical stimulation or intracoronary adenosine infusion, and 41% had their characteristic chest pain provoked by administration of edrophonium (Tensilon), infusion of hydrochloric acid (Bernstein test), or intraesophageal balloon distention during esophageal motility testing. The prevalence of abnormal cardiac or esophageal pain sensitivity was similar for men and women, and for patients with and patients without psychiatric diagnoses. Forty-seven patients underwent 24 hours of ambulatory pH monitoring with a probe positioned in the distal esophagus; the remaining 13 patients were intolerant of the probe. During the 24-hour recording period, 34 of 47 patients (72%) experienced one or more episodes of chest pain. However, of the 217 episodes of chest pain experienced, only 28 (13%) were preceded within one minute by acid reflux (pH<4.0). Similarly, of the 1436 episodes of acid reflux, only 28 (2%) were followed by chest pain within one minute.

During the treatment phase, patients who received imipramine demonstrated a statistically significant 52% reduction in chest pain episodes, as opposed to no change in chest pain frequency in the placebo group when the treatment phase was compared to the placebo phase of the study. Clonidine-treated patients experienced a 39% reduction in chest pain episodes that was not significantly different from the placebo group response. There was also a trend towards the reduction in the intensity of pain in the clonidine and imipramine-treated patients. The symptom benefit of imipramine was noted equally in men and women. The response to imipramine was not dependent on results of cardiac, esophageal, or psychiatric testing at baseline (Figure 3), or on changes in psychiatric profile as assessed at baseline, following the placebo phase, and following the treatment phase of the study. Repeat assessment of esophageal motility at the end of the treatment phase showed no overall changes among treatment groups, although inspection of baseline and treatment phase motility test results in the placebo group showed that motility patterns are not reproducible. However, repeat assessment of cardiac sensitivity while on treatment showed significant improvement in the imipramine group only. Thus, we concluded that imipramine improves symptoms in patients with chest pain and normal coronary angiograms, probably because of a visceral analgesic effect of this drug.

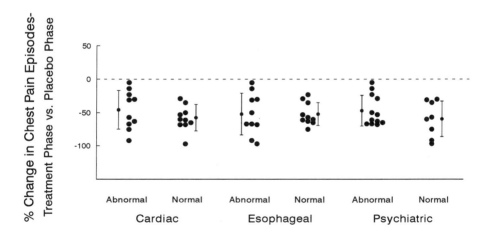

Figure 3. Percent change in the frequency of chest pain from the placebo phase to the treatment phase in patients randomized to imipramine, with a comparison in the symptom response between patients with normal and patients with abnormal results on baseline cardiac, esophageal, and psychiatric testing. From JAMA 1995;273:883-887, with permission of the American Medical Association.

Chest pain and the esophagus

Although chest pain in patients with normal coronary angiograms is often considered to be gastrointestinal in etiology, we did not find esophageal testing to be helpful in identifying the cause of pain in most patients in our study. Indeed, many groups are rethinking the value of routine esophageal testing in these patients. Frobert and coworkers [10] performed upper endoscopy with distal esophageal biopsies and 24 hour pH monitoring in 49 consecutive patients with chest pain and normal coronary angiograms. Evidence of esophagitis was found in 18 patients, with no differences in the presence of ischemic-appearing versus normal exercise testing between patients with esophagitis and those without. Twenty-four hour pH monitoring showed reflux patterns similar to 22 asymptomatic controls. Although 38% of the patients were treated with acid inhibitor therapy, symptoms were benefited in only 4%. The authors concluded that routine endoscopy and pH monitoring are of limited value in patients with chest pain and normal coronary angiograms. The same group performed 24 hour esophageal manometric and 2 channel pH monitoring in 63 consecutive patients with chest pain and normal coronary angiograms and in 22 healthy controls [11]. They found no differences in esophageal motility patterns between patients and controls, and in patients before and during episodes of spontaneous chest pain.

Approach to patient management

The management recommendations that follow are predicated on determination of normal cardiac pressures and angiograms during cardiac catheterization, a normal echocardiogram showing absence of hypertrophy or valvular heart disease, and no evidence of coronary artery spasm either by testing during catheterization (ergonovine, acetylcholine) or absence of characteristic ST segment changes during spontaneous episodes of chest pain. Given this constellation of findings, the patient should be reassured that he or she has a chest pain syndrome that poses no cardiovascular morbidity or mortality risk [12,13]. The one exception might be patients with a left bundle branch block conduction abnormality on their electrocardiograms, who may have an occult cardiomyopathy which requires further follow-up [14]. Although mitral valve prolapse has been considered in the past to be an ischemic syndrome, the etiology of pain in patients that with mitral valve prolapse is likely no different than the larger group of patients with chest pain and normal coronary angiograms without mitral prolapse. In some, reassurance alone will sufficiently alleviate symptoms, and thus no further evaluation is necessary.

Should symptoms persist despite reassurance, features of the history may direct subspecialty referral. For example, should a patient report dysphagia or regurgitant symptoms, gastrointestinal evaluation should be considered for performance of motility testing and endoscopy to exclude conditions such as achalasia. Should the patient have evidence of reassurance-resistant anxiety or panic disorders, psychiatric assessment and management should be considered. Performance of exercise or dobutamine echocardiography can provide evidence for or against inducible myocardial ischemia. Should a wall motion abnormality or diminished transmural contractility be induced, a trial of anti-ischemic therapy should be considered with drugs such as calcium channel blockers or beta blockers. However, the majority of patients will likely demonstrate a uniform increase in contractility [1]. If this is associated with chest pain, trials of tricyclic antidepressant therapy coupled with beta blockers may be of symptom benefit. Nitrates may also be of benefit, not because of anti-ischemic effects of this therapy, but because of antinociceptive effects of nitric oxide, as shown in animal models [15]. For those patients who demonstrate a uniform increase in contractility without provocation of chest pain, a trial of omeprazole may be considered for acid inhibition. If chest pain persists despite these therapeutic trials, gastrointestinal evaluation may be necessary with endoscopy to rule out chronic gastritis or ulceration, perhaps of an infectious etiology (e.g., H. pylori).

Should these evaluations and therapeutic trials fail to control chest pain symptoms, referral to a pain clinic may be necessary for a multi-disciplinary approach to the problem. Regardless of the path taken, sympathetic appreciation by the physician of the deleterious impact of chronic pain on the patient's quality of life can go a long way towards reassuring the patient that the physician is making an earnest attempt to help alleviate symptoms.

References

1. Panza JA, Lorienzo JM, Curiel RV, Unger EF, Quyyumi AA, Dilsizian V, Cannon RO. Investigation of the mechanism of chest pain in patients with angiographically normal coronary arteries using transesophageal dobutamine stress echocardiography. J Am Coll Cardiol 1997;29:293-301.
2. Sawada SG, Segar DS, Ryan T, Brown SE, Dohan AM, Williams R, Fineberg NS, Armstrong WF, Feigenbaum H. Echocardiographic detection of coronary artery disease during dobutamine infusion. Circulation 1991;81:1605-14.
3. Mazeika OK, Nadazdin A, Oakley CM. Dobutamine stress echo for detection and assessment of coronary artery disease. J Am Coll Cardiol 1992;19:1203-11.
4. Panza JA, Laurienzo JM, Curiel RV, Quyyumi AA, Cannon RO. Transesophageal dobutamine stress echocardiography for evaluation of patients with coronary artery disease. J Am Coll Cardiol 1994;24:1260-7.
5. Cannon RO, Quyyumi AA, Schenke WH, Fananapazir L, Tucker EE, Gaughan AM, Gracely RH, Cattau EL, Epstein SE. Abnormal cardiac sensitivity in patients with chest pain and normal coronary arteries. J Am Coll Cardiol 1990;16:1359-1366.
6. Cannon RO, Quyyumi AA, Mincemoyer R, Stine AM, Gracely RH, Smith WB,Geraci MF, Black BC, Uhde TW, Waclawiw MA, Maher K, Benjamin SB. Imipramine in patients with chest pain despite normal coronary angiograms. N Engl J Med 1994;330:1411-1417.
7. Richter JE, Barish CF, Castell DO. Abnormal sensory pain perception in patients with esophageal chest pain. Gastroenterology 1986;71:845-52
8. Lynn RB, Friedman LS. Irritable bowel syndrome. N Engl J Med 1993;329:1940-5.
9. Beitman BD, Mukerji V, Lamberti JW, Schmid L, De Rosear L, Kushner M, Flaker G, Basha I. Panic disorder in patients with chest pain and angiographically normal coronary arteries. Am J Cardiol 1989;63:1399-1403.
10. Frobert O, Funch-Jensen P, Jacobsen NO, Kruse A, Bagger JP. Upper endoscopy in patients with angina and normal coronary angiograms. Endoscopy 1995;27:365-370.
11. Frobert O, Funch-Jensen P, Bagger JP. Diagnostic value of esophageal studies in patients with angina-like chest pain and normal coronary angiograms. Ann Intern Med 1996;124:959-969.
12. Kemp HG, Kronmal RA, Vliestra RE, Frye RL. Seven year survival of patients with normal or near normal coronary arteriograms: A CASS registry study. J Am Coll Cardiol 1986;7:479-483.
13. Kaski JC, Rosano GMC, Collins P, Nihoyannopoulos P, Maseri A, Poole-Wilson PA. Cardiac Syndrome X: Clinical characteristics and left ventricular function. J Am Coll Cardiol 1995;25:807-814.
14. Opherk D, Schuler G, Wetterauer K, Manthey J, Schwarz F, Kubler W. Four-year follow-up study in patients with angina pectoris and normal coronary arteriograms ('syndrome X'). Circulation

1989;80:1610-1616.
15. Zhou M, Meller ST, Gebhart GF. Endogenous nitric oxide is required for tonic cholinergic inhibition of spinal mechanical transmission. Pain 1993;54:71-78

Chapter 21

ABNORMAL AUTONOMIC NERVOUS CONTROL OF THE CARDIOVASCULAR SYSTEM

Giuseppe M.C. Rosano, Gabriele Fragasso, Sergio L. Chierchia

The pathogenetic mechanisms underlying chest pain in patients with angina and normal coronary arteriograms are controversial and there is no consensus regarding the cause of symptoms in these patients. The identification of a pathogenetic mechanism for syndrome X is complicated by the heterogeneity of patients encompassed by this syndrome. In fact, syndrome X is a true syndrome and not a disease. As such it is based on clinical features such as chest pain and normal coronary arteriograms. These may be the expression of various, often unrelated, disorders.

A series of clinical studies have suggested that sympathetic drive is increased in patients with angina and normal coronary arteriograms. Early studies by Mammohansigh and Parker [1] have shown that some patients with angina and normal coronary arteriograms have an increased left ventricular contractility. Studies have shown that patients with angina and normal coronary arteriograms have a higher heart rate during 24h continuous ambulatory electrocardiographic monitoring [2], increased coronary artery tone [3] and increased plasma levels of catecholamines during exercise [4], compared to either normal individuals or patients with coronary artery disease. These studies suggest that, in at least a subgroup of patients, increased sympathetic drive may be associated with the syndrome. Interestingly, it has been suggested that most of the metabolic features of patients with angina and normal coronary arteriograms may be the consequence of increased sympathetic activity [5]. This increased sympathetic tone, however, may be only one of the manifestations of a more complex imbalance of the autonomic nervous system, which may affect the control of the cardiovascular system either directly or via neurohumoral changes.

In a 6 year follow up study, Romeo et al [6] observed that 50% of syndrome X patients who showed an increased sympathetic drive in response to exercise stress testing developed systemic hypertension whilst the other 50% developed dilated cardiomyopathy. Their results suggest that, in patients with syndrome X, a link may exist between an exaggerated sympathetic response to exercise and the development of systemic hypertension or incipient cardiomyopathy. Rosano et al [7] have also reported that syndrome X patients whose systolic blood pressure increases >20 mm Hg during the first stage of the modified Bruce exercise protocol are at a higher risk of developing systemic hypertension during long term follow up.

Findings during ambulatory electrocardiographic monitoring

Using ambulatory electrocardiographic monitoring Galassi *et al* [8] showed that patients with syndrome X have a higher mean diurnal heart rate than patients with coronary artery disease and healthy subjects. This may be regarded as evidence of an increased sympathetic drive in patients with syndrome X. Moreover, it has been shown that conditions associated with increased sympathetic activity and/or increased catecholamine levels are usually associated with an increased heart rate. In the study of Galassi *et al* [8] no differences in plasma catecholamine levels were observed between patients with syndrome X, patients with coronary artery disease and normal subjects. However, not all patients in this study underwent determination of plasma catecholamine levels and a single blood sample was obtained for the assessment of catecholamine status in these patients. In another study, Galassi *et al* [9] showed that α-receptor blockade with prazosin and/or clonidine did not reduce the frequency of the anginal episodes or improved effort-induced myocardial ischemia in patients with syndrome X. However, preliminary studies by Camici *et al* [10] using doxazosin (a novel α_1-blocker) seem to suggest that α-blockade may improve coronary flow reserve in syndrome X. These controversial findings require further investigation.

Studies using ambulatory electrocardiographic monitoring showed that during ordinary daily life most of the episodes of ST segment depression in patients with syndrome X are effort-related and that 60-95% of the episodes are preceded by an increase of heart rate [2]. Borghi *et al* [11] recently suggested that patients with syndrome X may have periods when the symptomatology is active and periods when there is a (partial) resolution of the symptoms. These periods are associated with variations in ischemic threshold and changes in sympathetic activity. During the "active" phase of the disease most patients showed abnormalities in the blood pressure response to sustained handgrip and positional maneuvers. During the "inactive" phases most patients had normal cardiovascular responses.

Heart rate variability

It is accepted that the autonomic nervous system modulates coronary artery tone and abnormalities in its control may result in a reduction of coronary blood flow [12-20]. In recent years, evidence has accumulated which suggests that changes in the beat to beat interval (RR interval) depend predominantly on the autonomic nervous system, and the study of the variability of the RR interval (heart rate variability) is a useful and accurate non invasive method for the assessment of the autonomic control of the cardiovascular system [21]. Rosano *et al* [22-23] have evaluated autonomic responses in patients with syndrome X and in a group of age and sex matched controls using heart rate variability analysis. These authors found that patients with syndrome X have an imbalance of the sympatho-vagal control of the cardiovascular system, with a shift toward sympathetic predominance. This increased sympathetic drive is more evident in those patients with an increased mean heart rate.

Rosano *et al* [22,23] reported that patients with syndrome X who also have increased heart rate on ambulatory electrocardiographic monitoring had depressed values of SDRR, pNN50, rMSSD and high values of low frequency/high frequency ratio associated with low high frequency values on heart rate variability analysis. SDRR is commonly used for the assessment of changes in the autonomic control of the cardiovascular system. Although it has been shown to be of some clinical value, this measurement is influenced by external factors and therefore does not provide satisfactory insight into the physiologic mechanisms controlling heart rate. In contrast, rMSSD and pNN50, which are dependent upon the analysis of successive RR intervals, are more sensitive indices of parasympathetic activity. On average, patients with syndrome X showed lower values of SDRR and pNN50. Patients with higher mean heart rates also showed reduced values of rMSSD, suggesting that the autonomic control of the cardiovascular system may be abnormal in these patients. The high frequency power is considered to be a pure index of parasympathetic activity since it reflects the influence of the respiratory sinus arrhythmia. The clinical importance of low frequency (LF) power remains controversial. On the 24 hour ambulatory electrocardiographic monitoring the LF power is influenced by both sympathetic and parasympathetic activity. The finding of depressed values of spectral components of heart rate variability in patients with syndrome X and higher heart rates further confirms the presence of an imbalance of the autonomic control of the cardiovascular system in these patients. β-blockade is associated with low values of low frequency/high frequency ratio together with greater values of high frequency, and the combination of these two indices is a sensible indicator of sympathetic activity. These findings seem to support the hypothesis of increased sympathetic drive as a pathogenic mechanism in patients with syndrome X. An imbalance of the sympathovagal activity shifted towards sympathetic predominance may explain the common findings of increased mean heart rate and increased rate pressure product response to exercise in some patients with syndrome X. However, separating sympathetic and vagal activities, as if they worked independently from each other, appears to be artificial and mainly depending upon the crudeness of artificial models and subtractive logics. Furthermore, since the sympathetic and the vagal system are strongly associated as a consequence of central integration, an alteration of both systems is likely to occur. It is therefore possible that the alterations found in this study are features of a widespread disturbance of the autonomic nervous control of the cardiovascular system with a shift towards sympathetic predominance. Ponikowski et al [24], also using analysis of heart rate variability, evaluated whether an alteration of the autonomic control of the cardiovascular system may be responsible for episodes of silent ST segment depression in syndrome X. They found that most of the episodes of silent ST segment depression occurring without an increase in heart rate were associated with changes in heart rate variability parameters indicative of an increased sympathetic activity. If ST segment depression episodes in syndrome X are due to myocardial ischemia then the findings of the study of Ponikowski et al [24] suggest that increased sympathetic drive may be responsible for episodes of myocardial ischemia at rest in these patients.

Assessment of the QT interval and its dispersion allows evaluation of the sympathovagal balance in normal subjects and in patients with cardiac diseases. Rosen et al [25] and Mammana et al [26] reported that in patients with syndrome X the corrected QT interval (QTc) is significantly prolonged. Rosen et al [25] speculated that QT prolongation in syndrome X patients was due to increased sympathetic activity. More recently, Leonardo et al [27] observed that both QT interval and QT dispersion, indices of sympathetic activity, are increased in patients with syndrome X compared to normal controls. Of interest, these electrocardiographic markers of sympathetic activity are normalized by ß-blocker therapy. As the normalization of both the QT interval and dispersion in Leonardo's study was associated with a parallel improvement of symptoms, the authors suggested that the increased sympathetic tone may be of importance in determining episodes of chest pain.

Autonomic control of coronary vasomotor tone

The sympathetic nervous system modulates coronary vasomotion at the microcirculation level (vessels <100 microns in diameter) and also influences dynamic behavior of the large epicardial vessels. Alpha-adrenergic stimulation causes constriction of epicardial coronary arteries through activation of α_1 adrenergic receptors. The effects of α adrenergic stimulation are complex since endothelial α_2 adrenergic receptor stimulation may cause release of EDRF, which may result in dilatation of epicardial vessels. On the contrary, β_1 and β_2 adrenergic stimulation causes dilation of large epicardial vessels and resistive vessels. Under physiological conditions sympathetic stimulation causes vasoconstriction, while increased myocardial metabolic demand triggers the release of vasoactive substances which cause coronary vascular relaxation. Coronary blood flow increases during exercise as a consequence of increased metabolic myocardial demand and autonomic nervous system mechanisms. During exercise, coronary blood flow can be further increased (by nearly 30%) by phentolamine (an α_1 blocker) infusion, suggesting that the increase in coronary blood flow is indeed modulated by concurrent sympathetic stimulation [28]. In patients with syndrome X, constrictor and dilator responses to non-endothelial dependent stimuli are similar to those observed in normal subjects [29]. Patients with syndrome X, however, may exhibit paradoxical constriction of distal epicardial coronary arteries in response to stimuli such as exercise or cold pressor test that cause vasodilatation in the presence of a normal endothelium [30-31]. Montorsi *et al* [31] found constriction of both epicardial and resistive vessels following cold pressor test in patients with syndrome X who had inverted T waves in their baseline electrocardiograms. The response to cold pressor testing may be related either to an increased neurohumoral discharge or to a hyper-reactivity of the coronary circulation to sympathetic stimulation. Bortone *et al* [30] measured coronary artery diameters and coronary blood flow before and during submaximal exercise in 13 patients with syndrome X. Two patterns of response were observed: 7 patients who had a normal increase in coronary blood flow showed epicardial coronary artery vasodilatation during exercise, while 6 patients showed both a reduced coronary flow reserve and vasoconstriction of distal epicardial vessels. This behavior of the distal coronary arteries in patients with syndrome X may be related to both abnormal endothelial function and abnormal neurohumoral regulation or altered reactivity to sympathetic stimulation of the small coronary arteries and resistance vessels. Small epicardial arteries have a distribution of α_2-receptors similar to that of the arterioles and small distal coronary arteries.

Neuropeptides in the modulation of coronary artery tone

The reason for the abnormal behavior of the coronary microcirculation observed in patients with angina and normal coronary arteriograms is still unknown. In patients with microvascular angina, the administration of ergonovine can exacerbate the limitation of coronary flow reserve observed during pacing. Vasoactive peptides belonging to the non-adrenergic, non-cholinergic system may also play a role in the modulation of vasomotor tone. Amongst these, neuropeptide Y (NPY), a 36 aminoacid residue peptide, endogenous to human coronary arteries, has been shown to cause a sustained reduction of coronary blood flow in both animals and humans [32]. Studies suggest that NPY is a potent vasoconstrictor which acts mainly on arterioles. NPY is a potent inhibitor of cardiac vagal activity and is released, like norepinephrine, after sympathetic stimulation. Clarke *et al* [32] suggested that exogenously administered NPY may induce transient myocardial ischemia in man by causing constriction at the microvascular level. Because of its biological activity and sites of action NPY, like other neuropeptides, may have a pathogenetic role in the syndrome of angina with normal coronary arteriograms. Kaski *et al* [33] compared the effect of NPY administration (0.2, 0.6 and 1.0 pmol/Kg/min) upon coronary artery flow in patients with syndrome X, normal controls and patients with chronic stable angina. The degree of proximal and distal epicardial coronary artery constriction was similar in the 3 groups following NPY infusion. Despite a similar contrast media run-off time (an indirect index of coronary microcirculatory resistance) at rest in the 3 groups, patients with syndrome X showed a significant prolongation of the run-off after NPY infusion (57% lengthening compared to baseline). In addition, some syndrome X patients developed chest pain and ischemic ST segment changes during NPY administration. This study showed that NPY causes significant constriction of small intramyocardial coronary arteries in patients with syndrome X. This constrictor response of the small coronary arteries in patients with syndrome X may be related to an increased sensitivity of these vessels to constrictor stimuli in general or to sympathetic stimulation, in particular.

Estrogen deficiency and increased sympathetic activity

Rosano *et al* [36] have suggested that syndrome X is more common in women with signs and symptoms of ovarian insufficiency. Estrogen deficiency states are often associated with increased sympathetic activity which is reversed almost completely by estrogen replacement therapy [37-39]. It is therefore possible that estrogen deficiency may trigger chest pain in women during premenopause by increasing sympathetic tone. Hormonal deficiency may be the link between increased sympathetic activity and chest pain in female patients with syndrome X.

The combination of increased demand and reduced vasodilator capacity may certainly promote the development of a supply/demand imbalance. This may not be severe enough to cause "full-blown" myocardial ischemia but may suffice to induce subtle alterations of various cardiac functions. This interpretation could explain, for instance, the presence of resting diastolic dysfunction, [40] the increase in regional glucose uptake [41] and the interstitial deposition of gadolinium DTPA [42] which have been reported in patients with angina and normal coronary arteriograms. These abnormalities were shown to improve with long term treatment with ß-blockers. The beneficial effects of ß-blockers may be the result of reduced myocardial oxygen consumption which improves the supply/demand ratio. However, it may be also speculated that prolonged administration of these agents may have reduced sympathetic tone.

Increased sympathetic tone and cardiac metabolism

Increased sympathetic activity induces several other effects that may affect cardiovascular function. Among these, excessive stimulation of myocardial ß-receptors that may increase intracellular calcium concentrations and cause a negative lusitropic effect which, in turn, may impair diastolic function. Some patients with syndrome X preferentially utilize lipid fuel for myocardial energy production and have a proportionally lower oxidation of carbohydrates. Increased sympathetic activity can, by itself, contribute to this phenomenon [43-44] and ß-blockers may, potentially, reverse it [45]. These agents reduce the levels of circulating free fatty acids that are typically increased during adrenergic stimulation [45].

Insulin resistance has also been suggested to contribute to the pathophysiology of cardiac syndrome [46] and, once again, excessive sympathetic activity may play a major role in this regard. Indeed, there are several mechanisms by which excessive sympathetic stimulation may lead to insulin resistance. Skeletal muscle vasoconstriction may increase the diffusion distance between the nutritional blood vessel and the metabolizing cell. This will impair delivery of glucose to the muscle cell, thereby creating a state of relative insulin resistance [47]. In addition to the effect of vasoconstriction, sympathetic stimulation can induce acute insulin resistance through ß-adrenergic receptor stimulation and their blockade can reinstate a normal glucose uptake [48]. Whatever the mechanism, insulin resistant states, such as diabetes and hypertension, have been linked with reduced activity of endothelium-derived relaxing factor [49-50]. Insulin has also been shown to prompt smooth muscle proliferation in man [51]. Such mechanisms may contribute to an abnormal vasoconstrictive response in syndrome X leading to microvascular dysfunction and myocardial ischemia.

Conclusions

Thus, current clinical evidence supports the notion that an alteration of the autonomic control of the cardiovascular system may play a role in patients with angina and normal coronary arteriograms. The increased sympathetic activity observed in syndrome X patients may affect coronary blood flow and also increase myocardial oxygen consumption and metabolism. Coronary hyper-reactivity to sympathetic stimulation and constrictor neuropeptides, such as neuropeptide Y may be present in patients with angina with normal coronary arteriograms, and this may result in a reduced coronary blood flow reserve. An increased sympathetic drive may also be of importance in the development of arterial hypertension and insulin resistance. The clinical recognition of an increased sympathetic drive may be pivotal to identify those patients at increased risk of developing hypertension and/or hyperinsulinemia, in addition to identifying a pathogenetic mechanism amenable of treatment.

References

1. Mammohansingh P, Parker JO: Angina pectoris with normal coronary arteriograms: hemodynamic and metabolic response to atrial pacing. Am Heart J 1975;90:555-561.
2. Kaski JC, Crea F, Nihoyannopoulos P, Hackett D, Maseri A: Transient myocardial ischemia during daily life in patients with syndrome X. Am J Cardiol 1986;58:1242-1247.
3. Montorsi P, Manfredi M, Loaldi A, Fabbiocchi F, Polese A, de Cesare N, Bartorelli A, Guazzi MD: Comparison of coronary vasomotor responses to nifedipine in syndrome X and in Prinzmetal's angina pectoris. Am J Cardiol 1989;63:1198-1202.
4. Ishihara T, Seki I, Yamada Y, Tamoto S, Fukai M, Takada K, Fujiwara M, Ashida H, Shimada T, Ohsawa N: Coronary circulation, myocardial metabolism and cardiac catecholamine flux in patients with syndrome X. J Cardiol 1990;20:267-274..
5. Camici PG, Marraccini P, Lorenzoni R, Buzzigoli G, Pecori N, Perissinotto A, Ferrannini E, L'Abbate A, Marzilli M: Coronary hemodynamics and myocardial metabolism in patients with syndrome X: response to pacing stress. J Am Coll Cardiol 1991;17:1461-1470.
6. Romeo F, Gaspardone A, Ciavolella M, Gioffrè P, Reale A: Verapamil versus acebutolol for syndrome X. Am J Cardiol 1988;62:312-313.
7. Rosano GMC, Kaski JC, Maseri A, Poole-Wilson PA: Early increase of blood pressure during exercise in patients with syndrome X predicts the development of systemic hypertension. Eur Heart J 1992;13:87
8. Galassi AR, Kaski JC, Crea F, Pupita G, Gavrielides S, Tousoullis D, Maseri A: Heart rate response during exercise testing and ambulatory ECG monitoring in patients with syndrome X. Am Heart J 1991;122:458-463.
9. Galassi AR, Kaski JC, Pupita G, Vejar M, Crea F, Maseri A: Lack of evidence for alpha-adrenergic receptor-mediated mechanisms in the genesis of ischemia in syndrome X. Am J Cardiol 1989;64:264-269.
10. Camici PG: Studies of coronary blood flow and myocardial metabolism in patients with chest pain and angiographically normal coronary arteries, in Kaski JC (ed): Angina pectoris with normal coronary arteries: syndrome X. London, Kluwer Academic Publishers, 1994, pp 149-164.
11. Borghi A, Di Clemente D, Puddu GM, Ruggeri A, Bugiardini R: Long-term clinical outcome of patients with angina pectoris, normal coronary angiograms and evidence of myocardial ischemia. J Am Coll Cardiol 1993;21:476A.
12. Buffington CW, Feigl EO: Adrenergic coronary vasoconstriction in the presence of coronary stenosis in the dog. Circ Res 1981;48:416-423.
13. Heusch G, Deussen A: The effects of cardiac sympathetic nerve stimulation on the perfusion of stenotic coronary arteries in dog. Circ Res 1983;53:8-15.
14. Nathan HJ, Feigl EO: Adrenergic vasoconstriction lessen transmural steal during coronary hypoperfusion. Am J Physiol 1986;250:H645-H653.
15. Chilian WM, Ackell PH: Transmural differences in sympathetic coronary constriction during exercise in the presence of coronary stenosis. Circ Res 1988;62:216-225.
16. Gwirtz PA, Stone HL: Coronary blood flow changes following activation of adrenergic receptors in the conscious dog. Am J Physiol 1982;243:H13-H19.
17. Heusch G: Control of coronary vasomotor tone in ischemic myocardium by local metabolism and neurohumoral mechanisms. Eur Heart J 1991;12:F99-F106.
18. Heusch G: Alpha-adrenergic mechanisms in myocardial ischemia. Circulation 1990;81:1-13.
19. Raizner AE, Chahine RA, Ishimori T, Verani MS, Zacca N, Jamal N, Miller RR, Luchi RJ: Provocation of coronary artery spasm by the cold pressor test. Circulation 1980;62:925-932.
20. Brown BG, Bolson EL, Dodge HT: Dynamic mechanisms in human coronary artery stenosis. Circulation 1984;70:917-922.
21. Pomeranz B, Macaulay RJB, Caudill MA, Kutz I, Adam D, Gordon D, Kilborn KM, Barger AC, Shannon DC, Cohen RJ, Benson H: Assessment of autonomic function in humans by heart rate spectral analysis. Am J Physiol 1985;248:H151-H153.

22. Rosano GMC, Kaski JC: Abnormal neurohumoral control in the pathogenesis of syndrome X, in Kaski JC (ed): Angina pectoris with normal coronary arteries: Syndrome X. Boston, Kluwer Academic Publishers, 1994, pp 211-224.

23. Rosano GMC, Ponikowski P, Adamopoulos S, Collins P, Poole-Wilson PA, Coats A, Kaski JC. Abnormal autonomic control of the cardiovascular system in syndrome X. Am.J.Cardiol. 73:1174-1179, 1994.

24. Ponikowski P, Rosano GMC, Amadi A, Collins P *et al.* Transient autonomic dysfunction precedes ST-segment depression in patients with syndrome X. Am J Cardiol 1996; 77:942-947.

25. Rosen SD, Dritsas A, Bourdillon PJ, Camici PG. Analysis of the electrocardiographic QT interval in patients with syndrome X. Am J Cardiol 1994; 73:971-972.

26. Mammana C, Salomone O, Kautzner J, Schwartzman R, Kaski JC. Heart rate-independent prolongation of QTc interval in women with syndrome X. Clin Cardiol 1997; 20:357-360.

27. Leonardo F, Fragasso G, Rosano GMC, Pagnotta P, Chierchia SL. Effect of atenolol on QT interval and dispersion in patients with syndrome X. Am J Cardiol 1997; 80: 789-90.

28. Bassenge E, Walter P, Doutheil U: Wirkungsumkehr der adrenergischen coronargefassreaction in abhangigkeit vom coronargefasstonus. Pflugers Arch 1969;297:146-155.

29. Maseri A, Crea F, Kaski JC, Crake T: Mechanisms of angina pectoris in syndrome X. J Am Coll Cardiol 1991;17:499-506.

30. Bortone AS, Hess OM, Eberli FR, Nonogi H, Marolf AP, Grimm J, Krayenbuehl HP. Abnormal coronary vasomotion during exercise in patients with normal coronary arteries and reduced coronary flow reserve. Circulation 79:516-527, 1989.

31. Montorsi P, Cozzi S, Loaldi A, Fabbiocchi F, Polese A, de Cesare N, Guazzi MD: Acute coronary vasomotor effects of nifedipine and therapeutic correlates in syndrome X. Am J Cardiol 1990;66:302-307.

32. Clarke J, Benjamin N, Larkin S, Webb D, Maseri A, Davies G: Interaction of neuropeptide Y and the sympathetic nervous system in vascular control in man. Circulation 1991;83:774-777.

33. Kaski JC, Tousoulis D, Rosano GMC, Clarke J, McFadden E, Davies GJ: Role of Neuropeptide Y in the pathogenesis of syndrome X. Circulation 1992;86, No 4:I527.

34. Cannon RO, Schenke WH, Leon MB, Rosing DR, Urqhart J, Epstein SE: Limited coronary flow reserve after dipyridamole in patients with ergonovine-induced coronary vasoconstriction. Circulation 1987;75:163-174.

35. Kaski JC, Tousoulis D, Galassi AR, McFadden E, Pereira WI, Crea F, Maseri A: Epicardial coronary artery tone and reactivity in patients with normal coronary arteriograms and reduced coronary flow reserve (syndrome X). J Am Coll Cardiol 1991;18:50-54.

36. Rosano GMC, Collins P, Kaski JC, Lindsay D, Sarrel PM, Poole-Wilson PA. Syndrome X is associated with oestrogen deficiency. Eur Heart J 1995; 16: 610-614.

37. Rees MC, Barlow DH: Absence of sustained reflex vasoconstriction in women with menopausal flushes. Hum Reprod 1988;3:823-825.

38. Rosano GMC, Peters N, Lefroy D, Lindsay D, Sarrel PM, Collins P, Poole-Wilson PA. 17-beta estradiol therapy lessens angina in postmenopausal women with syndrome X. J Am Coll Cardiol 1996; 28: 1500-5.

39. Kronenberg F, Cote LJ, Linkie DM, Dyrenfurth I, Downey JA: Menopausal hot flushes: thermoregulatory, cardiovascular and circulating catecholamine and LH changes. Maturitas 1984;6:31-43.

40. Fragasso G, Chierchia S, Pizzetti G, Rossetti E, Carlino M, Gerosa S, Carandente O, Fedele A, Cattaneo N: Impaired left ventricular filling dynamics in patients with angina pectoris and angiographically normal coronary arteries; effect of beta-adrenergic blockade. Heart 1997; 77: 32-39.

41. Fragasso G, Chierchia SL, Rossetti E, Landoni C, Lucignani G, Fazio F. Abnormal myocardial glucose handling in patients with syndrome X: effect of beta adrenergic blockade. Giorn It Cardiol 1997; 27: 1113-1120.

42. Rossetti E, Fragasso G, Vanzulli A *et al.* Magnetic resonance imaging in patients with angina and normal coronary angiograms. J Am Coll Cardiol 1994; 445A.

43. Newsholme EA, Start C. Regulation in metabolism. London: J Wiley and Sons, 1974: 329-37.

44. Van Zweiten PA. Interaction between alpha- and beta-adrenoceptor-mediated cardiovascular effects. J Cardiovasc Pharmacol 1986; 8 (4): S21-8.

45. Jackson G, Atkinson L, Oram S. Improvement of myocardial metabolism in coronary artery disease by beta-blockade. Br Heart J 1977; 39: 829-33.

46. Dean JD, Jones CJ, Hutchison SJ, Peters JR, Henderson AH: Hyperinsulinaemia and microvascular angina ("syndrome X"). Lancet 1991;337:456-457.

47. Julius S. Sympathetic hyperactivity and coronary risk in hypertension. Hypertension 1993; 21: 886-93.

48. Deibert DC, De Fronzo RA. Epinephrine-induced insulin resistance in man. J Clin Invest 1980; 65: 717-21.

49. De Tejada IS, Goldstein I, Azadzio K, Krane RJ, Cohen RA. Impaired neurogenic and endothelium-mediated relaxation of penile smooth muscle from diabetic men with impotence. N Engl J Med 1989; 320: 1025-30.

50. Panza JA, Quyyumi AA, Brush JE, Epstein SE. Abnormal endothelium-dependent vascular relaxation in patients with essential hypertension. N Engl J Med 1990; 323: 22-6.

51. Pfeide B, Ditschuneit H. Effect of insulin on growth of cultured human arterial smooth muscle cells. Diabetologia 1981; 20: 155-8.

Chapter 22

THE METABOLIC SYNDROME

Francisco Leyva and John C. Stevenson

The association between coronary heart disease (CHD), non-insulin dependent diabetes mellitus (NIDDM), hypertension and obesity has long been recognized by both clinicians and epidemiologists. In 1988, Reaven coined the term "Syndrome X" to denote the association of these disorders with metabolic disturbances such as low plasma high density lipoprotein (HDL) cholesterol and hypertriglyceridemia, hyperinsulinemia, hyperglycemia and insulin resistance [1]. However, the term "syndrome X", had been previously coined by Kemp in 1973 to denote the cardiological syndrome of angina and normal coronary arteries [2]. Regarding Reaven's syndrome X, further objection to the inclusion of insulin resistance in its description is that insulin resistance has not confidently been shown to be the key metabolic disturbance, despite the plausibility of the proposed mechanism in this respect. For now, the syndrome is best referred to as the "metabolic syndrome".

Interest in a metabolic syndrome of cardiovascular risk has been fuelled by the recognition that the classical cardiovascular risk factors, such as age, obesity, hypertension, smoking and hypercholesterolemia only partly explain the incidence of CHD [3]. The metabolic syndrome has served as a point of reference for investigations into alternative metabolic risk factors for CHD. It should be emphasized, however, that to date we have no threshold of measurement above or below which to diagnose the metabolic syndrome [4] and that its clinical significance is still debated. The syndrome does appear to predict the development of NIDDM, and limited data using surrogate measures suggests that insulin resistance may predispose to the development of CHD [5]. As it stands, the metabolic syndrome is an epidemiological entity and not a clinical condition which can be diagnosed [6] or treated in individual patients. It is therefore best viewed as a tendency [4].

Coronary heart disease, diabetes and hypertension

CHD, hypertension and NIDDM behave as mutually supporting conditions (Table 1). Patients with NIDDM are more likely to have CHD [7, 8], there being a two-fold increase of CHD in men and a four-fold increase in women [9-11]. Hypertension is also more common in patients with NIDDM [12-14]. Almost 50% of patients with newly-diagnosed NIDDM are hypertensive [15,16] and approximately 80% of diabetic patients aged 60 years have a blood pressure greater than 140/90 mmHg. The excess of hypertension in diabetics compared to non-diabetics is apparent at all ages [17], particularly in women [18].

Table 1. Excess of cardiovascular disease in diabetic patients

---

↑ Incidence of myocardial infarction (MI) [8,29-31]
↑ Infarct size [32] and infarct extension [33]
↑ Re-infarction [8]
↑ Acute complications of MI [8]
↑ Heart failure after MI [8,33]
↑ Mortality after MI, short- and long-term [34,35]
↑ Angina, silent and symptomatic [8]
↑ Angiographic CHD [36]
↑ Restenosis after coronary angioplasty [8]
↑ Incidence of systolic/diastolic and isolated systolic hypertension
↑ Left ventricular hypertrophy [37]?
↑ Microangiopathy (gangrene etc)

Reproduced with permission from Leyva F, Coats AJS. Practical management of hypertension. Blackwell Science, 1998 (In press).

As well as being more common in NIDDM, the mortality attributable to hypertension in NIDDM patients is also higher, by almost two-fold [19]. This increased mortality is apparent at all levels of blood pressure [20]. Moreover, the severity of cardiac disease is much increased when hypertension and diabetes co-exist [21]. This adverse synergistic effect of the combination of NIDDM and hypertension also applies to retinal, renal and peripheral vascular disease [22-25].

Histopathological studies reflect the epidemiological picture. Diabetic CHD is characterized by discrete and diffuse multi-vessel involvement. Salient features of myocardial infarction in diabetics include myocardial hypertrophy and diffuse, patchy fibrosis more frequently than macroscopic myocardial necrosis [26]; proliferative lesions in arterial branches and even venules [27]; and atherosclerotic lesions in intramural coronary artery branches [28]. There is evidently a conspicuous predilection for microvascular damage.

The metabolic syndrome

In 1988, Reaven proposed that resistance to insulin-stimulated glucose uptake (insulin resistance) and hyperinsulinemia may be involved in the development and progression of NIDDM, hypertension and CHD [1]. Reaven's concept of a metabolic syndrome emerged from the recognition that these diseases and their metabolic risk factors were highly intercorrelated. These originally included insulin resistance, hyperinsulinemia, glucose intolerance, increased plasma very low-density lipoprotein (VLDL) cholesterol and triglyceride concentrations, low plasma HDL cholesterol and elevated blood pressure. Since its description, many further components have been added [6,38-41] (Table 2). The salient components of the syndrome are considered below.

Table 2. Proposed components of a metabolic syndrome

↑ Non-insulin dependent diabetes mellitus
↑ Blood pressure
↑ Serum uric acid
↑ Plasma triglycerides
↑ Plasma LDL cholesterol
↓ Plasma HDL and HDL_2 cholesterol
↓ Glucose tolerance
↑ Proportion of central (android) fat
↓ Insulin sensitivity
↑ Plasma insulin
↑ Plasma insulin propeptides
↑ Plasma leptin
↑ Small dense LDL cholesterol particles
↑ Non-esterified fatty acid flux
↑ Plasminogen activator inhibitor-1
↓ Arterial wall compliance
↓ Arterial blood flow

↑ = increase; ↓ = decrease

Elevated blood pressure

In 1966 Welborn found that, compared to normotensive controls, hypertensive patients had higher insulin levels in the fasting state and after an oral glucose challenge, independent of age and antihypertensive therapy [42]. An early study of war-injured amputees demonstrated a strong association between diastolic blood pressure and the insulin response to oral glucose [43]. A study of 194 patients with glucose intolerance revealed that both fasting and post-glucose insulin levels were related to the level of blood pressure whilst sex, age and glucose levels were not [44]. The positive association between insulin and diastolic blood pressure has been confirmed by large-scale epidemiological studies [45]. It was subsequently shown that post-glucose insulin levels are elevated in hypertensive subjects compared to normotensive controls, and that this effect is independent of age, obesity, glucose intolerance and antihypertensive therapy [46]. In the same study, hyperinsulinemia was shown to be present in most hypertensive subjects, and the highest insulin levels were found in those who had a combination of obesity, hypertension and glucose intolerance. Findings such as these suggested that insulin may be important in the pathogenesis of hypertension. Experimental studies showing that insulin activates the sympathetic nervous system and enhances sodium reabsorption in the kidney [47] added further credence to this concept.

There has been debate as to whether obesity plays a modulating effect on the relationship between hyperinsulinemia and hypertension. In a study of obese, non-diabetic and non-hypertensive women, the association between fasting serum insulin levels and both systolic and diastolic blood pressure was independent of body mass index (BMI) [48]. In contrast, a study of obese hypertensive subjects revealed that although fasting serum insulin correlated with mean arterial blood pressure, this relationship was eliminated when body weight and body fat distribution were taken into consideration [49] . An attempt to control for the effect of obesity was made by Bonora *et al* [50], in the light of suggestions that the relationship between serum insulin and blood pressure may be largely explained by the mutual association with body composition and fat distribution [49]. This group showed that when obese and non-obese healthy subjects were analyzed separately, the association between post-glucose plasma insulin and systolic and diastolic blood pressure was only evident in the non-obese group. In this study, systolic and diastolic blood pressures tended to be higher in hyperinsulinemic subjects, whilst no such relationship was evident in obese, hyperinsulinemic subjects.

Insulin resistance and its surrogate measures, hyperglycemia and hyperinsulinemia

Numerous studies support the notion of a pathogenetic link between insulin resistance and CHD. An independent relationship between insulin resistance and arteriosclerosis (measured by ultrasound) has recently been demonstrated in healthy individuals [51] and in diabetic patients [52]. These findings are in accord with three major epidemiological studies in which hyperinsulinemia, a surrogate measure of insulin resistance, emerged as an independent predictor of CHD [53-55]. This adds to the finding that glucose intolerance, another surrogate measure of insulin resistance, is also predictive of CHD [23,56-58]. The increasing recognition that insulin resistance *per se* may be involved in the pathogenesis of atherosclerosis [59] has paralleled the finding from small-scale clinical studies that it also plays a pivotal role in the syndrome of metabolic disturbances with which it is commonly associated [4], such as hypertension, hypertriglyceridemia, glucose intolerance, hyperinsulinemia, obesity, low serum HDL cholesterol and hyperuricemia [60].

With regard to established disease, we have demonstrated that insulin sensitivity is significantly lower in non-obese men with angiographically-proven CHD compared with matched normals [61]. These men exhibited other features of the insulin resistance syndrome, with relative hyperinsulinemia in the absence of significantly impaired glucose tolerance, lower HDL and HDL_2 cholesterol concentrations together with lower concentrations of apolipoproteins AI and AII, higher triglycerides, higher systolic blood pressure, and greater proportions of android fat despite having the same total fat mass as the controls. We have also shown that heart failure is an insulin resistant state [61,62] in which insulin sensitivity is positively related to clinical parameters, including functional class [61] and muscle strength [63].

There are a number of ways in which insulin resistance may lead to the development of CHD. Its accompanying hyperinsulinemia may promote smooth muscle cell proliferation and arterial lipid deposition, and hence may be involved in the pathogenesis of atheroma [64]. Increased levels of insulin propeptides have been linked with CHD and atheroma, and increased concentrations of proinsulin have been found in young male survivors of myocardial infarction [65]. Increased proportions of insulin propeptides are found in patients with NIDDM. In other states of insulin resistance, these proportions may not be altered, but absolute levels of insulin propeptides are increased in association with the increased insulin concentrations [66]. Thus it may be necessary to consider whether increased insulin propeptide concentrations are a feature of the insulin resistance syndrome.

Assessment of insulin resistance. Insulin resistance is tissue resistance to insulin action, whether it is in terms of glucose or lipid metabolism, or the vasodilatory actions of insulin. Its traditional measure is the change in glucose elimination rate elicited by a unit change in insulin concentration. This measurement is by no means straightforward. Only two methods provide a true measure of insulin sensitivity (the inverse of insulin resistance).

1. The euglycemic hyperinsulinemic clamp utilizes a constant intravenous infusion of insulin and a varying intravenous infusion of glucose. The rate of glucose infusion is varied according to rapid and regular blood glucose estimations until basal glycemia can be maintained without changing the glucose infusion rate; this is usually achieved after 2 or 3 hours. The glucose infusion rate is then taken as the glucose elimination rate, and dividing this by the prevailing degree of hyperinsulinemia provides the measure of insulin sensitivity. The disadvantages of this technique are that it is non-physiological in that such sustained hyperinsulinemia does not normally occur. The transient elevations in insulin secretion seen in normal physiology elicit smaller increases in glucose elimination rate and thus the clamp overestimates insulin sensitivity. Another major disadvantage is that the procedure is very time-consuming and labor-intensive.

2. An alternative to the clamp technique is the use of minimal model analysis of glucose and insulin profiles during an intravenous glucose tolerance test (IVGTT). This technique utilizes the non-steady-state glucose and insulin responses to an intravenous glucose bolus to provide a measure of the constant which best relates change in glucose elimination to change in insulin concentration in the plasma. The advantages of this technique are that the clinical procedure is relatively straightforward, and the insulin response is physiological. However, it is reliant on a sufficient pancreatic insulin response and hence its appropriateness in diabetic patients is uncertain. Furthermore, the mathematical modeling is complex and requires skilled and experienced operators.

Because of the constraints of these procedures, prospective population studies of CHD have used surrogate measures for insulin resistance, either the fasting insulin concentration or the insulin response to an oral glucose load. It should be noted that such measures are also dependent on other parameters, such as pancreatic secretion and hepatic throughput of insulin. As such, they are weak surrogate measures of insulin resistance.

Dyslipidemia

Dyslipidemia is a consistent finding in the metabolic syndrome. The associations between insulin resistance, serum triglycerides and HDL cholesterol [67,68] are well characterized. These age and BMI-independent associations appear across different populations [69]. In the UK, clear associations between insulin and an atherogenic lipid profile have been reported in healthy, normoglycemic Asian men [70]. In the Bogalusa Heart Study of healthy young adults, elevated VLDL cholesterol (a marker of triglycerides) was associated with other components of the metabolic syndrome, including hyperinsulinemia, hypertension and obesity [71].

HDL may participate in reverse cholesterol transport whereby they remove cholesterol from tissues such as arterial walls and return it to the liver for excretion or resecretion. Thus HDL levels are inversely associated with CHD risk [72]. The HDL_2 subfraction is considered to be the subfraction which confers the major benefit, and HDL_2 can be catabolized by hepatic lipase. Conditions which increase hepatic lipase activity, such as increased adiposity or increased androgen activity, are associated with low HDL_2 levels. Triglyceride levels are inversely associated with HDL and HDL_2 levels [73]. Increased hepatic triglyceride production leads to increased levels of triglyceride-rich VLDL. Reduced VLDL clearance results in increased plasma residence of VLDL remnants, decreased HDL_2 and increased intermediate density lipoprotein (IDL) levels, an atherogenic lipoprotein profile. Thus low levels of HDL and HDL_2 may reflect a reduction in reverse cholesterol transport or a reduction in VLDL remnant clearance, and it is not clear as to which is more important. The role of the HDL_3 cholesterol subfraction is less clear. Animal model studies have shown that increased levels of apolipoprotein AI are associated with a decrease in the development of vascular fatty streaks [74] whereas increased levels of apolipoprotein AII are associated with an increase in their development. In humans, an increase in apolipoprotein AII would be associated more with an increase in HDL_3 whereas an increase in apolipoprotein AI would be associated more with an increase in HDL_2 concentrations. It therefore remains possible that high levels of HDL_3, in contrast to HDL_2, are disadvantageous in terms of CHD risk.

The relationship between HDL cholesterol and insulin-stimulated glucose uptake appears to be independent of plasma triglyceride levels [75,76]. Patients with high triglycerides and low HDL cholesterol tend to exhibit other metabolic abnormalities, such as increased overall and abdominal adiposity, and elevated fasting and post-glucose insulin levels [68]. In contrast, patients with high plasma triglycerides and normal HDL cholesterol do not exhibit other features of the insulin resistance syndrome, except for obesity. These observations support the concept that the combination of hypertriglyceridemia and low HDL cholesterol is an insulin resistant state, and that various mechanisms govern the relationship between these factors. The association between hepatic insulin metabolism and HDL_2 cholesterol suggests that hepatic lipase activity may be important [77]. This is supported by reports of increased hepatic lipase activity in insulin-resistant states [78,79].

The size of the LDL particle appears to be important in the pathogenesis of atherosclerosis. Patients with CHD, and particularly female patients, have an increased proportion of small dense LDL compared with healthy controls [80]. These smaller denser LDL particles are more atherogenic, perhaps because they are more readily cleared through scavenger mechanisms rather than by the $apoB_{100}$ receptors, and also because they may be more susceptible to oxidative damage [81]. Small dense LDL are found in individuals with raised triglycerides and low HDL [82] and are a feature of the metabolic syndrome [82].

There has been some debate as to whether hypercholesterolemia per se is an insulin resistant state. Patients with combined hyperlipoproteinemia have impaired glucose tolerance and higher fasting and post-glucose insulin levels, compared to normocholesterolemic subjects matched for other confounding factors [83]. However, patients with familial or non-familial hypercholesterolemia do not exhibit disturbances of insulin-mediated glucose uptake, nor suppression of free fatty acids during the euglycemic clamp [84]. This vies against the concept of hypercholesterolemia as an insulin resistant state.

Endothelial dysfunction

It is currently thought that endothelial dysfunction is the earliest antecedent of atherosclerosis. Signs of endothelial dysfunction can been observed in patients with CHD [85-87], hypercholesterolemia [88,89], diabetes mellitus [90], hypertension [91] and obesity.

The relationship between endothelial function and the metabolic syndrome is ill understood. It is well established, however, that insulin has a vasodilatory action [92] which is independent of its metabolic effects [93-95]. In addition, insulin causes sympathetic system activation, and promotes tissue capillarization and vascular conductivity. On this basis, the hypothesis has emerged that insulin normally promotes its own delivery into its target compartments, such as skeletal muscle. It has also been considered that, in a state of resistance to the vasodilatory actions of insulin, there may be reduced delivery of insulin to its target tissue and a resultant impairment of its metabolic actions. In this respect, it is noteworthy that endothelial denudation abolishes insulin-mediated vasodilation in aortic rings [96]. Furthermore, in healthy individuals insulin-stimulated blood flow correlates with nitric oxide-dependent blood flow [97]. Other studies have shown that insulin-induced blood flow responses are abolished by N^G-monomethyl-L-arginine (L-NMMA) [98-101]. These data indicate that insulin is an endothelium-dependent vasoactive agent, acting through endothelial nitric oxide synthesis-dependent pathways. We have recently shown that in healthy individuals forearm blood flow increases after intravenous glucose administration and that this response is paradoxically reduced in patients with CHD [102]. Although this evidence adds to the increasing recognition that endothelial dysfunction is associated with changes in insulin and glucose metabolism, it does not clarify whether this association is cause or effect.

Obesity

It has long been recognized that obesity is an insulin resistant state which frequently coexists with impaired glucose tolerance and hyperinsulinemia [103,104]. There is an increasing recognition that accumulation of fat in the abdominal region, in particular around the viscera, is more strongly associated with metabolic abnormalities than overall body obesity [105], although a degree of obesity is required for the expression of this relationship [106]. The android fat distribution is typical of the male whereas the gynoid fat distribution, particularly around the hips, thighs and buttocks, is typical of the female. In a study of over 100 healthy men, we found that android fat rather than overall adiposity was associated with adverse metabolic changes such as lower HDL_2 cholesterol, higher triglycerides, and increased insulin resistance [107], and hence with increased CHD risk. In a further study of non-obese men with CHD, they had higher proportions of android fat than matched healthy controls [108]. It may be that android obesity is also a CHD risk factor for women. Loss of ovarian hormones at the menopause results in a redistribution of body fat towards the male pattern with a relative increase in the proportion of android fat and a relative decrease in the proportion of fat in the female gynoid distribution [109]. This redistribution of body fat would therefore be expected to be associated with an increase in CHD risk.

The strong association between increasing visceral fat and metabolic abnormalities may relate to the fact that visceral fat has a higher lipolytic activity and lipid uptake, both of which increase fatty acid flux to the liver [110].

Hemostasis

The hemostatic system is a dynamic system which is designed to provide immediate clot formation at the site of hemorrhage whilst at the same time preventing intravascular clot formation. This is achieved by balances between coagulation and fibrinolysis which are in turn achieved by complex interplays between pro-thrombotic and anti-thrombotic factors and pro-fibrinolytic and anti-fibrinolytic factors. Since the recognition by Morris [111] in 1951 that an increase in the prevalence of CHD coincided with a disproportionately low prevalence of advanced atheroma, it has become apparent that CHD involves factors other than atherogenesis. Early reports of a beneficial effect of aspirin in the secondary prevention of myocardial infarction [112] have been supported by the findings of recent, large-scale mortality studies. It is now well recognized that acute thrombosis plays a critical role in the pathogenesis of unstable angina and myocardial infarction.

Of particular interest in CHD pathogenesis are the clotting factors VII and fibrinogen. Cross-sectional and prevalence studies have shown a higher factor VII levels in patients with CHD compared to controls. In addition, high serum levels of factor VII are predictive of CHD mortality [113] and recurrence of CHD events [114]. There is also a positive association between plasma fibrinogen levels and the onset and severity of peripheral vascular disease [115], and the stenosis rate of vein coronary bypass grafts [116]. With regard to fibrinolysis, elevated levels of plasminogen activator inhibitor-1 (PAI-1) have been reported in survivors of acute myocardial infarction and in patients with angiographical evidence of CHD [117,118]. In addition, plasma levels of PAI-1 correlate with the incidence of reinfarction in men [118,119].

Evidence is accumulating for a link between hemostatic and fibrinolytic factors and the insulin resistance syndrome. Recently, insulin levels have been shown to correlate positively with levels of factor VII antigen and activity in healthy individuals [120]. Insulin has been shown to stimulate the synthesis of PAI-1, and insulin sensitivity is inversely related to PAI-1 levels. In a study of 45 healthy men, we have recently shown that factor VII and PAI-1, as well as factor X and fibrinogen, correlate with plasma insulin levels [121]. In accord with the known ability of insulin to stimulate hepatic and endothelial PAI-1 release, the association between PAI-1 and insulin levels appears to be particularly strong [121].

Elevated serum uric acid

Gout, the principal disorder of urate metabolism, is associated with obesity [122,123], hypertension [124,125], hypertriglyceridemia [126-128], dyslipidemias [124,129,130] and, in some but not all studies, with diabetes mellitus [129,131]. Although the epidemiology of hyperuricemia is different to that of gout, it has similar cardiovascular associations. Elevated serum uric acid levels are associated with CHD and its metabolic risk factors, including glucose intolerance and hyperinsulinemia [46,124,132-135] and dyslipidemia [136,137].

Hyperuricemia is well established as a risk factor in the field of cardiovascular disease. However, most studies of uric acid in relation to cardiovascular disease have not examined why and how hyperuricemia develops. The observation that serum uric acid levels correlate with the plasma insulin response to an oral glucose challenge [136,138,139] has suggested that hyperinsulinemia may be an important contributor. In this respect, Ferrannini's group have recently shown that hyperinsulinemia acutely reduces urinary uric acid excretion [140]. However, this study did not include an assessment of uric acid production, and therefore no conclusions can be made as to whether the mechanism of hyperuricemia in hyperinsulinemic states relates to decreased renal excretion or to increased uric acid production.

Other mechanisms may be responsible for the hyperuricemia of the insulin resistance syndrome. Xanthine oxidase, which generates uric acid, is present in the microvasculature and in the heart [141,142], as well as in the liver [143]. Coronary artery-to-coronary sinus gradients of uric acid concentrations, indicating increased production, have been shown to occur in patients with CHD [144,145]. If xanthine oxidase is present in the capillary endothelium, processes that lead to endothelial cell injury might also be expected to lead to increased microvascular production of urate. This possibility has not been addressed in relation to the endothelial damage that accompanies cardiovascular disease. However, in pre-eclampsia, which is a microvascular disorder, serum urate levels correlate with circulating thrombomodulin levels [146]. In keeping with a link between endothelial cell activation and microvascular production of urate is our finding that chronic heart failure is a hyperuricemic condition in which circulating uric acid correlates with circulating interleukin-6, soluble tumor necrosis factor receptor-1 and -2, soluble intercellular adhesion molecule-1 (ICAM-1) and E-selectin [147]. These findings suggest that in certain situations the vascular endothelium is a focus for elevations in serum uric acid and a rise in the circulating markers of endothelial injury.

Hyperuricemia may in certain circumstances reflect a generalized derangement of endothelial cell metabolism, integrity and function. According to this hypothesis, hypoxia and/or insulin resistance lead activation of xanthine oxidase. Free radicals thus released cause an impairment of vascular function and immune activation in the vicinity of endothelial cells. This process is accompanied by upregulation of cytokine receptors, and release of pro-inflammatory cytokines and intercellular adhesion molecules into the circulation. These speculations offer a plausible explanation for the association of hyperuricemia with atherosclerosis and components of the metabolic syndrome.

Elevated plasma leptin levels

Plasma concentrations of the peptide leptin, a product of the *ob* gene, are directly related to body fat content [148-150]. There is evidence to suggest that hyperleptinemia in obese individuals reflects leptin resistance [149,150]. The finding of considerable inter-individual variations in plasma leptin levels amongst individuals with comparable degrees of obesity [151] suggests that factors other than adiposity influence the regulation of leptin production. A possible involvement of insulin is suggested by the finding that short-term [152] and long-term [153] hyperinsulinemia increases *ob* gene expression in mice. In humans, insulin is known to stimulates *ob* gene expression, but acute changes in plasma insulin do not increase plasma leptin concentrations [154-158]. Prolonged insulin infusions, however, appear to promote hyperleptinemia [157,159]. Other studies suggest that plasma leptin levels are inversely related to insulin sensitivity [160], whilst a positive correlation between plasma leptin and both fasting insulin and insulin sensitivity has been demonstrated by others [161,162]. Prominent amongst the links between leptin, adiposity and insulin are reports of mutations of the *ob* gene leading non-insulin dependent diabetes mellitus in obese *ob/ob* mice [163].

Pivotal abnormalities of the metabolic syndrome

Insulin resistance

Although insulin resistance has been considered as the key metabolic disturbance of the metabolic syndrome, its role in the coordination of the syndrome is based on small-scale experimental studies. Within the expanded definition of the syndrome, it is too early to assume that such is the case.

Leptin

Plasma leptin concentrations might constitute an additional and even pivotal component of the metabolic syndrome [40,164-166]. In a recent study, we have shown that inter-individual variations in plasma leptin concentrations are strongly related to the components of metabolic syndrome [40]. An important finding from this study was that plasma leptin levels were predominately related to both fasting and post-glucose insulin concentrations, suggesting that the insulin-leptin axis play a coordinating role in the expression of the metabolic syndrome.

Glycolytic metabolism

The possibility arises that glycolytic disturbances may be central to the expression of the metabolic syndrome [167] (Figure 1). This might be expected from the fact that uric acid production is linked to glycolysis, and that glycolysis is controlled by insulin. Phosphoribosyl pyrophosphate may be an important metabolite in this respect. Diversion of glycolytic intermediates towards ribose-5-phosphate, phosphoribosyl pyrophosphate and uric acid may occur if there is a reduction in the activity of glyceraldehyde-3-phosphate dehydrogenase (GA3PDH), a key glycolytic enzyme which is regulated by insulin. As a result, triglyceride production may also rise, as might be expected from accumulation of glycerol-3-phosphate. Thus, in this context, loss of the responsiveness of GA3PDH to insulin and a resultant accumulation of glycolytic intermediates may explain the association between insulin resistance, hyperuricemia and hypertriglyceridemia. This hypothesis has not been tested. Nevertheless the possibility that disturbances of a single glycolytic enzyme may be pivotal in the modulation of metabolic risk factors for CHD remains unresolved.

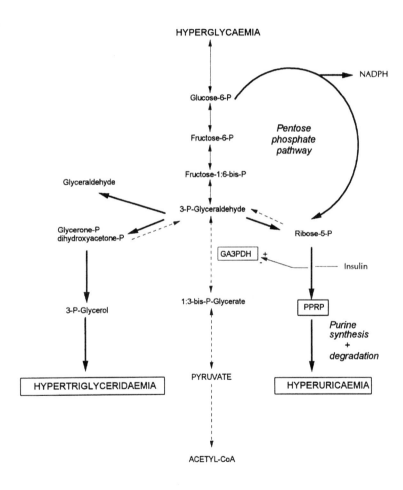

Figure 1. Possible consequences of decreased activity of glyceraldehyde-3-phosphate dehydrogenase. GA3PDH = glyceraldehyde-3-phosphate dehydrogenase, PPRP = phosphoribosyl pyrophosphate, P = phosphate.

Genes

Several genetic polymorphisms have been implicated in CHD risk. The DD genotype of the insertion deletion (I/D) polymorphism of the angiotensin 1-converting enzyme (ACE) gene been linked to a greater risk of CHD in several studies [168-173]. This finding may be considered in the context that NIDDM, an insulin resistant state, is associated with elevated plasma ACE levels [174,175] and that some ACE inhibitors improve insulin sensitivity [176,177]. Using intravenous glucose tolerance tests, we have recently shown that the I/D polymorphism of the ACE gene modulates insulin sensitivity and serum urate in healthy Caucasian white men [178]. This may be of pathogenetic importance in the increased risk of coronary heart disease associated with this genotype.

Several groups have reported an interaction on CHD risk between the I/D polymorphism of the ACE gene and the M235T polymorphism of the angiotensinogen (AGT) gene [179-181]. Moreover, the Trp64Arg polymorphism of the $_3$-adrenenoceptor gene has been shown to modulate insulin and glucose levels and adiposity [182,183]. These observations have paralleled the finding that Pima Indians, who are homozygous for the Trp64Arg $_3$-adrenenoceptor mutation, have an earlier onset of non-insulin dependent diabetes mellitus [184]. Another relevant genetic influence relates to the polymorphism of the apolipoprotein E 2/ 3/ 4 gene, which appears to modulate the strength of the relationship between insulin levels and triglyceride levels [185].

So far, no single gene has been identified as being responsible for the metabolic syndrome, though findings such as the above suggest some of its components have a genetic basis. However, it must be appreciated that an understanding of the pathogenetic mechanisms, rather than the genetic mechanisms, underlying the basis of the metabolic syndrome is more essential to clinical practice.

Coronary heart disease and the metabolic syndrome in women

Several aspects of cardiovascular disease are gender-related (Table 3). Cardiovascular disease is the most common cause of morbidity and mortality in postmenopausal women, with approximately 50% developing CHD in their lifetime, 30% dying from the disease and 20% developing a stroke [186-188].

The age-independent increase in CHD which is associated with the menopause [189-193] is paralleled by metabolic disturbances similar to those found in men. The observation that diabetic women have a higher incidence of CHD than diabetic men [35] is in keeping with the notion that the central metabolic disturbance of diabetes, namely insulin resistance, may be particularly important in women. In fact, most metabolic risk factors for CHD in women have now been linked to estrogen deficiency [73]. Protein glycosylation is a possible mechanism linking elevated glucose levels with CHD in diabetics, but the increased risk seen in those with lesser degrees of glucose tolerance are likely to be mediated through insulin resistance and hyperinsulinemia.

Table 3. Gender differences in aspects of cardiovascular disease

---

Disease-related aspects
Atypical symptoms of MI more common, particularly in older women
Higher in-hospital mortality from MI [194,195]
More acute complications of MI [196-198], even after thrombolytic therapy [199,200]
More complications [201,202] and mortality [203] from coronary artery bypass grafting (CABG)
Lower rates of CABG patency and more likely to require a second CABG [204]
More women eventually develop hypertension [205]

Management-related aspects
Women with MI present later to hospital
Less likely to receive thrombolytic treatment, beta-blockers and aspirin206
More likely to be older, have hypertension, hypercholesterolemia and NIDDM when referred for percutaneous transluminal coronary angioplasty207
Less likely to be referred for exercise rehabilitation after MI

Reproduced with permission from Leyva F, Coats AJS. Practical Management of hypertension. Blackwell Science, 1998 (In press).

Metabolic syndrome and cardiac syndrome X

Hyperinsulinemia has also been implicated in the pathogenesis of cardiac syndrome X - angina, positive ECG exercise test but no atheromatous blockage on coronary angiography - a condition which may result in some cases from coronary vascular dysfunction. We have studied both non-obese males [108,208] and females [209] with cardiological syndrome X. The men demonstrated many features of the metabolic syndrome, including lower insulin sensitivity, lower HDL and HDL_2 cholesterol concentrations together with lower concentrations of apolipoprotein AI, higher fasting and post-challenge insulin concentrations, higher triglycerides, higher systolic blood pressure and increased proportions of android fat. The women appeared not to exhibit all the features of the insulin resistance syndrome. They did, however, have significantly lower insulin sensitivity, and lower HDL cholesterol and apolipoprotein AI and AII concentrations, and higher post-challenge insulin responses. No significant differences emerged with respect to body fat distribution, systolic blood pressure or PAI-1 concentrations.

Conclusions

Features of the metabolic syndrome are found in patients with both atherosclerotic and non-atherosclerotic CHD, as well as in those with heart failure. In patients with cardiac syndrome X there may be a variable expression of the syndrome, consistent with underlying heterogeneity in the pathogenesis of cardiac syndrome X. The fact that similar metabolic disturbances may be seen in both atheromatous CHD and cardiac syndrome X (where there is no obvious atheroma) might suggest that further abnormalities need to be superimposed on an adverse metabolic milieu in order to result in atherogenesis. Such further abnormalities could conceivably involve processes such as endothelial function and vascular remodeling. The results of prospective population studies regarding an association between insulin resistance and CHD are still somewhat inconclusive, and studies incorporating true measures of insulin resistance are needed to clarify this issue.

There are currently no generally available therapies for improving insulin resistance, perhaps with the exception of certain hormone replacement therapies (HRT) in postmenopausal women. Whether new compounds, such as thiazolodinediones or imidazoline receptor agonists, will prove useful in modifying the metabolic syndrome remains to be seen.

References

1. Reaven GM. Banting Lecture: role of insulin resistance in human disease. Diabetes 1988;37:1595-607.
2. Kemp HG. Left ventricular function in patients with the anginal syndrome and normal coronary arteriograms. Am J Cardiol 1973;32:375-76.
3. Rose GA. CHD risk factors as a basis for screening. In: Oliver M, Ashley-Miller M, Wood D, eds. Screening for risk of coronary heart disease. Chichester: John Wiley & Sons, 1987:11-16.
4. Godsland IF, Stevenson JC. Insulin resistance: syndrome or tendency? Lancet 1995;346:100-3.
5. Yip J, Facchini FS, Reaven GM. Resistance to insulin-mediated glucose disposal as a predictor of cardiovascular disease. J Clin Endocrinol Metab 1998;83:2773-76.
6. Taskinen M-R. Strategies for the diagnosis of the metabolic syndrome. Curr Opin Lipidol 1993;4:434-43.
7. Jarrett RJ. The epidemiology of coronary heart disease and related factors in the context of diabetes mellitus and impaired glucose tolerance. In: Jarrett RJ, ed. Diabetes and heart disease. Amsterdam: Elsevier, 1984:1-24.
8. Pyorälä K, Laakso M, Uusitupa M. Diabetes and atherosclerosis: an epidemiologic view. Diabetes Metab Rev 1987;3:463-524.
9. Panzram G. Mortality and survival in type 2 (non-insulin-dependent) diabetes mellitus. Diabetologia 1987;30:123-31.
10. Pan W-H, Cedres LB, Liu K, et al. Relationship of clinical diabetes and asymptomatic hyperglycemia to risk of coronary heart disease mortality in men and women. Am J Epidemiol 1986;123:504-16.
11. Fontbonne A, Charles MA, Thibult N, et al. Hyperinsulinemia as a predictor of coronary heart disease mortality in a healthy population: the Paris Prospective Study, 15-year follow-up. Diabetologia 1991;34:356-61.
12. Weidmann P. Hypertension and diabetes. In: Kaplan N, ed. Metabolic aspects of hypertension. London: Science Press, 1994:2.1-2.23.
13. Weidmann P, Boehlen LM, de Courten M. Pathogenesis and treatment of hypertension associated with diabetes mellitus. Am Heart J 1993;125:1498-1513.
14. Simonsson DC. Etiology and prevalence of hypertension in diabetic patients. Diabetes Care 1988;11:821-27.
15. Turner RC, Mann J, Oakes S, et al. United Kingdom Prospective Diabetes Study, a multicenter study. Hypertension 1985;7 (Suppl II):8-13.
16. Tarnow L, Rossing P, Gall M, et al. Prevalence of arterial hypertension in diabetic patients after the JNC-V. Diabetes Care 1994;17:1247-51.
17. Krolewski AS, Warram JH, Cupples A, Gorman CK, Szabo AJ, Christlieb AR. Hypertension, orthostatic hypotension and the microvascular complications of diabetes. J Chron Dis 1985;38:319-26.
18. Ferrannini E, Natali A. Hypertension, insulin resistance and diabetes. In: Swales J, ed. Textbook of hypertension. London, Edinburgh, Boston, Melbourne, Paris, Berlin, Vienna: Blackwell Scientific Publications, 1994:785-97.
19. Morrish NJ, Stevens LK, Head J, et al. A prospective study of mortality among middle-aged diabetic patients (the London cohort of the WHO Multinational Study of Vascular Disease in Diabetics.) II: Associated risk factors. Diabetologia 1990;33:542-48.
20. Stamler J, Vaccaro O, Neaton JD, Wentworth D. Diabetes, other risk factors, and 12-yr cardiovascular mortality for men screened in the multiple risk factor intervention trial. Diabetes Care 1993;16:434-44

21. Giles TD, Sander GE. Myocardial disease in hypertensive-diabetic patients. Am J Med 1989;87 (Suppl 6A):235-85.
22. Kannel WB, McGee DL. Diabetes and cardiovascular risk factors: The Framingham study. Circulation 1979;59:8-13.
23. Fuller JH, Shipley MJ, Rose G, Jarrett RJ, Keen H. Mortality from coronary heart disease and stroke in relation to degree of glycemia: the Whitehall Study. Br Med J 1983;287:867-70.
24. Van Hoeven K, Factor S. A comparison of the pathological spectrum of hypertensive, diabetic, and hypertensive-diabetic heart disease. Circulation 1990;82:848-55.
25. Klein R, Klein BEK, Moss SE, et al. Is blood pressure a predictor of the incidence or progression of diabetic retinopathy? Arch Intern Med 1989;149:2427-32.
26. Rubler S, Dlugash J, Yuceoglu YZ, al et. New type of cardiomyopathy associated with diabetic glomerulosclerosis. Am J Cardiol 1972;30:595-602.
27. Kannel WB, McNamara PM, Feinlieb M, et al. The unrecognized myocardial infarction: 14 year follow-up experience in the Framingham study. Geriatrics 1970;25:75-8
28. Blumenthal HT, Alex M, Goldenbert S. A study of lesions of the intramural coronary artery branches in diabetes mellitus. Arch Pathol 1960;70:27-42.
29. Waller BF, Palumbo PJ, Lie JT, Roberts WC. Status of the coronary arteries at necropsy in diabetes mellitus with onset after age 30 years: Analysis of 229 diabetic patients with and without clinical evidence of coronary heart disease and comparison of 183 control subjects. Am J Med 1980;69:498-506.
30. Woods KL, Samanta A, Burden AC. Diabetes mellitus as a risk factor for acute myocardial infarction in Asians and Europeans. Br Heart J 1989;62:118-22.
31. Turner RC, Neil HAW, Stratton IM, et al. Risk factors for coronary artery disease in non-insulin dependent diabetes mellitus: United Kingdom prospective diabetes study (UKPDS:23). Br Med J 1998;316:823-28.
32. Rennert G, Saltz-Rennert H, Wanderman K, Weitzman S. Size of acute myocardial infarct in patients with diabetes mellitus. Am J Cardiol 1985;55:1629-30.
33. Stone PH, Muller JE, Hartwell T, et al. The effect of diabetes mellitus on prognosis and serial left ventricular function after acute myocardial infarction: contribution of both coronary disease and diastolic left ventricular dysfunction to adverse prognosis. J Am Coll Cardiol 1989;14:49-57.
34. Smith JW, Marcus FI, Serokman R. Prognosis of patients with diabetes mellitus after acute myocardial infarction. Am J Cardiol 1984;54:718-21
35. Abbott RD, Donahue RP, Kannel WB, Wilson PF. The impact of diabetes on survival following myocardial infarction in men vs women. The Framingham Study. J Am Med Assoc 1988;260:3456-60.
36. Vigorita VJ, Moore GW, Hutchins GM. Absence of correlation between coronary arterial atherosclerosis and severity or duration of diabetes mellitus of adult onset. Am J Cardiol 1980;46:535-42.
37. Hara-Nakamura N, Kohara K, Suminoto T, Lin M, Hiwada K. Glucose intolerance exaggerates left ventricular hypertrophy and dysfunction in essential hypertension. Am J Hypertens 1994;7:1110-14.
38. Reaven GM. Role of insulin resistance in human disease (Syndrome X): an expanded definition. Ann Rev Med 1993;44:121-31.
39. Frayn KN. Insulin resistance and lipid metabolism. Curr Opin Lipidol 1993;4:197-204.
40. Leyva F, Godsland IF, Ghatei M, et al. Hyperleptinemia as a component of a metabolic syndrome of cardiovascular risk. Arterioscl Thromb Vasc Biol 1998;18:928-33.
41. Després J-P, Marette A. Relation of components of insulin resistance syndrome to coronary disease risk. Curr Opin Lipidol 1994;5:274-89.
42. Welborn TA, Breckenridge A, Rubinstein AH, Dollery CT, Fraser TR. Serum insulin in essential hypertension and in peripheral vascular disease. Lancet 1966;i:1336-37.
43. Rose HG, Yalow RS, Schweitzer P, Schwartz E. Insulin as a potential factor influencing blood pressure in amputees. Hypertension 1986;8:793-800.
44. Fournier AM, Gadia MT, Kubrusly DB, Skyler JS, Sosenko JM. Blood pressure, insulin and glycemia in non-diabetic subjects. Am J Med 1986;80:861-64.
45. Schroll M, Hagerup L. Relationship of fasting blood glucose to prevalence of ECG abnormalities in men born in 1914: from the Gloserup population studies. J Chron Dis 1979;32:699-707.
46. Modan M, Halkin H, Almog S, et al. Hyperinsulinemia - a link between hypertension, obesity and glucose intolerance. J Clin Invest 1985;75:809-17.

47. Reaven GM, Hoffman BB. A role for insulin in the etiology and course of hypertension? Lancet 1987;ii:435-37.
48. Lucas CP, Estigarriba JA, Darga LL, Reaven GM. Insulin and blood pressure. Hypertension 1985;7:702-6.
49. Berglund G, Larsson B, Anderson O, et al. Body composition and glucose metabolism in hypertensive middle-aged males. Acta Med Scand 1976;200:163-69.
50. Bonora E, Zavaroni I, Alpi O, et al. Relationship between blood pressure and plasma insulin in non-obese and obese non-diabetic subjects. Diabetologia 1987;30:719-23.
51. Howard G, O'Leary DH, Zaccaro D, et al. Insulin sensitivity and atherosclerosis. The Insulin Resistance Atherosclerosis Study (IRAS) Investigators. Circulation 1996;93:1809-17.
52. Hosoi M, Nishizawa Y, Kogawa K, et al. Angiotensin-converting enzyme gene polymorphism is associated with carotid arterial wall thickness in non-insulin-dependent diabetic patients. Circulation 1996;94:704-7.
53. Pyörälä M, Miettinen H, Laakso M, Pyörälä K. Hyperinsulinemia predicts coronary heart disease risk in healthy middle-aged males. Circulation 1998;98:398-404.
54. Pyörälä K, Savolainen E, Kaukola S, Haapakoski J. Plasma insulin as coronary heart disease risk factor: relationship to other risk factors and predictive value during 91/2 year follow-up of the Helsinki Policemen Study population. Acta Med Scand 1985;701 (Suppl):38-52.
55. Ducimetière P, Eschwege E, Papoz L, Richard JL, Claude JR, Rosselin G. Relationship of plasma insulin levels to the incidence of myocardial infarction and coronary heart disease in a middle-aged population. Diabetologia 1980;19:205-10.
56. Welborn TA, Wearne K. Coronary heart disease incidence and cardiovascular mortality in Busselton with reference to glucose and insulin concentrations. Diabetes Care 1979;2:154-60.
57. Jarrett RJ, McCartney P, Keen H. The Bedford Survey: ten year mortality rates in newly diagnosed diabetics, borderline diabetics and normoglycemic controls and risk for coronary heart disease in borderline diabetics. Diabetologia 1982;22:79-84.
58. Donahue RP, Orchard TJ, Becker DJ, Kuller LH, Drash AL. Sex differences in the coronary heart disease risk profile: a possible role for insulin. Am J Epidemiol 1987;125:650-7.
59. Stout RW. Insulin and atheroma: 20-yr perspective. Diabetes Care 1990;13:631-54.
60. Leyva F, Godsland IF, Worthington M, Walton C, Stevenson JC. Factors of the metabolic syndrome. Baseline interrelationships in the first follow-up cohort of the HDDRISC study (HDDRISC-1). Arterioscl Thromb Vasc Biol 1998;18:208-214.
61. Swan JW, Anker SD, Walton C, et al. Insulin resistance in chronic heart failure: relation to severity and etiology of heart failure. J Am Coll Cardiol 1997;30:527-32.
62. Swan JW, Walton C, Godsland IF, Clark AL, Coats AJS, Oliver MF. Insulin resistance in heart failure. Eur Heart J 1994;15:1528-32.
63. Leyva F, Anker SD, Chua T-P, Godsland IF, Stevenson JC, Coats AJS. Muscle strength is related to insulin sensitivity and serum uric acid in chronic heart failure [abstract]. Heart Failure 1997. Cologne, Germany: Working Group of the European Society of Cardiology, 1997:P100.
64. Stout R W, Vallence-Owen J. Insulin and atheroma. Lancet 1969;i:1078-80.
65. Båvenholm P, Proudler A, Tornvall P, et al. Insulin, intact and split proinsulin and coronary artery disease in young men. Circulation 1995; 92: 1422-29.
66. Proudler AJ, Godsland IF, Stevenson JC. Insulin propeptides and conditions associated with insulin resistance in humans and their relevance to insulin measurements. Metabolism 1994;43:446-49.
67. Winocour PH, Kaluvya S, Ramaiya K, et al. Relation between insulinemia, body mass index, and lipoprotein composition in healthy, non-diabetic men and women. Arterioscler Thromb 1992;12:393-402.
68. Walton C, Godsland IF, Proudler AJ, Felton CV, Wynn V. Effect of body mass index and fat distribution on insulin sensitivity, secretion and clearance in nonobese, healthy men. J Clin Endocrinol Metab 1992;75:170-5.
69. Howard BV. Insulin, insulin resistance, and dyslipidemia. Ann N Y Acad Sci 1993;683:1-9.
70. Knight TM, Smith Z, Whittles A, et al. Insulin resistance, diabetes, and risk markers for ischemic heart disease in Asian men and non-Asian men in Bradford. Br Heart J 1992;67:343-50.
71. Srinivasan SR, Bao W, Berenson GS. Coexistence of increased levels of adiposity, insulin, and blood pressure in a young adult cohort with elevated very-low-density-lipoprotein cholesterol: the Bogalusa Heart Study. Metabolism 1993;42:170-76.

72. Miller NE. Associations of high-density lipoprotein subclasses and apolipoproteins with ischemic heart disease and coronary atherosclerosis. Am Heart J 1987;113:589-97.
73. Stevenson JC, Crook D, Godsland IF. Influence of age and menopause on serum lipids and lipoproteins in healthy women. Atherosclerosis 1993;98:83-90.
74. Rubin EM, Krauss RM, Spangler EA, Verstuyft JG, Clift SM. Inhibition of early atherogenesis in transgenic mice by human apolipoprotein AI. Nature 1991;353:265-67.
75. Abbott WHG, Lillioja S, Young AA. Relationships between plasma lipoprotein concentrations and insulin action in an obese hyperinsulinemic population. Diabetes 1987;36:897-904.
76. Laakso M, Sarlund H, Mykkänen L. Insulin resistance is associated with lipid and lipoprotein abnormalities in subjects with varying degrees of glucose intolerance. Arteriosclerosis 1990;10:223-31.
77. Godsland IF, Crook D, Walton C, Wynn V, Oliver MF. Influence of insulin resistance, secretion, and clearance on serum cholesterol, triglycerides, lipoprotein cholesterol, and blood pressure in healthy men. Arterioscler Thromb 1992;12:1030-5.
78. Kasim SE, Tseng K, Jen C, Khilnani S. Significance of hepatic triglyceride lipase activity in the regulation of serum high-density lipoproteins in type II diabetes mellitus. J Clin Endocrinol Metab 1987;65:183-87.
79. Baynes C, Henderson AD, Anyaoku V, et al. The role of insulin insensitivity and hepatic lipase in the dyslipidemia of type 2 diabetes. Diabetic Med 1991;8:560-66.
80. Austin MA, Breslow JL, Hennekens CH, Buring JE, Willett WC, Krauss RM. Low-density lipoprotein subclass patterns and risk of myocardial infarction. J Am Med Assoc 1988;260:1917-21.
81. Tribble DL, Holl LG, Wood PD, Krauss RM. Variations in oxidative susceptibility among six low-density lipoprotein subfractions of differing density and particle size. Atherosclerosis 1992;93:189-99.
82. Reaven GM, Chen YDI, Jeppesen J, Maheux P, Krauss RM. Insulin resistance and hyperinsulinemia in individuals with small, dense, low density lipoprotein particles. J Clin Invest 1993;92:141-146.
83. Paolisso G, Ferrannini E, Sgambato S, Varrichio M, D'Onofrio F. Hyperinsulinemia in patients with hypercholesterolemia. J Clin Endocrinol Metab 1992;75:1409-12.
84. Karphapää P, Voutilainen E, Kovanen PT, Laakso M. Insulin resistance in familial and non-familial hypercholesterolemia. Arterioscler Thromb 1993;13:41-47.
85. Sanz G, Castaner A, Betriu A, al et. Determinants of prognosis in survivors of myocardial infarction. A prospective clinical and angiographic study. N Eng J Med 1982;306:1065-70.
86. El-Tamimi H, Mansour M, Wargovich TJ, al et. Constrictor and dilator responses to intracoronary acetylcholine in adjacent segments of the same coronary artery in patients with coronary artery disease. Endothelial function revisited. Circulation 1994;12:56-62.
87. Reddy KG, Nair RN, Sheehan HM, Hodgson JMcB. Evidence that selective endothelial dysfunction may occur in the absence of angiographic or ultrasound atherosclerosis in patients with risk factors for atherosclerosis. J Am Coll Cardiol 1994;23:833-43.
88. Drexler H, Zeiher AM. Endothelial function in human coronary arteries in vivo. Focus on hypercholesterolemia. Hypertension 1991;18:II-90-II-99.
89. Egashira K, Hirooka Y, Kai H, al et. Reduction in serum cholesterol with pravastatin improves endothelium-dependent coronary vasomotion in patients with hypercholesterolemia. Circulation 1994;89:2519-24.
90. McVeigh GE, Brennan GM, Johnston DG, et al. Impaired endothelium-dependent and independent vasodilation in patients with type 2 (non-insulin-dependent) diabetes mellitus. Diabetologia 1992;35:771-6.
91. Vita JA, Treasure CB, Nabel EG, al et. Coronary vasomotor response to acetylcholine relates to risk factors for coronary artery disease. Circulation 1990;81:491-7.
92. Baron AD. Hemodynamic actions of insulin. Am J Physiol 1994;267:E187-E202.
93. Vollenweider P, Tappy L, Randin D, et al. Differential effects of hyperinsulinemia and carbohydrate metabolism on sympathetic nerve activity and muscle blood flow in humans. J Clin Invest 1993;92:147-54.
94. Mäkimattila S, Virkamäki A, Malmström R, et al. Insulin resistance in type 1 diabetes: a major role for reduced glucose extraction. J Clin Endocrinol Metab 1996;81:707-712.
95. McNulty PH, Pfau S. Insulin stimulates myocardial blood flow in humans by a direct effect within the coronary circulation. Circulation 1997;96:I-379.

96. Wu H-Y, Jeng Y-Y, Yue C-J, Chyu K-Y, Hsueh WA, Chan TM. Endothelial dependent vascular effects of insulin and insulin-like growth factor 1 in the perfused rat mesenteric artery and aortic ring. Diabetes 1994;43:1027-32.

97. Utrianen T, Mäkimattila S, Virkamäki A, Lindholm H, Sovijärvi A, Yri-Järvinen H. Physical fitness and endothelial function (nitric oxide synthesis) are independent determinants of insulin-stimulated blood flow in normal subjects. J Clin Endocrinol Metab 1996;81:4258-63.

98. Steinberg HO, Brechtel G, Johnson A, Fineberg N, Baron AD. Insulin-mediated skeletal muscle vasodilation is nitric oxide dependent. A novel action of insulin to increase nitric oxide release. J Clin Invest 1994;94:1172-79.

99. Scherrer YU, Randin D, Vollenweider P, Vollenweider L, Nicod P. Nitric oxide release accounts for insulin's vascular effects in humans. J Clin Invest 1994;94:2511-15.

100. Steinberg HO, Brechtel G, Johnson A, Baron AD. Insulin modulates endothelium derived relaxing factor / nitric oxide dependent vasodilation in skeletal muscle. Hypertension Dallas 1993;22:74-436.

101. Cardillo C, Kilcoyne CM, Quyyumi AA, Cannon RO, Panza JA. Nitric oxide-dependent vasodilator response to systemic but not to local hyperinsulinemia in the human forearm [abstract]. Circulation 1997;96:I-101.

102. Leyva F, Rauchhaus M, Proudler AJ, et al. Non-invasive assessment of vascular function: paradoxical vascular response to glucose in coronary heart disease [abstract]. Heart 1998;79:20.

103. Rabinowitz D, Zierler KL. Forearm metabolism in obesity and its response to intra-arterial insulin. Characterization of insulin resistance and evidence for adaptive hyperinsulinism. J Clin Invest 1962;41:2173-81.

104. Karam JH, Grodsky GM, Forsham PH. Excessive insulin response to glucose in obese subjects as measured by immunochemical assay. Diabetes 1963;12:197-204.

105. Després J-P, Moorjani S, Lupien PJ, Tremblay A, Nadeau A, Bouchard C. Regional distribution of body fat, plasma lipoproteins, and cardiovascular disease. Arteriosclerosis 1990;10:497-511.

106. Pouliot MC, Després J-P, Nadeau A, et al. Associations with glucose tolerance, plasma insulin, and lipoprotein levels. Diabetes 1992;41:826-34.

107. Walton C, Lees B, Crook D, Worthington M, Godsland IF, Stevenson JC. Body fat distribution, rather than overall adiposity, influences serum lipids and lipoproteins in healthy men independently of age. Am J Med 1995;99:459-64.

108. Ley C J, Swan J, Godsland IF, Walton C, Crook D, Stevenson JC. Insulin resistance, lipoproteins, body fat and hemostasis in nonobese men with angina and a normal or abnormal coronary angiogram. J Am Coll Cardiol 1994;23:377-83.

109. Ley CJ, Lees B, Stevenson JC. Sex- and menopause-associated changes in body-fat distribution. Am J Clin Nutr 1992;55:950-4.

110. Mårin P, Anderson B, Ottosson M, et al. The morphology and metabolism of intra-abdominal adipose tissue in men. Metabolism 1992;41:1242-48.

111. Morris JN. Recent history of coronary heart disease. Lancet 1951;ii:1053-1057.

112. Elwood PC, Cochrane AL, Burr ML, al et. A randomized controlled trial of acetylsalicylic acid in the secondary prevention of mortality from myocardial infarction. Br Med J 1974;1:436-40.

113. Meade TW, Brozovic M, Chakrabarti RR, et al. Hemostatic function and ischemic heart disease: principal results of the Northwick Park Heart Study. Lancet 1986;ii:533-37.

114. Haines AP, Howard D, North WRS, et al. Hemostatic variables and the outcome of myocardial infarction. Thromb Haemost 1983;50:800-3.

115. Dormandy JA, Hoare E, Khattab AH, Arrowsmith DE, Dormandy TL. Prognostic significance of rheological and biochemical findings in patients with intermittent claudication. Br Med J 1973;4:581-83.

116. Wiseman S, Kenchington G, Dain R, et al. Influence of smoking and plasma factors on patency of femoropopliteal vein grafts. Br Med J 1989;299:643-46.

117. Paramo JA, Colucci M, Collen D, van der Werf F. Plasminogen activator inhibitor in the blood of patients with coronary artery disease. Br Med J 1985;291:575-76.

118. Mehta J, Mehta P, Lawson D, Saldeen T. Plasma tissue plasminogen activator inhibitor levels in coronary artery disease: correlation with age and serum triglyceride concentrations. J Am Coll Cardiol 1987;9:263-8.

119. Hamsten A, Wiman B, DeFaire U, Blombäck M. Increased plasma levels of a rapid inhibitor of tissue plasminogen activator in young survivors of myocardial infarction. N Engl J Med 1985;313:1557-63.

120. Kario K, Matsuo T, BKobayashi H, Sakata T, Miyata T, Shimada K. Gender differences of disturbed hemostasis related to fasting insulin level in healthy very elderly Japanese aged > or = 75 years. Atherosclerosis 1995;116:211-9.
121. Godsland IF, Sidhu M, Crook D, Stevenson JC. Coagulation and fibrinolytic factors, insulin resistance and the metabolic syndrome of coronary heart disease risk. Eur Heart J 1996;17 (suppl):331.
122. Grahame R, Scott JT. Clinical survey of 354 patients with gout. Ann Rheum Dis 1970;29:461-68.
123. Emmerson BT. Alteration of urate metabolism by weight reduction. Aust NZ J Med 1970;3:410-12.
124. Emerson BT. Abnormal urate excretion associated with renal and systemic disorders, drugs and toxins. In: Kelley W, ed. Uric acid (Handbook of Experimental Pharmacology vol 51.). Berlin, Heidelberg, NewYork: Springer, 1978:287-324.
125. Messerli FH, Fröhlich ED , Dreslinski GR, Suarez DH, Aristimuno GG. Serum uric acid in essential hypertension: an indicator of renal vascular involvement. Ann Int Med 1980;93:817-21.
126. Berkowitz D. Blood lipid and uric acid interrelationships. J Am Med Assoc 1966;190:856-58.
127. Friedman EB, Wallace SL. Hypertriglyceridemia in gout. Circulation 1964;29:508-11.
128. Barlow KA. Hyperlipidemia in primary gout. Metabolism 1968;17:289-99.
129. Wyngaarden JB, Kelley WN. Gout and hyperuricemia. New York: Grune & Stratton, Inc, 1976.
130. Yu T, Dorph DJ, Smith H. Hyperlipidemia in primary gout. Semin Arthritis Rheum 1978;38:698-701.
131. Herman JB, Gouldbourt U. Uric acid and diabetes: observations in a population study. Lancet 1982;II:240-43.
132. Beard JT. Serum uric acid and coronary heart disease. Am Heart J 1983;106:397-400.
133. Yano K, Rhoads CG, Kagan A. Epidemiology of serum uric acid among 8000 Japanese-American men in Hawaii. J Chron Dis 1977;30:171-84.
134. Bergman RN, Finegood DT, Ader M. Assessment of insulin sensitivity in vivo. Endocrine Rev 1985;6:45-86.
135. DeFronzo RA, Ferrannini E. The pathogenesis of non-insulin dependent diabetes: an update. Medicine 1982;61:125-40.
136. Abrams ME, Jarrett RJ, Keen H. Oral glucose tolerance and related factors in a normal population sample. II Interrelationships of glycerides, cholesterol and other factors with glucose and insulin response. Br Med J 1969;1:599-602.
137. Fox IH, John D, DeBruyne S, Dwosh I, Marliss EB. Hyperuricemia and hypertriglyceridemia: metabolic basis for the association. Metabolism 1985;34:741-46.
138. Reaven GM, Chen YDI, Donner CC, Fraze E. How insulin resistant are patients with insulin dependent diabetes mellitus? J Clin Endocrinol Metab 1985;61:32-36.
139. Modan M, Halkin H, Karasik A, Lusky A. Elevated serum uric acid - a facet of hyperinsulinemia. Diabetologia 1987;30:713-18.
140. Quiñones-Galvan A, Natali A, Baldi S, et al. Effect of insulin on uric acid excretion in humans. Am J Physiol 1995;268:E1-E5.
141. Watts RWE, Watts JEM, Seegmiller JE. Xanthine oxidase activity in human tissues and its inhibition by allopurinol (4-hydroxypyrazodol [3,4-d] pyrimidine). J Lab Clin Med 1965;66:688-97.
142. Wajner M, Harkness RA. Distribution of xanthine dehydrogenase and oxidase activitites in human and rabbit tissues. Biochim Biophys Acta 1988;991:79-84.
143. Hellsten-Westing Y. Immunohistochemical localization of xanthine oxidase in human cardiac and skeletal muscle. Histochemistry 1993;100:215-222.
144. Becker BF, Permanetter B, Richardt G, et al. Coronary sinus uric acid as an index of chronic myocardial ischemia in man. Second International Meeting of the Working Group on Heart Failure. Cologne: European Society of Cardiology, 1997:10.
145. DeScheerder IK, van de Kraay AM, Lamers JMJ, Koster JF, de Jong J, Serruys PW. Myocardial malondialdehyde and uric acid release after short-lasting coronary occlusion during coronary angioplasty: Potential mechanisms for free radical generation. Am J Cardiol 1991;68:392-95.
146. Hsu CD, Iriye B, Johnson TR, Witter FR, Hong SF, Chan DW. Elevated circulating thrombomodulin in severe pre-eclampsia [published erratum appears in Am J Obstet Gynecol 1994;174:1165]. Am J Obstet Gynecol 1993;169:148-49.
147. Leyva F, Anker SD, Godsland IF, et al. Hyperuricaemia in chronic heart failure: marker of a chronic inflammatory response? Eur Heart J 1998;(In press).
148. Frederich RC, Hamann A, Anderson S , Loellmann B, Lowell BB, Flier JS. Leptin levels reflect body lipid content in mice: evidence for diet-induced resistance to leptin action. Nature Med 1995;1:1311-14.

240

149. Lonnqvist F, Arner P, Nordfors L, Schalling M. Overexpression of the obese (ob) gene in adipose tissue of human obese subjects. Nature Med 1995;1:950-53.
150. Hamilton BS, Paglia D, Kwan AYM, Deitel M. Increased obese mRNA expression in omental fat cells from massively obese humans. Nature Med 1995;1:953-56.
151. Saad MF, Damani S, Gingerich ERL, et al. Sexual dimorphism in plasma leptin concentration. J Clin Endocrinol Metab 1997;82:579-84.
152. Saladin R, De Vos P, Guerro-Milo M, al et. Transient increase in obese gene expression after food intake or insulin administration. Nature 1995;377:527-29.
153. Cusin I, Sainsbury A, Doyle P, Rohner-Jeanrenaud B. The ob gene and insulin. A relationship leading to clues to the understanding of obesity. Diabetes 1995;44:1467-70.
154. Considine RV, Sinha MK, Heiman ML, al et. Serum immunoreactive leptin concentrations in normal-weight and obese humans. N Engl J Med 1996;334:292-95.
155. Sinha MK, Ohannesian JP, Heiman ML, al et. Nocturnal rise of leptin in lean, obese, and non-insulin-dependent diabetes mellitus subjects. J Clin Invest 1996;97:1344-47.
156. Dagogo-Jack S, Fanelli C, Paramore D, Brothers J, Landt M. Plasma leptin and insulin relationships in obese and nonobese humans. Diabetes 1996;45:695-98.
157. Kolaczynski JW, Nyce MR, Considine RV, al et. Acute and chronic effect of insulin on leptin production in humans. Studies in vivo and in vitro. Diabetes 1996;45:699-701.
158. Ryan AS, Elahi D. The effects of acute hyperglycemia and hyperinsulinemia on plasma leptin levels: its relationship with body fat, visceral adiposity, and age in women. J Clin Endocrinol Metab 1996;81:4433-38.
159. Malmstrom R, Taskinen MR, Karonen SL, Yki-Jarvinen H. Insulin increases plasma leptin concentrations in normal subjects and patients with NIDDM. Diabetologia 1996;39:993-96.
160. Segal KR, Landt M, Klein S. Relationship between insulin sensitivity and plasma leptin concentration in lean and obese men. Diabetes 1996;45:988-91.
161. Haffner SM, Miettinen H, Mykkänen L, Karhappää P, Rainwater DL, Laakso M. Leptin concentrations and insulin sensitivity in normoglycemic men. Int J Obes 1997;21:393-99.
162. Widjaja A, Stratton IM, Horn R, Holman RR, Turner R, Brabant G. UKPDS 20: plasma leptin, obesity, and plasma insulin in type 2 diabetic subjects. J Clin Endocrinol Metab 1997;82:654-57.
163. Zhang Y, Proenca R, Maffei M, Barone M, Leopold L, Friedman JM. Positional cloning of the mouse obese gene and its human monologue. Nature 1994;372:425-32.
164. de Courten M, Zimmet P, Hodge A, et al. Hyperletinaemia: The missing link in the metabolic syndrome. Diabetic Medicine 1996;14:200-8.
165. Hodge AM, Westerman RA, de Courten MP, Collier GR, Zimmet PZ, Alberti KGGM. Is leptin sensitivity the link between smoking cessation and weight gain? Int J Obes 1997;21:50-53.
166. Zimmet PZ, Collins VR, de Courten MP, et al. Is there a relationship between leptin and insulin sensitivity independent of obesity? A population-based study in the Indian Ocean nation of Mauritius. Int J Obes 1998;22:171-77.
167. Leyva F, Wingrove C, Godsland IF, Stevenson JC. The glycolytic pathway to coronary heart disease: A hypothesis. Metabolism 1998;47:657-62.
168. Cambien F, Poirier O, Lecerf L, et al. Deletion polymorphism in the gene for angiotensin-converting enzyme is a potent risk factor for myocardial infarction. Nature 1992;359:641-44.
169. Samani NJ, Thompson JR, O'Toole L, Channer K, Woods KL. A meta-analysis of the association of the deletion allele of the angiotensin-converting enzyme gene with myocardial infarction. Circulation 1996;94:708-12.
170. Evans AE, Poirier O, Kee F, et al. Polymorphisms of the angiotensin-converting enzyme gene in subjects who die from coronary heart disease. Q J Med 1994;87:211-14.
171. Mattu RK, Needham EWA, Galton DJ, Frangos E, Clark AJL, Caulfield M. A DNA variant of the angiotensin-converting enzyme gene locus associates with coronary heart disease in the Caerphilly Heart study. Circulation 1995;91:270-74.
172. Ludwig E, Corneli PS, Anderson JL, Marshall HW, Lalouel J-M, Ward RH. Angiotensin-converting enzyme gene polymorphism is associated with myocardial infarction but not with development of coronary stenosis. Circulation 1995;91:2120-24.
173. Beohar N, Damaraju S, Prather A, et al. Angiotensin-1 converting enzyme genotype DD is a risk factor for coronary heart disease. J Invest Med 1995;43:275-80.
174. Lieberman J, Nosal A, Schlesser LA, et al. Serum angiotensin-converting enzyme for diagnosis and therapeutic evaluation of sarcoidosis. Am Rev Resp Dis 1979;120:329-35.

175. Lieberman J, Sastre A. Serum angiotensin-converting enzyme: Elevations in diabetes mellitus. Ann Intern Med 1980;93:825-26.
176. Pollare T, Lithell H, Berne C. A comparison of the effects of hydrochlorothiazide and captopril on glucose and lipid metabolism in patients with hypertension. N Engl J Med 1989;321:868-73.
177. Paolisso G, Gambardella A, Verza M, O'Amore A, Sgambato S, Varricchio M. ACE inhibition improves insulin-sensitivity in aged insulin-resistant hypertensive patients. J Hum Hypertens 1992;6:175-79.
178. Leyva F, Godsland IF, Villar J, et al. Influence of the insertion/deletion polymorphism of the ACE gene on insulin resistance and serum urate [abstract]. Eur Heart J 1998;19 (Abstr. Suppl.):44.
179. Ludwig EH, Boreck IB, Ellison RC, et al. Associations between candidate loci angiotensin-converting enzyme and angiotensinogen with coronay heart disease and myocardial infarction: The NHLBI family heart study. Ann Epidemiol 1997;7:3-12.
180. Kamitani A, Rakugi H, Higaki J, et al. Enhanced predictability of myocardial infarction in Japanese by combined genotype analysis. Hypertension 1995;25:950-53.
181. Katsuya T, Kotke G, Yee TW, et al. Association of angiotensinogen gene T235 variant with increased risk of coronary heart disease. Lancet 1995;345:1800-3.
182. Widén E, Lehto M, Kanninen T, Walston J, Shuldiner AR, Groop LC. Association of polymorphisms in the beta-3 adrenergic-receptor gene with features of the insulin resistance syndrome in Finns. N Eng J Med 1995;333:348-51.
183. Clément K, Vaisse C, Manning S StJ, et al. Genetic variation in the beta3-adrenergic receptor and an increased capacity to gain weight in patients with morbid obesity. N Eng J Med 1995;333:352-54.
184. Walston J, Silver K, Bogardus C, et al. Time of onset of non-insulin dependent diabetes mellitus and genetic variation in the beta 3-adrenergic-receptor gene. N Eng J Med 1995;333:343-47.
185. Després J-P, Verdon M-F, Moorjani S, et al. Apolipoprotein E polymorphism modifies relation of hyperinsulinaemia to hypertriglyceridaemia. Diabetes 1993;42:1474-81.
186. Kuhn FE, Rackley CE. Coronary artery disease in women: risk factors, evaluation, treatment and prevention. Arch Intern Med 1993;153:2626-36.
187. Cummings SR, Black DM, Rubin SM. Lifetime risks of hip, Colles' or vertebral fracture and coronary heart disease among white postmenopausal women. Arch Intern Med 1989;149:2445-48.
188. Grady D, Rubin SM, Petitti DB, et al. Hormone therapy to prevent disease and prolong life in postmenopausal women. Ann Intern Med 1992;117:1016-37.
189. Oliver MF, Boyd GS. Effect of bilateral ovariectomy on coronary heart disease and serum lipid levels. Lancet 1959;ii:690-92.
190. Sznajderman M, Oliver MF. Spontaneous premature menopause, ischaemic heart disease, and serum lipids. Lancet 1963;i:962-64.
191. Rich-Edwards JW, Manson JE, Hennekens CH, Buring JE. The primary prevention of coronary heart disease in women. N Engl J Med 1995;332:1758-66.
192. Kitler ME. Coronary disease: are there gender differences? Eur Heart J 1994;15:409-17.
193. Gordon T, Kannel WB, Hjortland MC, McNamara PM. Menopause and coronary heart disease. The Framingham Study. Ann Int Med 1978;89:157-61.
194. Kostis JB, Wilson AC, O'Dowd K, et al. Sex differences in the management and long-term outcome of acute myocardial infarction. A statewide study. Circulation 1994;90:1715-30.
195. Maynard C, Litwin PE, Martin JS, Weaver WD. Gender differences in the treatment and outcome of acute myocardial infarction. Results from the myocardial infarction triage and intervention registry. Arch Intern Med 1992;152:972-76.
196. Jenkins JS, Flaker GC, Nolte B, et al. Causes of higher in-hospital mortality in women than in men after acute myocardial infarction. Am J Cardiol 1994;73:319-22.
197. Clarke KW, Gray O, Keating NA, Hampton JR. Do women with acute myocardial infarction receive the same treatment as men? Br Med J 1994;309:563-66.
198. Adams JN, Jamieson M, Rawles JM, Trent RJ, Jennings KP. Women and myocardial infarction: agism rather than sexism? Br Heart J 1995;73:87-91.
199. Weaver WD, White HD, Wilcox RG, et al. Comparisons of characteristics and outcomes among women and men with acute myocardial infarction treated with thrombolytic therapy. J Am Med Assoc 1996;275:777-82.
200. Woodfield SL, Lundergan CF, Reiner JS, et al. Gender and acute myocardial infarction: is there a different response to thrombolysis? J Am Coll Cardiol 1997;29:35-42.

242

201. Bandrup-Wognsen G, Berggren H, Harford M, Hjalmarson Å, Karlsson T, Herlitz J. Female sex is associated with increased mortality and morbidity early, but not late, after coronary artery bypass grafting. Eur Heart J 1996;17:1426-31.
202. Khan SS, Nessim S, Gray R, Czer LS, Chaux A, Matloff J. Increased mortality of women in coronary artery bypass surgery: Evidence for referral bias. Ann Intern Med 1990;112:561-67.
203. Maynard C, Weaver WD. Treatment of women with acute MI: new findings from the MITI registry. J Myocard Ischemia 1992;4:27-37.
204. King BKB, Porter LA, Rowe MA. Functional, social, and emotional outcomes in women and men in the first year following coronary artery bypass surgery. J Wom Health 1994;3:347-54.
205. Anastos K, Charney P, Charon RA, et al. Hypertension in women: what is really known. Ann Intern Med 1991;115:287-93.
206. McLaughlin TJ, Soumerai SB, Willison DJ, et al. Adherence to national guidelines for drug treatment of suspected acute myocardial infarction. Evidence for undertreatment in women and the elderly. Arch Intern Med 1996;156:799-805.
207. Weintraub WAS, Wenger NK, Kosinski AS, et al. Percutaneous transluminal coronary angioplasty in women compared to men. J Am Coll Cardiol 1994;24:81-90.
208. Swan JW, Walton C, Godsland IF, Crook D, Oliver MF, Stevenson JC. Insulin resistance syndrome as a feature of cardiological syndrome X in non-obese men. Br Heart J 1994;71:41-44.
209. Godsland IF, Crook D, Stevenson JC, et al. The insulin resistance syndrome in postmenopausal women with cardiological syndrome X. Br Heart J 1995;74:47-52.

Chapter 23

TWO SYNDROMES X

Andrew Henderson

There are now two syndromes X of interest to cardiovascular physicians - (1) "cardiac" syndrome X - angina without coronary arteriographic explanation [1], and (2) "metabolic" syndrome X - the epidemiological association of hypertension, non-insulin-dependent diabetes (NIDDM), dyslipidemia and coronary artery disease as described by Reaven in 1988 [2]. Both seem for the present to remain appropriately, albeit confusingly named, for each at root remains something of an enigma.

The first born of the two, cardiac syndrome X, continues to frustrate and intrigue, elusive of identity in clinical practice and pathophysiology alike. The term is however democratically and usefully non-exclusive, thus keeping options open as applicant entities jostle for recognition with varied investigative identity cards - necessitating of course that each investigator then define the diagnostic criteria he employs. The majority of patients with angina-like chest pain and normal coronary arteriogram will have identifiable non-cardiac pain [3], but inclusion of a positive exercise test among the diagnostic criteria will reduce, though probably not abolish, the dilution by those with non-cardiac pain; the residue with cardiac pain may or may not represent a single entity of as yet unknown cause and controversial pathophysiology. The syndrome has for some 25 years attracted the interest of a relatively small band of cardiologists from many corners of the world, some of whom suspect that the condition will turn out to be of wider significance than for the relatively few patients who can presently be diagnosed as suffering from it.

The "arriviste" metabolic syndrome X describes a constellation of features, each long recognised as being a risk marker for CAD. It raises important questions about the inter-relationships between vascular and metabolic factors in the causation of coronary disease. Investigators of this syndrome are drawn from many disciplines other than cardiology - hence perhaps their choice of the term in 1988. It is coincidental that these two syndromes X of interest to cardiovascular physicians should share the same name. The coincidence however grows greater with recent evidence that they both may share also the presence of insulin resistance [4-7] and endothelial dysfunction [7-10] and possibly also the same dyslipidemic pattern [6]. Enhanced membrane sodium-hydrogen exchange has also been reported in both cardiac and metabolic syndrome X [11]. Without (necessarily) implying that they could represent different manifestations of the same fundamental disease, investigators of each may have something useful to learn from each other.

Metabolic syndrome X

The mechanisms underlying the association of features comprising this syndrome have been the subject of considerable speculation. Insulin resistance appears to be a seminal feature [7]. Insulin sensitivity has been shown to be inversely related to blood pressure (across a wide range embracing normal levels) and to age, but it is not directly related to high blood pressure in that it is found in normotensive first degree relatives of patients with essential hypertension, is unaffected by therapeutic lowering of blood pressure, and is not a feature of secondary hypertension. Insulin sensitivity is determined in large part by glucose uptake by skeletal muscle, and this has been shown to be influenced by insulin-stimulated increase in blood flow, which in turn appears to be endothelial NO-dependent [12-15]. Indirect support for a causal relationship between vascular factors and insulin resistance is provided by the demonstration that insulin sensitivity is related to capillary density in skeletal muscle [16] and can be increased by interventions such as exercise training which increase insulin- stimulated glucose uptake and blood flow. The insulin-stimulated increase in blood flow, moreover, is inversely related to blood pressure. Conversely, it has been suggested that hypertension could be the consequence of insulin resistance [7] in that this will lead progressively to hyperinsulinemia, which increases sympathetic activity through central control mechanisms, the increase in noradrenaline contributing to the development of hypertension and to centrally controlled energy expenditure. Epidemiologically, a correlation between adrenaline excretion and serum triglyceride and HDL levels has been observed which is the converse of the high triglyceride and low HDL levels which characterise this syndrome X - suggesting that the dyslipidemia and the associated central obesity might be related to reduced output of adrenaline by the adrenal medulla, as is found with obesity. Severe hyperinsulinemia and ultimate inadequacy of insulin production with consequent glucose intolerance and hyperglycaemia are probably secondary consequences of insulin resistance. It is difficult to discriminate between cause and effect in the various associations demonstrated, and to elucidate the causal chain of events.

Small baby syndrome

Recognition that fetal malnutrition may give rise to the identical constellation of features in adult life [17] is thus of particular interest. Not only does it imply that nutritional factors in early development could contribute significantly to the prevalence of these common and important adult conditions. It offers also a potentially useful experimental and clinical model with which to gain insight into their development.

Insulin resistance has been reported at as early an age as 4 years in low birth weight subjects [18] and the increased prevalence of NIDDM in adults of low birth weight appears to be mediated primarily by insulin resistance rather than hyposecretion of insulin [19]. Experimental evidence supports the concept of fetal programming. Prenatal exposure of rats to maternal dietary protein deprivation reduces neonatal beta-islet cell mass and vascularisation [20], irreversibly alters the expression and activity of key insulin-sensitive hepatic enzymes [21], and leads in young adult offspring to insulin resistance [22] and hypertension [23].

Low birth weight has also now been shown clinically to be associated with endothelial dysfunction in early life [24,25], before the development of any of the adult features of syndrome X and in the absence of any other known cause of endothelial dysfunction [25]. This adds to the list of conditions in which insulin resistance and endothelial dysfunction co-exist [26], which includes most known risk factors for CAD. The association is clearly strong and thus potentially causal, though its universality is still contentious [27]. This may reflect the contribution of other factors and that endothelial dysfunction is unlikely to be a single entity with respect to its mechanisms and manifestations. The spatial resolution of imaging methods which fail to show an increase in heterogenity of microvascular perfusion is also an issue.

Much has been learned in recent years about the role of the endothelium. Endothelial dysfunction is now recognised as seminal to atherogenesis and thus to CAD [28]. It will reduce distensibility of large arteries and increase resistance of small arteries, leading to increased relative cardiac workload, increased blood pressure and reduced vasodilator reserve. Of particular interest is the experimental observation that maintenance of microvascular distribution of flow is dependent on flow-mediated NO production [29,30]. Loss of integrative flow-mediated NO production with endothelial dysfunction could thus prejudice tissue perfusion even if overall flow were maintained, albeit with reduced flow reserve. Conversely, improvement in endothelial function would be expected to improve homogeneity of microvascular distribution and tissue perfusion relative to 'macro-flow'. It is possible therefore that flow-dependent glucose uptake could become locally rate-limiting and contribute to insulin resistance as a consequence of unrecognised heterogeneity of skeletal muscle perfusion [6], supporting the primacy of endothelial dysfunction as a cause of insulin resistance. Pancreatic beta-islet cell dysfunction, as evidenced by high serum levels of proinsulin in patients with insulin resistance, NIDDM and hypertension [31,32], and also in cardiac syndrome X [6] may perhaps represent a further consequence of impaired microvascular perfusion, in this case of the relatively poorly vascularised pancreatic beta-islet cells. In the context of the Small Baby Syndrome, insulin is a fetal growth factor [33] and fetal insulin deficiency [34] could contribute to prejudicing endothelium-dependent angiogenesis and normal microvascular development. Microvascular dysfunction may be developmental, secondarily structural or primarily functional in origin. Moreover functional disturbances in endothelial dysfunction do not exclude the development of chronic structural consequences [34].

Cardiac syndrome X

Controversy surrounding the cardiac syndrome X is alive and kicking. Studies with apparently conflicting evidence have tested our concepts of myocardial ischemia and its manifestations. It has become fashionable to consider there to be multiple causes of the syndrome to evade accommodating apparent conflicts of data, but this would seem far from certain and should be a refuge of last resort. Negative findings can bear false witness if due to dilution of study groups by those with non-cardiac pain or if they reflect investigative insensitivity, while positive findings will survive. Evidence of inducible myocardial ischemia from investigations of contraction, perfusion and metabolism is often not found in all patients studied [36-38], though it is commonly present in some. Despite the obvious possible explanations relating to sensitivity and resolution of the investigative methods used and of diagnostic specificity, this raises the possibility that some patients with the same syndrome do and some do not have myocardial ischemia. Most studies have however found evidence of limited coronary perfusion reserve, due by exclusion and inference to microvascular dysfunction [39-42] - hence the term "microvascular angina". Reversible thallium defects, often but not always found, suggest regional relative perfusion deficit, especially since "perfusion" scans using other agents have given comparable such evidence when sought, though the alternative possibility that it reflects a primary myocardial dysfunction in relation to deficient potassium homeostasis has been raised [43]. Extracellular accumulation of potassium has also been invoked as the cause of ST segment depression, not from any positive evidence to that end but as a potential alternative explanation to myocardial ischemia. Evidence of increased resting coronary flow [42,44,45] has also led to suggestions of a primary myocardial condition, possibly associated with increased contractility, itself possibly due to increased sympathetic tone. Enhanced pain perception has been proposed as the cause of the symptoms [46-48]. Many if not all of these features are consistent with a single unifying hypothesis, at least for the mechanism of the syndrome.

Loss of endothelium-dependent vasodilatation, as demonstrated in response to receptor-mediated stimulation in the coronary arteries [9,49] and in response to flow in the brachial artery (after excluding all known causes of endothelial dysfunction) [50] points strongly to endothelial dysfunction as an integral feature of the syndrome. Heterogeneity of microvascular flow distribution, shown experimentally to result from endothelial dysfunction [29,30], has been modelled experimentally by coronary microembolisation and shown to result in increased adenosine production and resting flow, attributable to adenosine-mediated "steal", with myocardial ischemia occurring only with heavier loads of microemboli [51]. This accords with evidence that when endothelial NO production is experimentally blocked, whole heart adenosine output increases to mediate the increased flow required to meet increased energy consumption, within the overall ceiling of coronary reserve [52]. Endothelial dysfunction might indeed account for many of the apparently conflicting findings in this syndrome X. These include (i) increased resting coronary flow [42,44,45], (ii) enhanced perception of pain [46-48], attributable to adenosine [51,53,54] (which could also lower the threshold to other painful stimuli within the same neuronal distribution) even in the absence of ischemia, (iii) ST segment depolarisation shifts consequent on potassium efflux stimulated by adenosine [55], (iv) insulin resistance [6,15], (v) the frequent absence of confirmatory evidence of ischemic changes [36-38], which may reflect either a real absence of ischemia or lack of investigative sensitivity in demonstrating its widespread dissemination as microfoci of dysfunction in contrast to the more familiar regionally massed dysfunction with atheromatous coronary disease and (vi) perfusion-ventilation mismatch as pulmonary flow increases during exercise [56,57]. Abnormal production or responsiveness to adenosine in this syndrome X has been suggested previously [58-60]. A recent study measuring transmyocardial intermediary metabolite levels convincingly excluded myocardial ischemia at pacing-induced angina but interestingly confirmed inducible myocardial ischemia in some patients (personal communication, J.P. Bagger). Myocardial ischemia could thus be not an intrinsic feature of the syndrome but a feature of the more severe end of its spectrum.

The underlying causes of such endothelial dysfunction remain to be established. Whether endothelial dysfunction is sufficient to cause this syndrome or is part of a more widespread pathological disorder of unknown aetiology likewise remains to be resolved.

..... and the future?

The two syndromes X are likely to continue under their provocative common name for some years yet, hopefully towards mutual enlightenment and resolution of the X factors.

References

1.   Kemp HG. Editorial: Left ventricular function in patients with the anginal syndrome and normal coronary arteriograms. Am J Cardiol 1973; 32:375-376.
2.   Reaven GM. Role of insulin resistance in human disease. Diabetes1988;37:1595-1607.
3.   Dart AM, Davies HA, Dalal J, Ruttley M, Henderson AH. "Angina" and normal coronary arteriograms: a follow-up study. Eur Heart J 1980; 1:97-100.
4.   Dean JD, Jones CJH, Hutchison SJ, Peters JR, Henderson AH. Hyperinsulinemia and microvascular angina ("Syndrome X"). Lancet 1991; 337:456-457.
5.   Botker HE, Moller N, Oversen P, et al. Insulin resistance in microvascular angina (syndrome X). Lancet 1993; 342:136-140.
6.   Goodfellow J, Owens DR, Henderson AH. Cardiovascular Syndromes X, endothelial dysfunction and insulin resistance. Diabetes res clin pract 1996; 31(Suppl):S163-S171.
7.   Reaven GM, Lithell H, Landsberg L. Hypertension and associated metabolic abnormalities - the role of insulin resistance and the sympathoadrenal system. N Engl J Med 1996; 334:952-957.
8.   Henderson AH. Endothelial dysfunction: a reversible clinical measure of atherogenic susceptibility and cardiovascular inefficiency. Int J Cardiol 1997; 62(Suppl l):S43-S48.
9.   Egashira K, Inou T, Hirooka Y, Yamada A, Urabe Y, Takeshita A. Evidence of impaired endothelium-dependent coronary vasodilatation in patients with angina pectoris and normal coronary angiograms. N Engl J Med 1993; 328:1659-1664.
10. Vrints CJM, Bult H, Hitter E, Herman AG, Snoeck JP. Impaired endothelium-dependent cholinergic coronary vasodilatation in patients with angina and normal coronary arteriograms. J Am Coll Cardiol 1992; 19:21-31.
11. Koren W, Koldanov R, Peleg E, Rabinowitz B, Rosenthal T. Enhanced red cell sodium hydrogen exchange in microvascular angina. Eur Ht J 1997; 18:1296-1299.
12. Laakso M, Edelman SV, Brechtel G, Baron AD. Decreased effect of insulin to stimulate skeletal muscle blood flow in obese man. A novel mechanism for insulin resistance. J Clin Invest 1990; 85:1844-1852.
13. Steinberg HO, Brechtel G, Johnson A, Fineberg N, Baron AD. Insulin-mediated skeletal muscle vasodilatation is nitric oxide dependent. J Clin Invest 1994; 94:1172-1179.
14. Scherrer U, Randin D, Vollenweider P, Vollenweider L, Nicod P. Nitric oxide release accounts for insulin's vascular effects in humans. J Clin Invest 1994; 94:2511-2515.
15. Baron AD. The coupling of glucose metabolism and perfusion in human skeletal muscle. The potential role of endothelium-derived nitric oxide. Diabetes 1996; 45(Suppl l):S105-S109.
16. Lillioja S, Young AA, Culter CL, et al. Skeletal muscle capillary density and fiber type are possible determinants of in vivo insulin resistance in man. J Clin Invest 1987; 80:415-424.
17. Barker DJP, Hales CN, Fall CHD, Osmond C, Phipps K, Clark PMS. Type 2 (non-insulin-dependent) diabetes mellitus, hypertension and hyperlipidaemia (syndrome X): relation to reduced fetal growth. Diabetologia 1993; 36:62-67.
18. Yajnik CS, Fall CHD, Vaidya U, et al. Fetal growth and glucose and insulin metabolism in four-year-old Indian children. Diabet Med 1995; 12:330-336.
19. Phillips DIW, Hirst S, Clark PMS, Hales CN, Osmond C. Fetal growth and insulin secretion in adult life. Diabetologia 1994; 37:592-596.
20. Snoeck A, Remacle C. Reussens B, Hoet JJ. Effect of a low protein diet during pregnancy on the fetal rat endocrine pancreas. Biol Neonate 1990; 57:107-118.
21. Desai M, Byrne CD, Zhang J, Petry CJ, Lucas A, Hales CN. Programming of hepatic insulin-sensitive

248

enzymes in offspring of rat dams fed a protein-restricted diet. Am J Physiol 1997; 272:G1083-G1090.

22. Dahri S, Snoeck A, Reusens-Billen B, Remacle C, Hoet JJ. Islet function in offspring of mothers on low protein diet during gestation. Diabetes 1991; 40:115-120.

23. Langley SC, Jackson AA. Increased systolic blood pressure in adult rats induced by fetal exposure to maternal low protein diets. Clin Sci 1994; 86:217-222.

24. Leeson CPM, Whincup PH, Cook DG, et al. Flow mediated dilatation in 9- to 11-year-old children. The influence of intrauterine and childhood factors. Circulation 1997; 96:2233-2238.

25. Goodfellow J, Bellamy MF, Ramsey MW, Lewis MJ, Davies DP, Henderson AH. Endothelial function is impaired in fit young adults of low birth weight. Cardiovasc Res (in press).

26. Henderson AH. St Cyre's Lecture: Endothelium in control. Br Heart J 1991; 65:116-125.

27. Utriainen T, Nuitila P, Takalala T, et al. Intact insulin stimulation of skeletal muscle blood flow, its heterogeneity and redistribution but not of glucose uptake in non-insulin-dependent diabetes mellitus. J Clin Invest 1997; 100:777-785.

28. Ross R. The pathogenesis of atherosclerosis: a perspective for the 1990's. Nature 1993; 362:801-809.

29. Griffith TM, Edwards DH, Davies RU, Harrison TJ, Evans KT. EDRF co-ordinates the behaviour of vascular resistance vessels. Nature 1987; 329:442-445.

30. Griffith TM, Edwards DH. EDRF supresses chaotic pressure oscillations in an isolated resistance artery without influencing their intrinsic complexity. Am J Physiol 1994; 266:H1786-1800.

31. Nagi DK, Hendra TJ, Ryle AJ, et al. The relationships of concentrations of insulin, intact proinsulin, and 32-33 split proinsulin with cardiovascular risk factors in type II (non-insulin-dependent) diabetic subjects. Diabetologia 1990; 33:532-537.

32. Haffner SM, Mykkanen L, Valdez RA, et al. Disproportionately increased proinsulin levels are associated with the insulin resistance syndrome. J Clin Endocrin Metab 1994; 79:1806~1810.

33. Fowden AL. The role of insulin in prenatal growth. J Devel Physiol 1989;12:173~182.

34. Godfrey KM, Robinson S, Hales CN, Barker DJP, Osmond C, Taylor KP. Nutrition in pregnancy and the concentration of proinsulin, 32-33 split proinsulin, insulin and C-peptide in cord plasma. Diabetic Med 1997; 13:868-873.

35. Ito A, Egashira K, Kadokami T, et al. Chronic inhibition of endothelium-derived nitric oxide synthesis causes coronary microvascular structural changes and hyperreactivity to seotonin in pigs. Circulation 1995; 92:2636-2644.

36. Nihoyannopoulos P, Kaski JC, Crake T, Maseri A. Absence of myocardial dysfunction during stress in patients with syndrome X. J Am Coll Cardiol 1991; 18:1463-1470.

37. Rosen SD, Uren NG, Kaski JC, Tousoulis D, Davies GJ, Camici PC. Coronary vasodilator reserve, pain perception, and sex in patients with syndrome X. Circulation 1994; 90:50-60.

38. Panza JA, Laurenzio JM, Curiel RV, et al. Investigation of the mechanism of chest pain in patients with angiographically normal coronary arteries using transoesophageal dobutamine stress echocardiography. J Am Coll Cardiol 1997; 29:293-301.

39. Opherk D, Zebe H, Schuler C, Weihe E, Mall C, Kubler W. Reduced coronary dilatory capacity and ultrastructural changes of the myocardium in patients with angina pectoris but normal coronary angiograms. Circulation 1981; 63:817-825.

40. Cannon RO, Watson RM, Rosing DR, Epstein S. Angina caused by reduced vasodilator reserve of the small coronary arteries. J Am Coll Cardiol 1983; 1:1359-1373.

41. Hutchison SJ, Poole-Wilson PA, Henderson AH. Angina with normal coronary arteries: a review. Q J Med 1989; 72:677-688.

42. Galassi AR, Crea F, Araujo LI, et al. Comparison of regional myocardial blood flow in syndrome X and one-vessel coronary artery disease. Am J Cardiol. 1993; 72:134-139.

43. Poole-Wilson PA. Potassium and the heart. Clin Endocrinol Metab 1984;13:249-268.

44. Geltman EM, Henes CC, Sennef MJ, Sobel BE, Bergman SR. Increased myocardial perfusion at rest and diminished perfusion reserve in patients with angina and angiographically normal coronary arteries. J Am Coll Cardiol 1990; 16:586-597.

45. Botker HE, Sonne HS, Bagger JP, Nielsen TT. Impact of impaired coronary flow reserve and insulin resistance on myocardial energy metabolism in patients with syndrome X. Am J Cardiol 1997; 79:1615-1622.

46. Shapiro LM, Crake T, Poole-Wilson PA. Is altered cardiac sensation responsible for chest pain in patients with normal coronaries? Clinical observation during cardiac catheterization. Br Med J 1988; 296:170-171.

47. Cannon RO, Quyyumi AA, Schenke W, et al. Abnormal cardiac sensitivity in patients with chest pain and normal coronary arteries. J Am Coll Cardiol 1990; 16:1359-1366.

48. Chauhan A, Mullins PA, Thuraisingham SI, Taylor G, Petch MC, Schofield PM. Abnormal cardiac pain perception in syndrome X. J Am Coll Cardiol 1994; 24:329-335.
49. Egashira K, Hirooka Y, Kuga T, Mohri M, Takeshita A. Effects of Larginine supplementation on endothelium-dependent coronary vasodilation in patients with angina pectoris and normal coronary angiograms. Circulation 1996; 94:130-134.
50. Bellamy MF, Goodfellow J, Tweddel AC, Lewis MJ, Henderson AH. Syndrome X and endolthelial dysfunction. Cardiovasc Res (in press).
51. Hori M, Inoue M, Kitakaze M, et al. Role of adenosine in hyperaemic response of coronary blood flow in microembolisation. Am J Physiol 1986; 250:H509-H518.
52. Kostic MM, Schrader J. Role of nitric oxide in reactive hyperaemia of the guinea pig heart. Circulation Res 1992; 70:208-212.
53. Sylven C, Jonzon B, Edlund A. Angina pectoris-like pain provoked by i.v. bolus of adenosine: relationship to coronary sinus blood flow, heart rate and blood pressure in healthy volunteers. Eur Heart J 1989; 10:48-54.
54. Burnstock G. A unifying purinergic hypothesis for the initiation of pain. Lancet 1996; 347:1604-1605.
55. Dart C, Standen NB. Adrenosine-activated potassium current in smooth muscle cells isolated from the pig coronary artery. J Physiol 1993; 471:767-786.
56. Lewis NP, Hutchinson SJ, Willis N, Henderson AH. Syndrome X and hyperventilation. Br Heart J 1991; 65:94-96.
57. Banning AP, Lewis NP, Northridge DB, Elborn JS, Henderson AH. Perfusion/ventilation mismatch during exercise in chronic heart failure: an analysis of circulatory determinants. Br Ht J 1995; 74:27-33.
58. Emdin M, Picano E, Lattanzi F, L'Abatte A. Improved exercise capacity with acute aminophylline administration in patients with syndrome X. J Am Coll Cardiol 1989; 14:1450-1453.
59. Maseri A, Crea F, Kaski JC, Crake T. Mechanisms of angina pectoris syndrome X. J Am Coll Cardiol 1991; 17:499-506.
60. Inobe Y, Kugiyama K, Morita E, et al. Role of adenosine in pathogenesis of syndrome X: assessment with coronary haemodynamic measurements and thallium -201 myocardial single-photon emission computed tomography. J Am Coll Cardiol 1996; 28:890-896.

Chapter 24

HYPERLIPIDEMIA AND ENDOTHELIAL VASODILATOR DYSFUNCTION: THE PATHOGENETIC LINK TO MYOCARDIAL ISCHEMIA

Andreas M. Zeiher

The endothelium is a crucial vascular structure, not only because of its strategically important barrier function as the interface between the flowing blood and the vascular wall, but also because it is a source of a variety of mediators regulating vascular growth, platelet function and coagulation. In addition, the endothelium plays a critical role in the control of vasomotor tone by synthesizing and metabolizing vasoactive substances including an endothelium-derived hyperpolarizing factor, prostacyclin, and, most notably, endothelium derived relaxing factor (EDRF), which has been identified as nitric oxide (NO) or a related compound [1]. NO, which is formed from L-arginine by the action of a constitutive form of the enzyme nitric oxide synthase [2], has been shown to inhibit platelet aggregation and adhesion, to modulate smooth muscle cell proliferation, to attenuate the generation of endothelin, and to modulate leukocyte and monocyte adhesion to the endothelium, all of which are cardinal features in the pathogenesis of atherosclerosis. Thus, in addition to the vasorelaxing effects of NO caused by stimulating guanylate cyclase to increase cyclic GMP levels in the vascular smooth muscle cell layer, NO appears to exert potent antiatherosclerotic functions.

The endothelium has been recognized long ago to be central to the pathogenesis of atherosclerosis; however, the assumption that endothelial desquamation preceded lesion development had to be revised and was replaced by the concept of „dysfunction" of the endothelium, since even advanced lesions may be covered by an intact, albeit morphologically altered endothelial cell layer. In recent years, evidence has been accumulating that atherosclerosis might be viewed as an inflammatory disease. Most notably, the metabolic stress imposed on the endothelium by various well-known risk factors and the concomitant excessive production of reactive oxygen species by the endothelium itself appear to play a key role for the recruitment of inflammatory cells into the atherosclerotic vascular wall via stimulation of a number of redox-sensitive genes [3]. Thus, the endothelium is not only a target for, but also a mediator of atherosclerosis. Importantly, NO - being a radical itself - avidly reacts with oxygen free radicals and, thereby, interferes with redox-sensitive mechanisms. Indeed, we have previously shown that NO inhibits the activation of NF-KappaB-like transcriptional regulatory proteins, which are activated by reactive oxygen species and mediate transcription of numerous genes implicated in the pathogenesis of atherosclerosis [4]. These findings pointed towards a molecular link between endothelial NO synthesis and oxidant-sensitive transcriptional regulatory mechanisms involved in the protective effects of preserved endothelial function. Excessive endothelial reactive oxygen species production may also account for the impaired endothelial vasodilator function characteristic of atherosclerotic and/or risk factor-exposed vessels, since scavenging of oxygen radicals by NO will reduce the bioavailability of NO to mediate vascular relaxation. These data led to the hypothesis that the abnormal redox state in the vascular endothelium, as the fundamental metabolic feature of atherosclerosis, not only contributes to the pathogenesis of atherosclerotic lesion development, but also mediates the impaired control of vasomotor tone in coronary artery disease thus establishing a mechanistically unifying relation between atherosclerosis and endothelial vasodilator dysfunction. It is the aim of the present chapter to discuss recently developed concepts of the mechanisms and consequences of coronary endothelial vasodilator dysfunction to the ischemic manifestations of coronary artery disease, with a focus on differentiating causal relationships from epiphenomena which merely accompany the presence of atherosclerosis.

Early in the '80s, it became apparent that myocardial ischemia is not necessarily the consequence of a failure of coronary blood flow to increase in response to an augmented demand, but quite commonly caused by a transient impairment of coronary blood supply implicating a possible pathogenetic role of increased coronary arterial tone due to inappropriate vasoconstriction [5]. The observation reported by Furchgott and Zawadzki [6] that vascular tone can be modulated by a factor released from the endothelium - now identified as NO or a related compound - opened new avenues for investigating the regulation of coronary blood flow. The demonstration that NO mediates the vasodilation produced by a number of neurohumoral substances, platelet-derived products and coagulation factors, while attenuating vasoconstriction caused by other mediators suggested that endothelial vasodilator function may represent a negative feedback mechanism to prevent vasoconstriction and thrombus formation at sites of normal endothelium. Indeed, experimentally, removal or injury of the endothelium reversed the vasodilator into vasoconstrictor effects supporting the notion that endothelial dysfunction may play an important role for inappropriate vasoconstriction.

Clinically, progressive impairment in endothelial dilator functions is observed with different early stages of coronary atherosclerosis [7]. In addition, numerous studies could demonstrate that local evidence of endothelial vasodilator dysfunction of atherosclerotic or even risk factor-exposed coronary arteries correlated with inappropriate vasoconstriction in response to several clinically relevant stimuli, e. g. exercise, pacing, cold pressor testing, mental stress, and intracoronary thrombus formation [8], which all are known to precipitate angina and myocardial ischemia in patients with coronary artery disease. Thus, the hypothesis was quickly put forward that endothelial vasodilator dysfunction of atherosclerotic epicardial arteries - unbalancing vascular tone towards vasoconstriction - is responsible for transient impairment of coronary blood supply.

The mechanisms underlying impaired endothelial vasodilator function in atherosclerosis appears to be related to a decreased bioactivity of NO rather than a reduced production of NO or alterations of the NO-synthase itself. Enhanced destruction of NO has been shown to be related to the increased endothelial synthesis of free radicals, especially superoxide anions [9]. Importantly, both experimental and preliminary clinical data demonstrated that scavenging superoxide anions ameliorates endothelial vasodilator dysfunction of atherosclerotic epicardial vessels. Thus, the extent of endothelial vasodilator dysfunction might reflect the oxidative stress imposed on the endothelium by risk factors and by the atherosclerotic process itself, again pointing towards a molecular link between vasomotor dysfunction and the pathogenesis of atherosclerosis.

Although epicardial conductance vessels, where atherosclerotic lesions develop and inappropriate vasoconstriction is observed, contribute only 10 - 15 % to total coronary vascular resistance, impaired endothelial vasodilator function superimposed on even a moderate stenosis might be an important mechanism contributing to myocardial ischemia. Luminal diameter reductions produced by clinically relevant stimuli in the presence of endothelial vasodilator dysfunction are usually less than 20 %. However, this increase in arterial tone might be enough to convert a hemodynamically insignificant lesion into a flow-limiting stenosis, since for example the resistance to flow offered by a stenosis is expected to quadruple as the degree of diameter narrowing increases from 70 to 90 % with ensuing reductions in resting blood flow. Thus, there clearly appears to be a pathogenetic link between endothelial vasodilator dysfunction and the variation in ischemic threshold in patients with moderate coronary stenoses.

However, in the absence of moderate-to-severe stenoses, inappropriate vasoconstriction of epicardial arteries due to endothelial vasodilator dysfunction is insufficient to explain transient impairment of coronary blood flow. In addition, the atherosclerotic process itself is associated with both structural and functional alterations of the vascular wall, which will counteract vasoconstriction in the presence of endothelial vasodilator dysfunction. Atherosclerosis leads to atrophy of the medial smooth muscle layer and increased stiffness of the vascular wall, which both are structural alterations favoring hyporeactivity to vasoconstrictor stimuli. Atherosclerotic coronary arteries undergo a structural remodeling process characterized by compensatory enlargement of atherosclerotic vessel segments to preserve the luminal diameter despite an increase in the size of the atherosclerotic plaque [10]. Moreover, there is also a functional remodeling process in atherosclerotic coronary arterial segments, characterized by a decrease in coronary vasomotor tone with increasing atherosclerotic plaque load [11]. In the aggregate, the effects of atherosclerosis in vivo are clearly different from those of simple removal of the endothelium. Thus, it is not justified to postulate that paradoxical vasoconstriction of epicardial conductance vessels due to endothelial vasodilator dysfunction will generally contribute to the ischemic manifestations of coronary artery disease.

The culprit lesion in acute coronary syndromes is characterized by an exaggerated constrictor response to a variety of stimuli. It has been suggested that endothelial vasodilator dysfunction might importantly contribute to the vasospastic propensity of these lesions. However, recent evidence indicates that localized chronic inflammatory processes within the atherosclerotic plaque rather than the endothelium appear to be responsible not only for plaque rupture itself leading to acute ischemic syndromes, but also for the hyperreactivity of these plaques in response to vasoconstrictor stimuli [12].

Finally, there is now compelling evidence that the syndrome of variant angina, which is characterized by frank coronary spasm and might be viewed as the extreme end of the spectrum of inappropriate epicardial artery constriction, is due to hyperreactivity of the smooth muscle cells, but not due to endothelial vasodilator dysfunction. Thus, endothelial vasodilator dysfunction of epicardial arteries does not appear to play a causal role in eliciting acute ischemic syndromes.

However, endothelial vasodilator dysfunction is not only confined to epicardial conductance vessels, where atherosclerotic lesions develop, but may also extend into the coronary microcirculation, where no overt atheroma develop, but where coronary blood flow and, hence, myocardial perfusion is determined. Endothelial vasodilator dysfunction of coronary resistance vessels appears to be a major determinant for the development of myocardial ischemia during increased metabolic demand. Inhibition of NO synthesis increases coronary vascular resistance in humans by > 20 % indicating that basal production of NO considerably contributes to the regulation of myocardial perfusion. However, it is likely that other endothelial mediators also affect the regulation of resistance vessel tone. Impaired endothelial vasodilation of the coronary microcirculation has been demonstrated in some patients with normal coronary arteries, but evidence of myocardial ischemia as detected by myocardial lactate production [13]. More importantly, in some patients with atherosclerosis, the endothelial vasodilator capacity of the coronary microcirculation is impaired indicating that the functional consequences of atherosclerosis extend into the coronary microcirculation. It is exactly those patients, who also demonstrate a paradoxical decrease in coronary blood flow during increased metabolic demand as well as exercise-induced thallium-perfusion defects indicative of myocardial ischemia [14]. These findings suggest a crucial role for endothelium-dependent vasodilation of coronary resistance vessels in coupling metabolic demand and coronary blood flow. Indeed, Quyyumi et al [15] recently established that, in humans, coronary blood flow regulation during increased myocardial demand is largely mediated by NO. However, neither the mechanism involved nor the precise site or vessel size of the resistance vasculature affected have been elucidated, so far. Moreover, we do not know whether the impaired dilator response originates from functional alterations of the microvascular endothelium itself or is mediated by factors released upstream in the atherosclerotic conductance vessels and acting downstream in the resistance vasculature. Interestingly, hypercholesterolemia, advanced age, and diabetes selectively impair endothelial dilator functions not only of coronary, but also of forearm resistance vessels suggesting a generalized functional impairment [16].

Hypercholesterolemia is an important cause of coronary artery disease in humans, and raised plasma concentrations of low density lipoproteins (LDL) are associated with accelerated atherogenesis [17]. As the first step of atheroma formation apoB-containing lipoproteins (VLDL, LDL, chylomicron remnants) are entrapped in the subendothelial space where they undergo an oxidative modification. Mild oxidation results in minimally oxidized LDL (MM-LDL) which can induce factors that cause monocyte chemotaxis and adhesion [3]. This results in binding of monocytes to the endothelial cells, their migration into the subintimal space, and their differentiation to macrophages [3]. The macrophages release reactive oxygen species and active aldehydes. Hypercholesterolemia imposes a significant oxidative stress upon the vessel wall.

Hypercholesterolemia has been shown to impair endothelial vasodilator function in large conduit vessels as well as in resistance vessels in experimental studies and in humans [7,16]. It has been suggested that enhanced destruction of NO is the cause of defective endothelium-dependent vascular relaxation. Enhanced destruction of NO in hypercholesterolemia seems to be related to increased production of free radicals, especially super-oxide anions [9]. In addition to impairing endothelial vasodilator function by oxidative stress, hypercholesterolemia may interfere with receptor-operated signal transduction mechanisms linked to the formation of EDRF. Hypercholesterolemia and advanced age have both been shown to impair selectively the endothelial vasodilator function of coronary resistance vessels in humans [16]. There appears to be a close correlation between the extent of impaired endothelium-dependent vasodilator function of coronary resistance vessels and serum cholesterol concentrations [16].

Cholesterol lowering trials have demonstrated a decrease of non-fatal myocardial infarction and total mortality [17]. However, improvement of clinical outcome occurred despite only minimal regression of coronary atherosclerosis determined by angiography, suggesting that factors other than the reduction of atherosclerotic plaque size might be important for the benefit of cholesterol lowering therapy [17]. Improvement of endothelial function probably contributes to the beneficial effects of cholesterol lowering therapy. In patients with angiographically normal coronary arteries, Leung et al [18] showed that a six month cholesterol lowering diet and cholestyramine therapy with a reduction in cholesterol concentration by 29%, reversed the initial vasoconstrictor response to acetylcholine, indicating an improvement of endothelial function of the coronary conductance vessels. Egashira et al [19] extended this observation to the coronary microcirculation in patients with coronary artery disease: after six months of treatment with pravastatin, resulting in a cholesterol reduction of 31%, coronary blood flow in response to acetycholine increased by about 60%.

However, regardless of the mechanisms involved, endothelial vasodilator function of coronary resistance vessels will not only contribute to ischemic manifestations of coronary artery disease in the absence of hemodynamically significant stenoses, but might also aggravate ischemic episodes in patients with advanced coronary artery disease, e. g. during plaque rupture-mediated epicardial artery thrombus formation with subsequent release of platelet-derived vasoconstrictors acting downstream on the vascular wall of resistance vessels.

Further insights into the pathogenetically important role of endothelial vasodilator dysfunction of coronary resistance vessels for the ischemic manifestations of coronary artery disease can be derived from recent therapeutic intervention studies aiming to improve endothelial vasodilator function. Effective lipid lowering normalizes endothelial vasodilator function of the coronary microcirculation and ameliorates vasoconstrictor responses of epicardial conductance vessels [17]. This functional improvement in the regulation of coronary vasomotor tone is accompanied by improved myocardial perfusion during increased myocardial demand and associated with a reduction in transient myocardial ischemia during daily life activities as assessed by ST-analysis of holter recordings. Importantly, the additive beneficial effect of an antioxidant treatment strategy [20] provides further support for the pivotal role of an abnormal redox state in the vascular endothelium to mediate impaired control of vasomotor tone in atherosclerotic coronary arteries. However, further studies will ultimately be necessary in order to demonstrate that the extent of endothelial vasodilator dysfunction of atherosclerotic vessels not only reflects the oxidative stress imposed on the endothelium by risk factors and by the atherosclerotic process itself, but, more importantly, that amelioration of endothelial vasodilator dysfunction suggestive of improved redox equilibrium by risk factor modification will eventually translate into a reduction of ischemic events indicative of plaque stabilization or even regression [21]. Such proof would establish the assessment of endothelial vasodilator function as an indispensable diagnostic tool to evaluate the prognostic significance of therapeutic interventions in patients with coronary artery disease.

References

1.   Bassenge E, Busse R. Endothelial modulation of coronary tone. Prog Cardiovasc Dis   1988; 349-380.
2.   Palmer RMJ, Ashton DS, Moncada S. Vascular endothelial cells synthesize nitric oxide from L-arginine. Nature 1988; 333: 664-666.
3.   Berliner JA, Navab M, Fogelman AM, Frank JS, Demer LL, Edwards PA, et al. Atherosclerosis: basic mechanisms. Oxidation, inflammation, and genetics. Circulation 1995; 91: 2488-2496.
4.   Zeiher AM, Fisslthaler B, Schray-Utz B, Busse R. Nitric oxide modulates the expression of monocyte chemoattractant protein 1 in cultured human endothelial cells. Circ Res 1995; 76: 980-986.
5.   Epstein SE, Talbot TL. Dynamic coronary tone in precipitation, exacerbation and relief of angina pectoris. Am J Cardiol 1981; 48: 797-803.
6.   Furchgott RF, Zawadzki JV. The obligatory role of endothelial cells in the relaxation   of arterial smooth muscle by acetylcholine. Nature 1980; 288: 373-376.
7.   Zeiher AM, Drexler H, Wollschläger H, Just H. Modulation of coronary vasomotor tone in humans: progressive endothelial dysfunction with different early stages of coronary atherosclerosis. Circulation 1991; 83: 391-401.
8.   Meredith IT, Yeung AC, Weidinger FF, Anderson TJ, Uehata A, Ryan TJ, et al. Role of impaired endothelium-dependent vasodilation in ischemic manifestations of coronary artery disease. Circulation 1993; 87: V-56-V-66.
9.   Ohara Y, Peterson TE, Harrison DG. Hypercholesterolemia increases endothelial superoxide anion production. J Clin Invest 1993; 91: 2546-2551.
10. Gibbons GH, Dzau VJ. The emerging concept of vascular remodeling. N Engl J Med 1994; 330: 1431-1438.
11. Schächinger V, Zeiher AM. Quantitative assessment of coronary vasoreactivity in humans in vivo: importance of baseline vasomotor tone in atherosclerosis. Circulation 1995; 2087-2094.
12. Zeiher AM, Goebel H, Schächinger V, Ihling C. Tissue endothelin-1 immuno-reactivity in the active coronary atherosclerotic plaque: a clue to the mechanism of increased vasoreactivity of the culprit lesion in unstable angina. Circulation 1995; 91: 941-947.
13. Egashira K, Inou T, Hirooka Y, Yamada A, Urabe Y, Takeshita A. Evidence of impaired endothelium-dependent coronary vasodilation in patients with angina pectoris and normal coronary angiograms. N Engl J Med 1993; 328: 1659-1664.
14. Zeiher AM, Krause T, Schächinger V, Minners J, Moser E. Impaired endothelium-dependent vasodilation of coronary resistance vessels is associated with exercise- induced myocardial ischemia. Circulation 1995; 91: 2345-2352.
15. Quyyumi AA, Dakak N, Andrews NP, Gilligan DM, Panza JA, Cannon RO, III. Contribution of nitric oxide to metabolic coronary vasodilation in the human heart. Circulation 1995; 92: 320-326.
16. Zeiher AM, Drexler H, Saurbier B, Just H. Endothelium-mediated coronary blood flow modulation in humans. Effects of age, atherosclerosis, hypercholesterolemia, and hypertension. J Clin Invest 1993; 92: 652-662.
17. Levine GN, Keaney JF, Jr., Vita JA. Cholesterol reduction in cardiovascular disease. Clinical benefits and possible mechanisms (comment). N Engl J Med 1995; 332: 512-521.

18. Leung WH, Lau CP, Wong CK.   Beneficial effect of cholesterol-lowering therapy on coronary endothelium-dependent relaxation in hypercholosterolaemic patients. Lancet 1993; 341:1496-1500.

19. Egashira K, Hirooka Y, Kai H, Sugimachi M, Suzuki S, Inou T, *et al.* Reduction in serum cholesterol with pravastatin improves endothelium-dependent coronary vasomotion in patients with hypercholesterolemia. Circulation 1994; 89:2519-24.

20. Anderson TJ, Meredith IT, Yeung AC, Frei B, Selwyn AP, Ganz P. The effect of cholesterol-lowering and antioxidant therapy on endothelium-dependent coronary vasomotion (see comments). N Engl J Med 1995; 332: 488-493.

21. Benzuly KH, Padgett RC, Kaul S, Piegors DJ, Armstrong ML, Heistad DD. Functional improvement precedes structural regression of atherosclerosis. Circulation 1994; 89: 1810-1818.

Chapter 25

MICROVASCULAR DYSFUNCTION IN PATIENTS WITH SYSTEMIC HYPERTENSION WITHOUT LEFT VENTRICULAR HYPERTROPHY: THE ROLE OF NITRIC OXIDE

Julio A. Panza

Essential hypertension is a disease characterized, in its established form, by increased systemic vascular resistance with normal cardiac output. The fundamental abnormality of this process resides at the level of small arteries, those with a diameter ranging between 50 and 400 microns that create resistance to blood flow. Although the precise mechanism accounting for the abnormality of the microvasculature that leads to increased systemic vascular resistance and elevated blood pressure is unknown, and likely heterogenous, microvascular dysfunction is at the core of the hypertensive process and constitutes the pathophysiological basis for the most clinically relevant complications of hypertension. Further, microvascular dysfunction may also be responsible for symptoms of chest pain in patients with essential hypertension, possibly secondary to myocardial ischemia that results from an imbalance between vasoconstrictor and vasodilator forces in the coronary microcirculation [1,2]. Finally, the microvascular abnormality is ultimately responsible for the structural phase of the hypertensive process that characterizes the end stage of the disease, including central nervous system damage, hypertensive nephropathy, and congestive heart failure as a result of hypertensive cardiomyopathy. This chapter will review the evidence for and speculate on the mechanisms of microvascular dysfunction in patients with essential hypertension with a focus on the role and potential mechanisms of decreased activity of endothelial nitric oxide in the hypertensive vasculature.

Heart disease in hypertension

The most conspicuous cardiac abnormality in essential hypertension is the presence of left ventricular hypertrophy, which occurs in a substantial number of patients with hypertension as a compensatory mechanism for the increased vascular resistance. However, not all patients with hypertension will develop an enlarged cardiac mass. The explanation for this variability in the presence of left ventricular hypertrophy or in the apparent lack of relation between its magnitude and the severity of hypertension in certain patients is unclear. It is possible that genetic factors predispose some patients to develop myocyte hypertrophy in response to elevated afterload.

The two most common cardiac symptoms reported by patients with essential hypertension are dyspnea and chest pain. Dyspnea occurs secondary to pulmonary venous congestion as a consequence of elevated left ventricular filling pressures. This is related to diastolic dysfunction that may lead to heart failure with or without associated systolic dysfunction. The presence of chest pain in patients with hypertension constitutes a diagnostic dilemma. Clearly, angina pectoris in a patient with a history of elevated blood pressure may be a manifestation of underlying obstructive coronary artery disease. Hypertension is a well established risk factor for the development of atherosclerosis [3] and a number of important complications of the hypertensive process are not directly related to the elevation in systemic blood pressure *per se*, but to the associated risk of atherosclerotic vascular disease, such as sudden death, arrhythmias, stroke, and peripheral vascular disease. In addition, hypertensive patients may also be at an increased risk of silent myocardial infarction and ambulatory episodes of silent myocardial ischemia [4]. Despite this increased prevalence of atherosclerosis in hypertension, the presence of angina-like chest pain is often not the reflection of significant stenoses of the epicardial coronary arteries but, instead, constitutes part of the syndrome of chest pain with angiographically normal coronary arteries. In these patients, chest pain has been proposed to be an expression of myocardial ischemia resulting from abnormal behavior of the coronary microvessels: those too small to be imaged during angiography. Several studies have demonstrated structural and functional abnormalities of the coronary microcirculation in hypertensive animals and humans with left ventricular hypertrophy; these are discussed in a separate chapter. However, it is clear that hypertensive patients without a recognizable enlargement of cardiac mass also have functional abnormalities of the coronary microvasculature that may impact significantly on the regulation of myocardial blood flow. For example, Brush *et al* [5] showed that patients with hypertension without left ventricular hypertrophy undergoing cardiac catheterization because of complaints of chest pain had an abnormal coronary microvascular response to ergonovine. This abnormal behavior of the coronary microvasculature may be related to endothelial dysfunction [6]. The significance of these observations has been underscored by the recent findings of Quyyumi *et al* [7] who demonstrated that hypertensive patients with no or minimal left ventricular hypertrophy had impaired coronary microvascular dilator responses to acetylcholine (an endothelium-dependent vasodilator) that correlated with the physiological blood flow increase in response to atrial pacing. Importantly, the endothelium-independent response to sodium nitroprusside did not, however, correlate with the response to pacing. These findings suggest that endothelial function of the coronary microvasculature importantly regulates changes in blood flow in response to physiological stimuli.

Microvascular dysfunction in essential hypertension

As mentioned above, the fundamental abnormality of the hypertensive process is an increase in systemic (or peripheral) vascular resistance. This abnormality, coupled with a preserved or slightly increased cardiac output, leads to an elevation in blood pressure. Mechanisms leading to increased vascular resistance are not well understood, but can be approached, at least conceptually, from the perspectives of two different, albeit related, abnormalities: structural alterations of small resistance arteries and functional abnormalities of the microcirculation. Both of these defects are related to each other in important ways. For example, as proposed by Folkow [8], an initial pressor mechanism (functional in nature) may initially lead to an increase in blood pressure that eventually results in vascular hypertrophy (structural abnormality) which, in turn, creates a vicious cycle by which the structural defect leads to a greater elevation in systemic blood pressure. In addition, the presence of abnormalities in vascular morphology may lead to the occurrence of impairment in the functional responses of microvessels [9,10].

Structural abnormalities of the microvasculature

Studies have shown that hypertensive resistance arteries have an increased media thickness relative to the vessel lumen size (i.e., increased wall:lumen ratio) compared to normotensive controls [11,12]. It has been proposed that this abnormal geometry of the microvessels of hypertensive patients has a profound impact on vascular resistance and hemodynamics. According to this concept, not only vascular resistance is increased as a consequence of this deranged structure in the microvasculature, but also the response to vasoconstrictor stimuli would be exaggerated by the increased media thickness encroaching upon the vascular lumen [9,10]. Of note, the increased wall:lumen ratio of hypertensive arteries may not necessarily be the result of hypertrophy or hyperplasia (or both) of the vascular smooth muscle. Instead, as demonstrated by *in vitro* studies of human subcutaneous resistance vessels, myocyte cell size is normal and the degree of growth is small. Based on these observations, it has been suggested that the process leading to structural abnormalities of the microvasculature is one of remodeling of normal elements in the vascular wall rearranged around a reduced lumen [13].

A different abnormality in the microcirculation of hypertensive patients is that of a reduction in the number of perfused capillaries, or rarefaction. This defect could be either functional (i.e., the vessels are temporarily not recruited for perfusion) or anatomical (i.e., the microvessels are not present). Thus, previous studies have demonstrated rarefaction of the conjunctival microvessels of patients with essential hypertension with a reduction in arteriolar density and diameter [14]. A reduction in capillary density has also been reported in the nailfold microcirculation of essential hypertensive patients [15]. Sullivan *et al* [16] reported capillary rarefaction but not arteriolar rarefaction in young patients with borderline hypertension, and proposed that this initial stage of the hypertensive process is characterized by increased cardiac output with reduction in the number of capillaries recruited for perfusion without a significant abnormality in the structure or behavior of resistance arteries. Finally, previous studies have shown that small resistance vessels of hypertensive patients have a reduced distensibility (another form of structural abnormality) as measured by applying transmural pressures to maximally vasodilated segments of hypertensive vessels [17].

The presence of this structural alteration in the resistance vasculature of hypertensive patients may have important implications of the natural course of the disease. First, even as a secondary phenomenon, the existence of structural changes may participate in the creation of a vicious circle in which vascular hypertrophy leads to elevated blood pressure which, in turn, potentiates the extent of structural abnormalities. Second, these changes may not only be responsible for the pathophysiology of elevated blood pressure, but also have prognostic implications. Thus, previous studies [18] have shown a relation between structural abnormalities in concentric hypertrophy and the development of target organ damage as shown by fundoscopic examination and renal function test in patients with hypertension.

Functional abnormalities of the microvasculature

Innumerable previous studies have shown that the small resistance arteries of patients with essential hypertension have abnormal vasodilator responses to certain stimuli. It is important to understand that, despite the presence of structural changes of the microvasculature in hypertension, arterioles of hypertensive patients can indeed dilate and lower vascular resistance to levels that are well below those observed in the vasculature of normotensive patients during baseline conditions. Thus, in addition to structural changes, there must be functional alterations of the microvessels that impose an elevated vascular resistance during resting conditions. Consequently, irrespective of the presence of structural alterations in the human microvasculature, functional abnormalities play a critical role in the pathophysiology of the hypertensive process. Of all the different methods used for the investigation of the behavior of small resistance vessels in hypertension, the forearm perfusion technique has been the most widely used. With this method, drugs are infused intra-arterially into the forearm circulation at small doses and the response of the vasculature is measured by strain gauge plethysmography. The technique offers the advantage that, because only small doses of the different agents are used, these drugs do not reach the systemic circulation and therefore do not activate counter-regulatory mechanisms that would obscure the interpretation of the results.

Nitric oxide dysfunction in essential hypertension

An important breakthrough in our understanding of the factors that modulate vascular tone was made by the observation of Furchgott and Zawadzki that the presence and integrity of the endothelium determines the contractile state of the underlying vascular smooth muscle [19]. This regulatory function of the endothelium is exerted through the release of several factors, the most important of which is nitric oxide (NO), a soluble molecule that stimulates guanylate cyclase in vascular smooth cells to produce vascular relaxation [20].

Basal release of NO has been shown to be critical for the maintenance of vascular tone. Thus, when the synthesis of NO *in vivo* is blocked by inhibitors of NO synthase, significant vasoconstriction ensues [21]. Because NO has a very short half-life, these findings are consistent with continuous basal release of NO as an important part of the physiology of the vascular system. This role of NO in vascular homeostasis has also been demonstrated in both the resistance and conductance arteries of the coronary vascular tree. In addition to regulation of vascular tone, NO has other important antiatherogenic actions (including inhibition of platelet aggregation, monocyte migration, and lipid oxidation).

Several studies have shown that patients with essential hypertension have abnormal endothelium-mediated vasodilation to acetylcholine in the peripheral or coronary vasculature [6,22-28]. Because the regulation of vascular tone involves many substances and a complex interplay among numerous cellular mechanisms, an impaired response to acetylcholine does not identify the nature of endothelial dysfunction.

The role of endothelium-derived NO, which is synthesized from L-arginine, has received extensive study in humans. In particular, the arginine analogue N^G-monomethyl-L-arginine (L-NMMA), which inhibits endothelial synthesis of NO, has been used to investigate the role of endothelium-derived NO in the abnormal endothelium-dependent vasodilation observed in patients with hypertension [29,30]. In normotensive controls, basal release of NO has been indicated by a reduction in blood flow and an increase in vascular resistance during infusion of L-NMMA [21,29,30]. Patients with hypertension also showed a significantly blunted vasoconstrictor response to L-NMMA, indicating that less NO is produced/released by hypertensive vessels in the basal state [29,30]. Further, L-NMMA effectively blunts the vasodilator response to acetylcholine in normotensive humans [21,29], whereas in hypertensive patients no significant change is observed during infusion of L-NMMA in the already blunted response to acetylcholine [29].

Potential mechanisms of reduced nitric oxide activity

The impaired NO activity of patients with essential hypertension could be related to one or more abnormalities along the NO system. As mentioned previously, NO is formed using the amino acid L-arginine as a substrate in response to a variety of physiological and pharmacological stimuli, and is broken down primarily by superoxide anions originated both intracellularly and extracellularly [31]. Several mechanisms that may potentially account for decreased vascular activity of NO have been investigated in patients with essential hypertension.

One potential defect in the NO system that could contribute to the decreased bioactivity of NO is a decreased availability of its precursor, L-arginine. Studies of the vasodilator response to acetylcholine in normotensive controls showed that infusion of L-arginine into the brachial artery augmented endothelium-dependent vascular relaxation; however, no change was observed in patients with hypertension [32]. These findings indicate that the defect in the endothelium-derived NO system in hypertensive vessels is likely not due to decreased availability of its precursor, L-arginine.

Another postulated defect in the endothelium-derived NO system that might contribute to decreased NO activity involves an abnormality of the muscarinic receptor, which is stimulated by acetylcholine and methacholine. Some evidence has suggested that atherosclerotic coronary arteries with abnormal responses to acetylcholine may demonstrate normal vasodilation in response to substance P, a non-muscarinic, endothelium-dependent vasodilator [33], acting on a different endothelial cell receptor, a tachykinin receptor. If the defect in NO activity of the hypertensive vasculature were located at the level of the muscarinic receptor, then the response to substance P would be similar between patients with hypertension and normotensive controls. However, forearm blood flow studies showed a significant reduction in blood flow and vascular resistance responses to substance P in patients with hypertension compared with normotensive controls [34], suggesting that the cause of endothelial dysfunction in patients with hypertension is not limited to a defect at the muscarinic receptor level.

Previous studies in animal models of dyslipidemia using pertussis toxin (a selective inhibitor of certain G proteins) have demonstrated that initially only endothelium-mediated responses that require the activation of pertussis toxin-sensitive G proteins are abnormal. Later in the course of disease, responses mediated by pertussis toxin-insensitive G proteins also become affected [35]. These observations suggest that the endothelial dysfunction in dyslipidemia may progress through different stages and have been recently confirmed in patients with hypercholesterolemia without clinical evidence of atherosclerosis [36]. However, in contrast to hypercholesterolemic patients, patients with hypertension show a significant reduction in the responses to both acetylcholine and bradykinin compared to normotensive controls [37], indicating that endothelial dysfunction in hypertension is likely due to a more generalized abnormality within the endothelial cell rather than a defect in a single G protein-dependent intracellular signal-transduction pathway.

A principal mechanism of NO inactivation is by superoxide anions produced by various radical-generating systems [31]. Superoxide dismutase is a superoxide anion scavenger that may thus block the inactivation of NO. Observations from animal models of hypercholesterolemia suggest that excess generation of superoxide anion may be responsible for increased inactivation of NO resulting in impaired endothelium-dependent vascular relaxation in atherosclerotic vessels [38]. Similar observations have been reported in different models of hypertension suggesting that a similar mechanism may be operative in this condition [39]. If this were the case in hypertensive patients, then administration of superoxide dismutase would be expected to improve their impaired response to acetylcholine. However, vascular responses to acetylcholine were similar before and after administration of copper zinc superoxide dismutase in both hypertensive patients and normotensive controls [40]. It must be noted that this form of the enzyme has poor intracellular penetrance. Therefore, one cannot rule out the possibility that enhanced production of oxygen free radical species formed within the intracellular space may contribute to a decreased bio-availability of NO.

An important intracellular source of superoxide radical is the xanthine oxidase system, which can be blocked by administration of oxypurinol. In an animal model, administration of oxypurinol normalized production of superoxide anion and improved acetylcholine-induced relaxation in hypercholesterolemic but not in normal vessels [38]. These findings suggest that endothelial cell production of superoxide anion may inactivate endothelium-derived NO, leading to endothelial dysfunction. We recently conducted an investigation in which acetylcholine-induced vascular relaxation in hypercholesterolemic patients was improved following oxpurinol administration [41], an observation in agreement with the results in hypercholesterolemic animal models. However, in hypertensive patients, the response to acetylcholine was not modified by administration of oxypurinol [41], suggesting that the xanthine oxidase system does not significantly contribute to their endothelial dysfunction.

Effect of antihypertensive treatment on endothelial dysfunction

The observation that induction of hypertension in animal models resulted in impaired endothelium-dependent vasodilation [42] led to the hypothesis that effective antihypertensive therapy may normalize or at least improve endothelial vasodilator function. Indeed, in spontaneously hypertensive rats, treatment with an ACE inhibitor or a calcium channel blocker reduced blood pressure and improved endothelial dysfunction in resistance vessels [43]. Long-term, but not short-term, treatment with an ACE inhibitor or a calcium channel blocker improved endothelial dysfunction in a rat model of NO-deficient hypertension [44]. These studies further suggested a beneficial effect on endothelial function with antihypertensive treatment. Studies in humans of the effects of antihypertensive treatment, including studies specifically related to the use of angiotensin-converting enzyme (ACE) inhibitors, have yielded negative results [28,45,46].

Summary

Microvascular dysfunction plays a critical part in the pathophysiology of the hypertensive process and thus determines the clinical course of patients with essential hypertension. This abnormal behavior of the small resistance vessels may be related to structural defects, functional alterations, or to the interplay between these two factors. Hypertensive patients have endothelial dysfunction of the microvasculature with reduced activity of NO. The functional and structural derangements associated with diminished bio-availability of NO may importantly contribute to the clinical presentation and complications of essential hypertension. Therefore, continued research to identify the intracellular mechanisms of endothelial dysfunction may lead to the development of novel therapies to forestall the natural course of hypertensive disease.

References

1. Opherk D, Mall G, Zeve H, et al: Reduction of coronary reserve: a mechanism for angina pectoris in patients with arterial hypertension and normal coronary arteries. Circulation 1984; 69:1-7.
2. Houghton JL, Frank MJ, Carr AA, et al: Relations among impaired coronary flow reserve, left ventricular hypertrophy, and thallium perfusion defects in hypertensive patients without obstructive coronary artery disease. J Am Coll Cardiol 1990; 15:43-51.
3. MacMahon S, Peto R, Cutler J, et al. Blood pressure, stroke, and coronary heart disease: I. Prolonged differences in blood presuure: Prospective observational studies corrected for the regression dilution bias. Lancet 1990;335:765.
4. Hedblad B, Janzon L. Hypertension and ST segment depression during ambulatory electrocardiographic recording: Results from the prospective population study "men born in 1914" in Malm, Sweden. Hypertension 1992;20:32.
5. Brush JE, Cannon RO, Schenke WH, et al: Angina due to coronary microvascular disease in hypertensive patients without left ventricular hypertrophy. N Engl J Med 1988; 319:1302-1307.
6. Brush JE Jr, Faxon DP, Salmon S, Jacobs AK, Ryan TJ. Abnormal endothelium-dependent coronary vasomotion in hypertensive patients. J Am Coll Cardiol 1992;19:809-15.
7. Quyyumi AA, Cannon RO, Panza JA, et al: Endothelial dysfunction in patients with chest pain and normal coronary arteries. Circulation 1992; 86:1864-1871.
8. Folkow B, Grimby G, Thulesius O: Adaptive structural changes of the vascular walls in hypertension and their relation to the control of the peripheral resistance. Acat Physiol Scand 1958, 44:255-272.
9. Sivertsson R: The hemodynamic importance of structural vascular change in essential hypertension. Acta Physiol Scand Suppl 1970, 343:1-56.
10. Folkow B: 'Structural factor' in primary and secondary hypertension. Hypertension 1990, 16:89-101.
11. Aalkjaer C, Heagerty AM, Peterson KK, Mulvany MJ: Evidence for increased media thickness, increased neuronal amine uptake and decreased excitation-contraction coupling in isolated resistance vessels from essential hypertensives. Circ Res 1987, 61:181-186.
12. Schiffrin EL, Deng LY, Larochelle P: Blunted effects of endothelin upon small subcutaneous resistance arteries of mild essential hypertensive patients. J Hypertens 1992, 10:437-444.
13. Heagerty AM, Aalkjaer C, Bund SJ, Korsgaard N, Mulvany MJ: Small artery structure in hypertension: dual processes of remodeling and growth. Hypertension 1993;21:391-397.
14. Harper RN, Moore MA, Marr MC, Watts LE, Hutchins PM: Arteriolar rarefaction in the conjunctiva of human essential hypertensives. Microvasc Res 1978, 16:369-372.
15. Gasser P, Buhler FR: Nailfold microcirculation in normotensive and essential hypertensive subjects, as assessed by video-microscopy. J Hypertens 1992, 10:83-86.
16. Sullivan JM, Prewitt RL, Joesephs JA: Attenuation of the microcirculation in young patients with high-output borderline hypertension. Hypertension 1983, 5:844-851.
17. Hartling O, Svendsen TL, Nielsen PE, Trap-Jensen J: The distensibility of the resistance vessels of skeletal muscle in hypertensive patients. Acata Physiol Scand 1978, 103:430-436.
18. Shigematsu Y, Hamada M, Mukai M, Matsuoka H, Sumimoto T, Hiwada K: Clinical evidence for an association between left ventricular geometric adaptation and extracardiac target organ damage in essential hypertension. J Hypertens 1995, 13:155-160.
19. Furchgott RF, Zawadzki JV. The obligatory role of endothelial cells in the relaxation of arterial smooth

muscle by acetylcholine. Nature 1980; 288: 373-6.

20. Palmer RMJ, Ferrige AG, Moncada S. Nitric oxide release accounts for the biological activity of endothelium-derived relaxing factor. Nature 1987;327:524-526.

21. Vallance P, Collier J, Moncada S. Effects of endothelium-derived nitric oxide on peripheral arteriolar tone in man. Lancet 1989;ii:997-1000.

22. Panza JA, Quyyumi AA, Brush JE Jr, Epstein SE. Abnormal endothelium-dependent vascular relaxation in patients with essential hypertension. N Engl J Med 1990;323:22-7.

23. Linder L, Kiowski W, Buhler FR, Luscher TF. Indirect evidence for release of endothelium-derived relaxing factor in human forearm circulation in vivo. Blunted response in essential hypertension. Circulation 1990;81:1762-7.

24. Yoshida M, Imaizumi T, Ando S, Hirooka Y, et al. Impaired forearm vasodilatation by acetylcholine in patients with hypertension. Heart Vessels 1991;6:218-23.

25. Treasure CB, Manoukian SV, Klein JL, Vita JA, et al. Epicardial coronary artery responses to acetylcholine are impaired in hypertensive patients. Circ Res 1992;71:776-81.

26. Taddei S, Virdis A, Mattei P, Salvetti A. Vasodilation to acetylcholine in primary and secondary forms of human hypertension. Hypertension 1993;21:929-33.

27. Falloon BJ, Heagerty AM. In vitro perfusion studies of human resistance artery function in essential hypertension. Hypertension 1994;24:16-23.

28. Creager MA, Roddy MA. Effect of captopril and enalapril on endothelial function in hypertensive patients. Hypertension 1994;24:499-505.

29. Panza JA, Casino PR, Kilcoyne CM, Quyyumi AA. Role of endothelium-derived nitric oxide in the abnormal endothelium-dependent vascular relaxation of patients with essential hypertension. Circulation 1993;87:1468-1474.

30. Calver A, Collier J, Moncada S, Vallance P. Effect of local intra-arterial N^G-monomethyl-L-arginine in patients with hypertension: the nitric oxide dilator mechanism appears abnormal. J Hypertension 1992;10:1025-1031.

31. Gryglewski RJ, Palmer RM, Moncada S. Superoxide anion is invovled in the breakdown of endothelium-derived vascular relaxing. Nature (Lond) 1986;320:454-456.

32. Panza JA, Casino PR, Badar DM, Quyyumi AA. Effect of increased availability of endothelium-derived nitric oxide precursor on endothelium-dependent vascular relaxation in normal subjects and in patients with essential hypertension. Circulation 1993;87:1475-1481.

33. Egashira K, Inou T, Yamada A, Hirooka Y, Urabe Y, Nagasawa K, Takeshita A. Heterogeneous effects of the endothelium-dependent vasodilators acetylcholine and substance P on the coronary circulation of patients with angiographically normal coronary arteries. Coronary Artery Dis 1992;3:945-952.

34. Panza JA, Casino PR, Kilcoyne CM, Quyyumi AA. Impaired endothelium-dependent vasodilation in patients with essential hypertension: evidence that the abnormality is not at the muscarinic receptor level. J Am Coll Cardiol 1994;23:1610-1616.

35. Flavahan NA. Atherosclerotic or lipoprotein-induced endothelial dysfunction: potential mechanisms underlying reduction in EDRF/nitric oxide activity. Circulation 1992;85:1927-1938.

36. Gilligan DM, Guetta V, Panza JA, García CE, Quyyumi AA, Cannon RO. Selective loss of microvascular endothelial function in human hypercholesterolemia. Circulation 1994;90:35-41.

37. Panza JA, Garcia CE, Kilcoyne CM, Quyyumi AA, Cannon RO III. Impaired endothelium-dependent vasodilation in patients with essential hypertension: evidence that nitric oxide abnormality is not localized to a single signal transduction pathway. Circulation 1995;91:1732-1738.

38. Ohara Y, Peterson TE, Harrison DG. Hypercholesterolemia increases endothelial superoxide anion production. J Clin Invest 1993;92:2546-2551.

39. Nakazono K, Watanabe N, Matsuno K, Sasak J, Sato T. Does superoxide underlie the pathogenesis of hypertension ? Proc Natl Acad Sci 1991;88:1045-1048.

40. Garcia CE, Kilcoyne CM, Cardillo C, Cannon RO, Quyyumi AA, Panza JA. Effect of copper-zinc superoxide dismutase on endothelium-dependent vasodilation in patients with essential hypertension. Hypertension 1995;26:863-868.

41. Cardillo C, Kilcoyne CM, Cannon RO, Quyyumi AA, Panza JA. Xanthine oxidase inhibition improves endothelium-dependent vasodilation in hypercholesterolemic but not in hypertensive patients. Hypertension 1997;30:57-63.

42. Miller MJS, Pinto A, Mullane KM. Impaired endothelium-dependent relaxations in rabbits subjected to aortic coarctation hypertension. Hypertension 1987;10:164-170.

43. Dohi Y, Criscione L, Pfeiffer K, Lüscher TF. Angiotensin blockade or calcium antagonists improve endothelial dysfunction in hypertension: studies in perfused mesenteric resistance arteries. J Cardiovasc Pharmacol 1994;24:372-379.

44. Takase H, Moreau P, Küng CF, Nava E, Lüscher TF. Antihypertensive therapy prevents endothelial

dysfunction in chronic nitric oxide deficiency: effect of verapamil and trandolapril. Hypertension 1996;27:25-31.

45. Panza J, Quyyumi AA, Callahan TS, Epstein SE. Effect of antihypertensive treatment on endothelium-dependent vascular relaxation in patients with essential hypertension. J Am Coll Cardiol 1993;21:1145-1151.

46. Kiowski W, Linder L, Nuesch R, Martina B. Effects of cilazapril on vascular structure and function in essential hypertension. Hypertension 1996;27(part 1):371-376.

Chapter 26

MICROVASCULAR ANGINA AND HYPERTENSIVE LEFT VENTRICULAR HYPERTROPHY

Wolfgang Motz and Sibylle Scheler

Chronic arterial hypertension induces specific functional and structural alterations of both the myocardium and the coronary microcirculation which can be summarised as hypertensive remodelling. Hypertensive remodelling reflects the fundamental reorganisation of the heart at the level of [1] the myocytes, [2] the extracellular matrix and [3] the vascular structure and endothelial cells.

Even in the absence of visible alterations of the epicardial coronary arteries, coronary flow reserve (CFR) its reduced in hypertensive patients. Impaired CFR in these patients is associated with structural alterations of the intramyocardial arterioles. These alterations are also found in the right septal subendocardium, which is not exposed to increased pressure load. Growing evidence suggests that structural remodelling of the vessels is caused by the interrelationship between mechanical stretch i. e. vascular wall stress, hormonal stimulation and growth factors. In particular the renin-angiotensin system modulates the growth of vascular smooth muscle cells and reinforces the process of hypertensive cardiac remodelling via induction of protooncogenes and growth factors mediated by angiotensin II. Other growth factors have been found to modulate medial hypertrophy through smooth muscle cell hypertrophy or hyperplasia.

Another factor potentially leading to myocardial ischemia is the loss of capillary pathways and an increase in the distance between capillaries, which may lead to limitations of oxygen diffusion into the myocardium. Both hypertensive perfusion and cardiac hypertrophy seem to decrease capillary density and increase the heterogenety of capillary spacing limiting the supply of oxygen to myocardial cells.

Apart from structural alterations of coronary resistance arteries, the extravascular component of coronary resistance i.e. the "myocardial factor" contributes to the impaired CFR in chronic arterial hypertension. The myocardial factor of coronary resistance comprises all forces which occur during the process of myocardial contraction and relaxation.

These extravascular factors which are active even in the normotensive healthy heart are amplified by the process of adaptive left ventricular hypertrophy (LVH) as such. Adaptive LVH describes the numeric amplification of sarcomeres without any change in myocardial composition. When additional qualitative changes in the myocardial structure occur due to activation of non-myocytic cells such as cardiac fibroblasts, this leads to an augmentation of interstitial collagen content. Ventricular and myocardial stiffness are increased consequently. Therefore, the myocardial component of coronary resistance is increased, which contributes to the impaired blood flow reserve.

The extravascular compression forces reflect all physical forces which act, principally, on the endocardial regions of the myocardium. Since coronary perfusion takes place mostly during diastole, diastolic wall stress represents the main determinant of the extravascular compression forces. In conditions associated with an increment in diastolic wall stress such as eccentric i. e. dilated LVH, severe concentric LVH with increased chamber and myocardial stiffness, forces further augment the extravascular component of coronary flow reserve.

In the presence of LVH, limitations also exist in endothelium-mediated control of coronary resistance vessels and vasomotion of the epicardial conductance arteries. Endothelial cells enzymatically synthesize nitric oxide. Compared with normotensive controls, hypertensive patients with LVH have markedly impaired endothelial dependent flow responses. The activity of cardiac NO synthase is up regulated in arterial hypertension and parallels the development of arterial hypertension. This speaks in favour of the hypothesis that in arterial hypertension the production of NO is not decreased, but the degradation of nitric oxide is increased, possibly by free radicals.

Left ventricular hypertrophy is the principal structural mechanism of adaptation of the myocardium to a chronic pressure or volume load in the course of arterial hypertension, aortic stenosis and incompetence of the aortic or mitral valve [1, 2]. Also, after regional loss of contractile substance following myocardial infarction, compensatory hypertrophy of the "surviving" myocardium occurs [3]. In the course of primary or secondary myocardial diseases, again, a hypertrophy of the surviving myocardial cells will develop as a consequence of permanent functional impairment of the contractile apparatus or loss of contractile material [4].

Initially, systolic wall stress or LV afterload is increased due to systolic pressure overload or LV dilatation. The emerging process of LV hypertrophy normalises systolic wall stress per cross-sectional area of the myocardium and enables the left ventricle to eject a normal cardiac output at the expense of a normal myocardial energy demand per weight unit myocardium in spite of a hypertensive systolic pressure in the left ventricle. Therefore, at least in the initial stages, LVH can be considered a desired adaptation to pressure overload [1, 2, 5].

In contrast to these pathophysiological considerations, clinical experience shows that LVH is an independent cardiovascular risk factor in the long run. Hypertensives with echocardiographic evidence of LVH show a higher cardiovascular mortality than hypertensives without LVH [6]. Furthermore, the Framingham data clearly indicate that the cardiovascular risk increases along with echocardiographic LV mass, equally in men and women [7].

These epidemiologic data suggest that only in the early stages of myocardial hypertrophy represents a beneficial mechanism of adaptation as it initially leads to normalisation of systolic wall stress. In the long run, adaptive compensatory hypertrophy becomes a process of disease ultimately leading to myocardial insufficiency and clinical heart failure. Accordingly, myocardial hypertrophy is not a permanent beneficial mechanism of adaptation, but rather a maladaption process overload cardiomyopathy [8] (Figure 1).

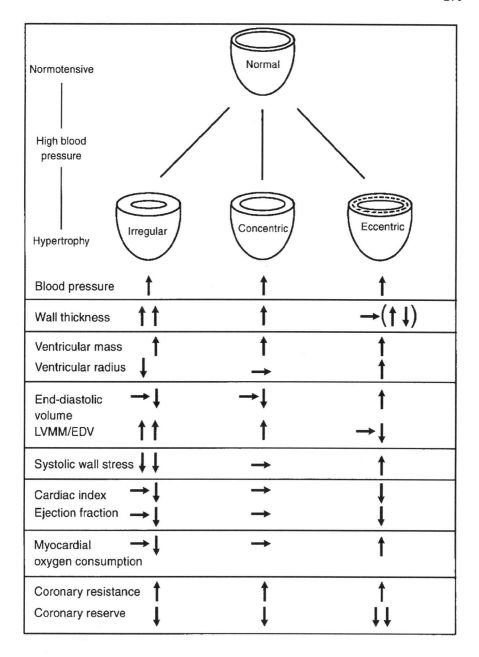

Figure 1. Development of concentric hypertrophy due to arterial hypertension. Persistent hypertension leads to irregular or eccentric hypertrophy. →, normal, ▲ raised; ↓ lowered; LVMM/EDV, mass: volume ratio. Redrawn from [8] with permission.

Molecular mechanisms of myocardial hypertrophy

Initially, the rise in systolic pressure in the left ventricle leads to an increase in systolic wall stress within the myocardial texture. The resulting increment in passive stretch of the myocardial cells activates phospholipase C, which results in increased intracellular concentration of inositolphosphates and diacylglycerol and increased intracellular calcium concentration. These steps activate protein kinase C and MAP2-kinase. Finally, the proto-oncogenes c-fos, c-jun and c-myc will be activated, which regulate the transcription of other genes towards protein synthesis after take-up of the cell nucleus. The induction of proto-oncogenes in the cell nucleus starts a series of events, which end at the division of the cell. Since adult cardiomyocytes have lost their ability of cell division, only myocardial cell hyperplasia will result instead of a terminally differentiated myocardial parenchyma [9].

The process of myocardial hypertrophy resembles fetal or postnatal development. In LVH there is a re-expression of isoforms of contractile proteins such as ß-myosin-heavy chain (MHC), ß -troponin and skeletal-actin. These proteins are expressed in the fetal state only and are later replaced by adult isoforms. Accordingly, from the molecular point of view, LVH reflects a process of myocardial growth similar to the fetal state rather than a quantitative augmentation of myocardial mass [9].

Angiotensin II plays a major part in the process of myocardial hypertrophy. Experimental studies have shown that myocardial ACE-activity is enhanced and the intracardiac conversion of angiotensin I to angiotensin II is stimulated due to an enhanced expression of angiotensinogen-mRNA and ACE-mRNA [4, 10, 11]. Angiotensin II promotes cardiac growth via induction of proto-oncogenes and stimulation of myocardial protein synthesis. The primary location of cardiac angiotensin II formation is the extensive microvascular capillary network. Due to the fact that cardiac ACE is located in the capillaries, a rapid conversion of angiotensin I to angiotensin II can occur. Angiotensin II will then be transported to both the interstitial space and the myocyte AT1-receptor [10].

There is also evidence that angiotensin II can be synthesised from angiotensinogen through the enzyme chymase independent from ACE. Chymase is localised in the vesicles of mast cells. The clinical relevance of this mode of formation, which is completely independent from the renin-angiotensin-system, is a subject for further studies [12].

Qualitative alterations in myocardial structure largely involve non-myocytic cells. There is ample evidence that the non-myocytic component of the myocardium represents the major determinant of hypertensive hypertrophy. The activation of cardiac fibroblasts leads to reactive fibrosis, which severely alters myocardial tissue structure and stiffness, as well as the diastolic and systolic function of the left ventricle [13-15].

In contrast to replacement fibrosis which restores structural integrity after parenchymal cell injury, reactive fibrosis is a condition where interstitial collagen and perivascular collagen surrounding small intramural arterioles are increased. This disproportionate increment in collagen concentration, which seems to be caused by circulating hormones such as aldosterone and angiotensin II rather than by the pressure load alone, was found to adversely influence myocardial stiffness [15, 16].

Consequently, hypertensive hypertrophy is completely different from the so called "plain myocardial hypertrophy", which represents an adaptive condition without any alteration in myocardial composition and structure as seen in trained athletes. In plain LVH there is quantitative augmentation of sarcomeres due to increased myocyte workload without any growth, or altered metabolism, of nonmyocyte cells (i.e. fibroblasts, vascular smooth muscle cells and endothelial cells). In this condition no change in the ratio between contractile and noncontractile proteins exist [16].

Structural changes of coronary microcirculation

Structural hypertensive remodelling of the coronary microcirculation includes alterations in the composition of the vessel wall [17, 19, 21] and a reduction in the number of parallel intramyocardial vessels or capillaries [2, 5] leading to a decreased vasodilator capacity. This can be caused by a disproportionate growth response of the myocyte compartment without a corresponding growth adaptation of coronary resistance vessels or capillaries or by a disproportionate loss of resistance vessels not accompanied by alterations in the myocyte compartment.

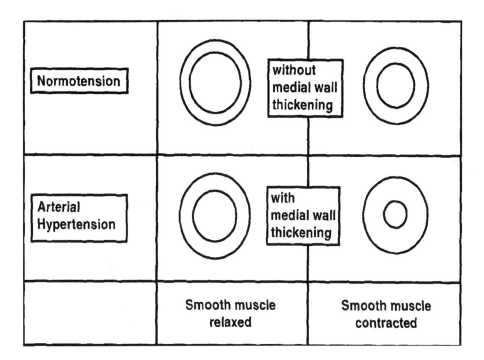

Figure 2. Folkow's concept of structural changes of myocardial vessels includes that the normotensive vessel without wall thickening shows a greater lumen when contracted, while the hypertensive altered vessel (with wall thickening) shows a decreased lumen.

The intramyocardial arterioles constitute a large part of coronary vascular resistance and play an important role in the autoregulation of myocardial perfusion. According to Folkow [22], structural changes of resistance vessels, such as vascular smooth muscle hypertrophy, are the consequence of hypertensive tissue perfusion. In experimental hypertension, arterial medial hypertrophy reduces the luminal diameter even when vascular smooth muscle is fully relaxed. In the presence of a high vessel wall-lumen ratio, every contraction of vascular smooth muscle leads to a more progressive luminal encroachment than the same smooth muscle contraction if the vessel wall-lumen ratio is low. This increment in the wall-lumen ratio of resistance vessels causes an increased vascular resistance (Figure 2). Recently, medial thickening of intramural coronary arteries in vivo has been demonstrated in hypertensive patients by morphometric evaluation of transvenous endomyocardial biopsies [19, 20]. Remodelling of the hypertrophied vascular wall leads to an increase in percent wall area, reducing the relative lumen and correlating with the increased minimal coronary resistance and the reduced coronary reserve.

These structural alterations of intramyocardial arterioles are found in the right septal subendocardium, which is not exposed to the pressure load [19, 20]. Consequently, wall thickening seems to be caused by high vascular wall stress due to hypertensive coronary perfusion or circulating and tissue-based growth hormones rather than by the direct cardiomyocytic load.

There is growing evidence that structural remodelling of the coronary vasculature in arterial hypertension is determined by the interrelationship of mechanical stretch, i.e. vascular wall stress exerted upon the vascular smooth muscle and activation of growth promoting hormones which exert their action in an endocrine, paracrine or autocrine way. Particularly the renin-angiotensin-system modulates the growth processes of the vascular smooth muscle and enhances the process of hypertensive remodeling due to induction of proto-oncogenes and other growth factors [10, 11, 23].

Several mechanisms are involved in the growth promoting processes of angiotensin II. Angiotensin II activates cellular growth processes of the vascular smooth muscle through activation of protein kinase C. Besides the expression of proto-oncogenes such as c-fos, c-myc and c-jun in the vascular smooth muscle cells growth factors such as the basic fibroblast growth factor (bFGF) and the transforming growth factor ß 1 (TGF ß 1) are activated [10, 23].

These structural abnormalities of the coronary microvessels lead to an impairment of coronary vascular conductance capacity which is clinically expressed by a reduced coronary vasodilator reserve. Maximal achievable coronary blood flow after dipyridamole administration (0.50-0.75 mg/kg body weight) is reduced by 30-50% and coronary resistance is accordingly elevated. Coronary reserve, which is defined as the ratio between coronary resistance under baseline conditions and that observed under maximal vasodilation due to dipyridamole, is likewise reduced relative to that seen in normotensive individuals (Figure 3) [21, 24, 25]. In hypertensive patients with dilated LV hypertrophy coronary reserve is also metabolically impaired by enhanced blood flow requirements under basal conditions due to increased myocardial oxygen consumption as a consequence of high afterload or systolic wall stress [1, 25].

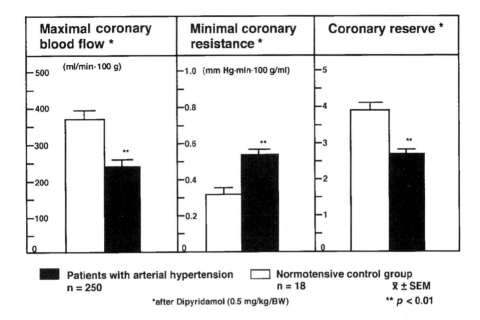

Figure 3. Maximal coronary blood flow, minimal coronary resistance and coronary reserve in hypertensive patients and normotensive controls. Coronary blood flow was measured using the argon gas chromatography. Maximal coronary blood flow was achieved using intravenous dipyridamole (0.5 mg/kg body weight).

Functional endothelial alterations of the coronary microculation

In addition to structural vascular and myocardial factors that contribute to impairment of coronary reserve in arterial hypertension, attenuations in endothelium-mediated control of coronary resistance vessels and vasomotion of the epicardial conductance arteries also play a role [26 29, 31-33].

Endothelial cells enzymatically synthesize (from L–arginine) the endothelial-derived-relaxing-factor nitric oxide (NO) [29, 30, 34]. Baseline endothelial NO production can be stimulated by bradykinin, acetylcholine (ACh) and physical forces such as shear stress [35]. Pharmacological blockade of endothelial NO synthesis results in an increase in total peripheral resistance [35]. Thus, endothelium-derived NO critically influences the tone of coronary and systemic resistance vessels.

Impaired endothelium-dependent coronary vasodilation of epicardial arteries to acetylcholine has been observed in studies in patients with essential hypertension, indicating an alteration of the NO system in human hypertension [33]. According to these findings an impaired endothelial NO metabolism seems to be present also at the level of coronary microcirculation. However, such a definitely blunted flow response to acetylcholine as described by Treasure and co-workers [33] is not generally seen in hypertensive patients with microvascular angina pectoris [31].

Aside from a defect in endothelial NO metabolism a diminished sensitivity of the vascular smooth muscle to NO, an impaired NO diffusion from the endothelial cell to the smooth muscle and a facilitated luminal ACh diffusion to the vascular smooth muscle due to endothelial denudation can also be the underlying cause for vasoconstriction under ACh. Consequently, one should be cautious in interpreting the altered acetylcholine response to ACh as a clear defect in the metabolism of endothelial NO. However, it is an interesting speculation that the altered acetylcholine response to ACh found in some hypertensive patients might indicate early endothelial dysfunction at coronary "macrocirculation" level and be a precursor of atherosclerotic heart disease. An alternative mechanism would be the production of endothelial constrictive factors. Angiotensin II diminishes endothelial NO release due to an enhanced degradation of bradykinin [36].

Therapeutical considerations

Main targets in the treatment of hypertensive heart disease are the prevention of structural myocardial and vascular complications which lead to myocardial ischemia and diastolic and systolic dysfunction of the left ventricle.

Therapy of hypertensive heart disease regarding "cardiac reparation" consists of: a) regression of cardiac hypertrophy, b) normalisation of myocardial structure through regression of newly formed interstitial collagen, and c) reversal of structural and functional alterations of the coronary microvasculature. Such a differentiated cardioreparative therapy differs significantly from the traditional blood pressure reduction only antihypertensive therapy [16, 37].

In recent years, experimental and clinical studies have shown [37, 40] that reduction of circulating and local levels of the growth factors angiotensin II and noradrenaline with ACE-inhibitors and antisympathicotonic drugs - induce regression of LVH. ACE-inhibition leads also to a reduction of myocardial collagen in experimental animals [13] and in hypertensive patients [41]. After treatment with calcium channel blockers, regression of both collagen and LVH was also found [37]. Antihypertensive treatment with diuretics and vasodilators do not usually improve LVH most likely due to activation of neurohumoral counterregulatory systems by these agents [37].

However, these observations are only based on uncontrolled consecutive studies and meta-analysis [42]. Prospective controlled studies which scientifically compare the ability of different antihypertensive agents in respect of regression of LVH are lacking.

From a therapeutic point of view based mostly on pathophysiological considerations, antihypertensive drugs which lower local and circulating angiotensin II and noradrenaline - ACE-inhibitors and probably also A II -receptor-blockers and antisympathotonic substances - are first-line drugs in the treatment of LVH (Figure 4).

Probably due to the widespread use of antihypertensive substances, the prevalence of dilated LVH has been reduced compared to 20 years ago. In the Framingham Study about 70% of all persons who developed heart failure were hypertensives during the follow-up period between 1949 and 1964 [43]. Nowadays, hypertension is considered to be the cause of heart failure in 10% of cases only [44]. Thus, modern antihypertensive therapy had a great impact on mortality from heart failure.

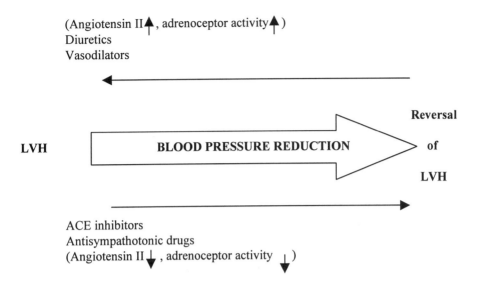

Figure 4. The current concept of reversal of LVH is shown; diuretics and vasodilators increase left ventricular muscle mass in spite of blood pressure reduction, while ACE inhibitors and antisympathotonic drugs decrease left ventricular hypertrophy (LVH) parallel to blood pressure reduction.

References

1. Strauer BE. Ventricular function and coronary hemodynamics in hypertensive heart disease. Am J Cardiol 1979; 44: 999-1006.
2. Tomanek RJ. Capillary and pre-capillary coronary vascular growth during left ventricular hypertrophy. Can J Cardiol 1986; 2:114-119.
3. Pfeffer MA, Braunwald E. Ventricular remodelling after myocardial infarction. Experimental observations and clinical implications. Circulation 1990; 81:1161.
4. Schunkert H, Riegger AJG. Molekularbiologie der adaptiven Myokardhypertrophie. Dtsch Med Wshr 1992; 117:1406-1412.
5. Turek Z, Rakusan K. Lognormal distribution in normal and hypertrophic rat heart as estimated by the method of concertric circles: its effect on tissue oxygenation. Pflügers Arch 1981; 391:17 - 31.
6. Koren MJ, Devereux RB, Caslae PN, Savage DD, Laragh JH. Relation of left ventricular mass and geometry to morbidity and mortality in uncomplicated essential hypertension. Ann Int Med 1991; 114:345-352.
7. Levy D, Garrison RJ, Savage DD, Kannek WB, Castelli WP. Prognostic implications of echocardiographically determined left ventricular mass in the Framingham Heart Study. N Engl J Med 1990; 322:1561-1566.
8. Katz AM. Physiology of the I-Ieart. Raven Press, New York 1992; 2nd Edition.
9. Nadal-Giner B, Mahdavi V. Molecular mechanisms of cardiac gene expression. In: Grobecker H, Heusch G, Strauer BE (Eds.). Angiotensin and the Heart. Springer Verlag, NewYork 1993:65-80.
10. Dzau VJ. Local expression and pathophysiological role of renin-angiotensin in the blood vessels and heart. In: Grobecker H, Heusch G, Strauer BE (Eds), Angiotensin and the Heart. Springer Verlag, New York 1993:1-14.
11. Lindpainter K, Ganten D. The cardiac renin-angiotensin system. Circ Res 1991; 68:905-920.
12. Urata H, Healey B, Stewart RW, Bumpus FM, Husain A. Angiotensin 11 formatting pathways in normal and failing human hearts. Circ Res 1990: 883-890.

278

13. Brilla CG, Janicki JS, Weber KT. Cardioreparative effects of lisinopril in rats with genetic hypertension and left ventricular hypertrophy. Circulation 1991; 83: 1771-1779.
14. Caulfield JB, Borg TK. The collagen network of the heart. Lab Invest 1979; 40:364-372.
15. Weber KT, Brilla CG. Pathological hypertrophy and the cardiac interstitium: Fibrosis and the renin-angiotensin-aldosterone system. Circulation 1991; 83:1849-1865.
16. Weber KT, Anversa P, Armstrong PW et al. Remodeling and reparation of the cardiovascular system. J Am Coll Cardiol 1992; 20:3-16.
17. Mulvany MJ, Baandrup U, Gundersen HJG. Evidence for hyperplasia in mesenteric resistance vessels of spontaneously hypertensive rats using a three-dimensional dissector. Circ Res 1985; 57:794-800.
18. Tanaka M, Fujiwara H, OnoderaT, HamashimaY, Kawai C. Quantitative analysis of narrowings of intramyocardial small arteries in normal hearts, hypertensive hearts and hearts with hypertrophic cardiomyopathy. Circulation 1987; 75:1130-1139.
19. Schwartzkopff B, Motz W, Frenzel H, Vogt M, Knauer S, Strauer BE. Structural and functional alterations of the intramyocardial coronary arterioles in patients in patients with arterial hypertension. Circulation 1993; 88:993-1003.
20. v Hoeven KH, Factor S. Endomyocardial biopsy diagnosis of small vessel disease: a clinicopathologic study. Int J Cardiol 1990; 26:103-110.
21. Strauer BE. The significance of coronary reserve in clinical heart disease. J Am Coll Cardiol 1990; 15: 775-783.
22. Folkow B. Physiological aspects of primary hypertension. PhysioL Rev 1982; 62:347-467.
23. Naftilan AJ, Pratt RE, Dzau VJ. Induction of platelet-derived growth factor A-chain and c-myc gene expression by angiotensin 11 in cultured rat vascular smooth muscle cells. J Clin Invest 1989; 83:1419-1424.
24. Brush JE, Cannon 111 RO, Schencke WH et al. Angina due to coronary microvascular disease in hypertensive patients without left ventricular hypertrophy. N Engl J Med 1988; 319:1302.
25. Strauer BE. Myocardial oxygen consumption in chronic heart disease: role of wall stress, hypertrophy and coronary reserve. Am J Cardiol 1979; 44:730-740.
26. Brush JE, Faxon DP, Salmon S, Jacobs AK, RyanTJ. Abnormal endothelium-dependent coronary vasomation in hypertensive patients. J Am Coll Cardiol 1992; 19: 809-815.
27. Lüscher TF, Vanhoutte PM. Endothelium-dependent contraction to acetylcholine in the aorta of the spontaneously hypertensive rat. Hypertension 1989; 8:344-348.
28. LüscherTF, Aarhus LL,Vanhoutte PM. Indomethacin improves impaired endothelium-dependent relaxations in small mesenteric arteries of the spontaneously hypertensive rat. Am J Hypertens 1990; 3:55-58.
29. Moncada S, Palmer RMJ, Higgs EA. Nitric oxide: physiology, pathophysiology and pharmacology. Pharmacol Rev; 43:109-142.
30. Vita JA, Treasure CB, Nabel EG et al. Coronary vasomotive response to acetylcholine relates to risk factors for coronary heart disease. Circulation 1990; 81:495-497.
31. Motz W, Vogt M, Rabenau 0, Scheler S, Lückhoff A, Strauer BE. Evidence of endothelial dysfunction in coronary resistance vessels in patients with angina pectoris and normal coronary angiograms. Am J Cardiol 1991; 68: 996-1000.
32. Panza JA, Quyyumi AA, Brush JE Jr, Epstein SE. Abnormal endothelium-dependent vascular relaxation in patients with essential hypertension. N Engl J Med 1990; 323:22-27.
33. Treasure CB, Klein JL,Vita JA et al. Hypertension and left ventricular hypertrophy are associated with impaired endothelium-mediated relaxation in human coronary resistance vessels. Circulation 1993; 87:86-93.
34. Kelm M, Schrader J. Control of coronary vascular tone by nitric oxide. Circ Res 1990; 66:1561-1575.
35. Kelm M, Feelisch M, Deußen A, Trauer BE, Schrader J. Release of endothelium derived nitric oxide in relation to pressure and flow. Cardiovasc Res 1991; 10:831-836.
36. Holtz J. The cardiac renin angiotensin system. Physiological relevance and pharmacological modulation. Clin Invest 1993 (in press).
37. Motz W, Vogt M, Scheler S, Strauer BE. Pharmacotherapeutic effects of antihypertensive agents on myocardium and coronary arteries in hypertension. Eur Heart J; 13 (SuppL D):100-106.
38. Mall, Greber D, Gharebhaghi H, Wiest G, Mattfeldt T Ganten U. Myokardprotektion und Hypertrophieregression bei spontan hypertensiven Ratten durch Nifedipin und Moxonidin - stereologische Untersuchungen. In: Ganten D, Mall G (Eds), Herz-Kreislauf-Regulation, Organprotektion und Organschäden. Schattauer, Stuttgart, NewYork 1991:91-106.

39. Motz W, Vogt M, Scheler S, Schwartzkopff B, Strauer BE. Verbesserung der Koronarreserve nach hypertrophieregression durch blutdrucksenkende Thera-pie mit einem ß-Rezeptorenblocker. Dtsch Med Wschr 1993; 118:535-540.

40. Vogt M, Motz W, Pölitz B, Scheler S, Strauer BE. Improvement of coronary reserve by chronic treatment with ACE-inhibitors. Circulation 1991; 84:111- 136.

41. Motz W, Schwartzkopff B, Vogt M. Hypertensive heart disease: cardio-reparation by reversal of interstitial collagen in patients. Eur Heart J 1995; 16:69-73.

42. Dahlöf B, Pennert K, Hansson L. Reversal of left ventricular hypertrophy in hypertensive patients. A meta-analysis of 109 treatment studies. Am J Hypertens 1992; 5:95-110.

43. McKee P, Castelli W, McNamara PM, Kannel W. The natural history of congestive heart failure. N Engl J Med 1971; 285:1441-1446.

44. Gradman A, Deedwania P, Cody R, Massie B, Packer M, Pitt B, Goldstein D for the Captopril-Digoxin Study Group. Predictors of total mortality and sudden death in mild to moderate heart failure. J Am Coll Cardiol 1989; 14:564-570.

Chapter 27

MYOCARDIAL ISCHEMIA IN HYPERTROPHIC CARDIOMYOPATHY: CLINICAL ASSESSMENT AND ROLE IN NATURAL HISTORY

Perry M. Elliott

The cardiomyopathies are a group of primary heart muscle diseases, classified into hypertrophic, dilated, restrictive, and arrhythmogenic right ventricular forms according to specific morphological and physiological criteria. The pathophysiology of all cardiomyopathies is complex and remains incompletely understood, but myocardial ischemia is thought to play a role in the natural history of several types of cardiomyopathy, in particular the hypertrophic form. This chapter reviews the evidence for impaired myocardial blood flow in patients with hypertrophic cardiomyopathy and briefly discusses its potential role in the pathophysiology of this disease.

Hypertrophic cardiomyopathy

Hypertrophic cardiomyopathy is defined by the presence of left ventricular hypertrophy in the absence of any other discernible cardiac or systemic cause [1-2]. Although traditionally thought of as a rare disease, most studies in the United States and Japan suggest that its prevalence may be as high as 1 in 500 of the general population. Most cases are caused by inherited mutations in a number of genes that encode cardiac sarcomeric proteins; ß-myosin heavy chain on chromosome 14q11 (35%), cardiac troponin T on chromosome 1q3 (15%), α-tropomyosin on chromosome 15q2 (<5%), myosin binding protein C on chromosome 11p11.2 (15%), and essential and regulatory light chains on chromosomes 3 and 12 respectively (<1%) [1]. The latest mutation to be described occurs in the troponin I gene on chromosome 19p13 [3]. Sarcomeric protein mutations are usually inherited in an autosomal dominant fashion with variable penetrance and age related expression, but they can appear sporadically [4]. Most patients develop hypertrophy during adolescence and occasionally in infancy, but presentation after the age of 60 years with so-called "elderly" HCM is well recognized. The characteristically diverse pathology that results from sarcomeric protein mutations includes myocyte hypertrophy and disarray, interstitial fibrosis, small vessel disease and left ventricular outflow tract obstruction [1]. Together, these morphological abnormalities contribute to a spectrum of functional disturbance that includes cardiac arrhythmia, diastolic and systolic dysfunction, and abnormal vascular responses. While many patients have few or no symptoms, a substantial number present with a dyspnoea, syncope, palpitation, and chest pain. The latter is often qualitatively similar to ischemic cardiac pain, but differs from typical angina pectoris in that it can be prolonged and occurs at rest [1,5-7]. Precipitation by meals is another characteristic feature described by many patients [8]. The cause of chest pain in hypertrophic cardiomyopathy is probably multifactorial, but as the following clinical and pathological evidence demonstrates, myocardial ischemia is an important mechanism.

Mechanisms of myocardial blood flow limitation in hypertrophic cardiomyopathy

Several aspects of the pathophysiology of hypertrophic cardiomyopathy theoretically predispose to the development of microvascular angina. Left ventricular hypertrophy results in an increase in total myocardial oxygen demand and may also increase extravascular compressive forces [9-10]. In hypertensive dogs, left ventricular hypertrophy is associated with a decrease in the number of coronary arterioles per unit volume of myocardium [11], indicating that inadequate microvascular growth may also contribute to a reduction in coronary blood flow. At a microscopic level, hypertrophic cardiomyopathy is characterized by disruption of myocardial architecture with loss of normal myocyte to myocyte orientation, abnormal intercellular connections, increased connective tissue and myocardial fibrosis [12]. The precise functional consequences of these anatomical changes are the subject of ongoing investigation, but it is very likely that they result in inefficient myocardial contraction and thereby contribute to increased oxygen demand. Several studies have described medial thickening and apparent narrowing of small intramural vessels in hearts affected by hypertrophic cardiomyopathy [13-14] (figure 1), particularly in regions of myocardial scarring and in hearts affected by "end-stage" dilatation. This distribution has led to the suggestion that small vessel disease causes myocardial ischemia, but this hypothesis is impossible to test in individual patients. In most patients with hypertrophic cardiomyopathy, large coronary vessels are angiographically normal, but systolic compression of septal perforator vessels and epicardial coronary vessels is described [15-16]. The fact that most myocardial perfusion occurs during diastole makes the clinical significance of coronary vessel compression unclear, but it may explain the dramatic systolic flow reversal observed during intracoronary and transesophageal Doppler studies of proximal coronary vessel blood flow [17]. Finally, approximately 25% of patients with hypertrophic cardiomyopathy have obstruction to the left ventricular outflow tract caused by contact between the anterior mitral leaflet and the interventricular septum during ventricular systole [1,7]. In spite of 30 years of investigation the clinical significance of this phenomenon remains controversial, but the fact that considerable symptomatic improvement may occur following successful surgical septal reduction makes it likely that the increased left ventricular pressures and wall tension associated with substantial gradients cause or exacerbate myocardial ischemia in some patients.

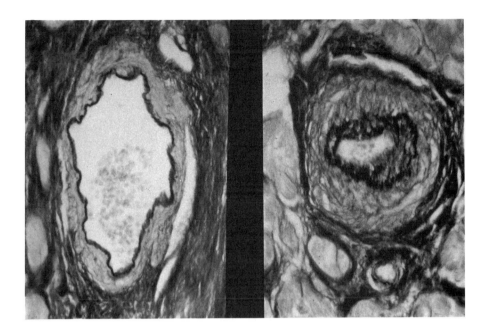

Figure 1. Sections thorough two intramural coronary blood vessels demonstrating normal anatomy (left panel) and medial thickening in a patient with hypertrophic cardiomyopathy (right panel) (Courtesy of Professor M. Davies, St. George's Hospital Medical School, London.

Clinical evidence for myocardial ischemia in hypertrophic cardiomyopathy

Electrocardiography

Patients with hypertrophic cardiomyopathy develop ST segment depression during symptom limited exercise testing, rapid atrial pacing, and 48 hour ambulatory electrocardiographic monitoring [18-21] (figure 2). ST segment depression is also described in isolated case reports preceding sudden cardiac death [21]. Although there are some studies describing associations between ST segment depression, symptomatic status [19], and low coronary flow reserve [22], data on the relationship between ST segment change and lactate extraction suggest that it is not a particularly sensitive or specific marker of myocardial ischemia [18,23]. This probably reflects the interpretative

284

difficulties caused by the presence of resting electrocardiographic abnormalities in many patients, and the influence of other factors such as exaggerated atrial repolarization on the ST segment.

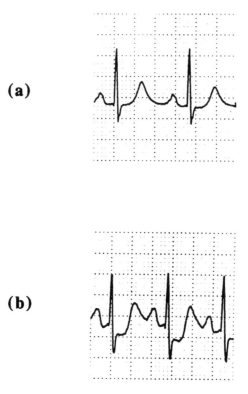

(a)

(b)

Figure 2. Ambulatory electrocardiograms from a 45 year patient with hypertrophic cardiomyopathy at rest (a) and during an episode of chest pain (b). From Elliott et al Eur Heart J 1996;17:1056-1064.

Thallium-201 perfusion abnormalities

A number of studies using both planar and SPECT thallium-201 myocardial perfusion imaging have determined the relation of clinical features to different types of perfusion defect in patients with hypertrophic cardiomyopathy [18,24-28]. Fixed defects are associated with increased left ventricular cavity dimensions, reduced shortening fraction and lower peak exercise oxygen consumption, suggesting they may represent areas of myocardial fibrosis [24-25]. Surprisingly, associations with reversible defects have been more elusive, with almost every study failing to demonstrate an association with a history of angina or dyspnoea [18,24-28]. This paradox has been explained by a high prevalence of "silent ischemia" and non-ischemic chest pain in hypertrophic cardiomyopathy, but the disparity between symptoms and reversible perfusion defects may also relate to the intrinsic limitations of single photon imaging. The fact that thallium-201 perfusion defects result from relative differences in myocardial thallium-201 uptake means that it is possible for a relatively homogeneous reduction in coronary vasodilator reserve to remain undetected by qualitative analysis of thallium-201 perfusion images [29], a situation that can rarely occur in patients with severe triple vessel disease. In addition, the limited resolution of conventional thallium-201 scanning means that this technique may not reliably detect subendocardial hypoperfusion. Finally, regional differences in tracer concentration secondary to factors such as the partial volume effect are more likely in hypertrophic cardiomyopathy. Thus, contrary to the situation in patients with coronary artery disease, the sensitivity and specificity of thallium-201 imaging in hypertrophic cardiomyopathy remains uncertain and requires further study.

Positron emission tomography

Positron emission tomography (PET) is theoretically superior to conventional single photon imaging in several respects, the most important of which are better resolution and the ability to quantitate myocardial blood flow. Studies using Nitrogen-13 ammonia as a flow tracer have shown that while baseline myocardial blood flow in the interventricular septum and the left ventricular free wall is similar to that of normal controls, coronary flow reserve during pharmacological coronary vasodilatation is much reduced in both hypertrophied and non-hypertrophied segments [22] (figure 3).

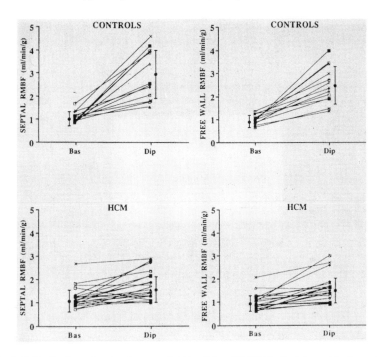

Figure 3. Individual values of regional myocardial blood flow (RMBF) in the interventricular septum and free left ventricular wall at baseline (Bas) and following dipyridamole infusion (Dip) in control subjects and patients with hypertrophic cardiomyopathy (HCM). From Camici et al. J Am Coll Cardiol 1991;17:879-86.

There are some data indicating that patients with chest pain have lower mean coronary flow reserve than patients without chest pain, although there is considerable inter-individual variation. PET has also been used to visualize subendocardial hypoperfusion across hypertrophied interventricular septa [30], and to investigate the relationship of myocardial blood flow abnormalities to myocardial metabolism using fluorine-18 labeled deoxyglucose (FDG) [31-32]. Areas of blood flow/FDG mismatch (thought to indicate the presence of ischemic myocardium) have been described at rest and during exercise in patients with hypertrophic cardiomyopathy. However, other studies have demonstrated only "matched" reductions in myocardial blood flow and FDG uptake. Therefore, further research is required before definitive conclusions on the significance of abnormal FDG uptake can be made in hypertrophic cardiomyopathy.

Myocardial lactate extraction in hypertrophic cardiomyopathy

The term myocardial ischemia is used to describe the physiological and metabolic consequences of an imbalance between myocardial blood flow and oxygen demand. Ideally, the clinical evaluation of myocardial ischemia should include an assessment of myocardial metabolism, but practical constraints dictate that most of the clinical tests used to detect myocardial ischemia use functional surrogates such as ST segment change and regional wall motion abnormality. This is not a problem when applying such tests to populations with a high prevalence of myocardial ischemia (e.g. middle aged male smokers with angina), but it is a potential confounding factor in diseases like hypertrophic cardiomyopathy in which the prevalence of myocardial ischemia is unknown. The implication of this Bayesian construct is that the sensitivity and specificity of "conventional" clinical markers of myocardial ischemia in hypertrophic cardiomyopathy should be established by the unequivocal demonstration of the metabolic consequences of ischemia in patients with the disease. Several papers have reported reduced lactate consumption in patients with hypertrophic cardiomyopathy in association with ST segment depression, reductions in coronary sinus blood flow and elevated left ventricular end-diastolic pressure [18] (figure 4). One study has also demonstrated that reversible thallium-201 perfusion defects, defined as regional perfusion abnormality and "apparent cavity dilatation", are more frequent in patients with net lactate production during rapid atrial pacing [23]. This latter observation has led to the belief that thallium-201 scans are a sensitive marker of myocardial ischemia in hypertrophic cardiomyopathy. However, careful analysis of the thallium-201 data reveals that the strongest association with lactate production was with apparent cavity dilatation rather than "regional' defects. While this interesting observation supports the hypothesis that apparent cavity dilatation is caused by subendocardial hypoperfusion, the limited ability of single photon imaging to resolve differential blood flow across the myocardium means that use of cavity dilatation as an "ischemic" marker is likely to be limited in routine clinical practice. The superior resolution of PET and other imaging techniques may in the future provide a more reliable method for detecting subendocardial flow limitation.

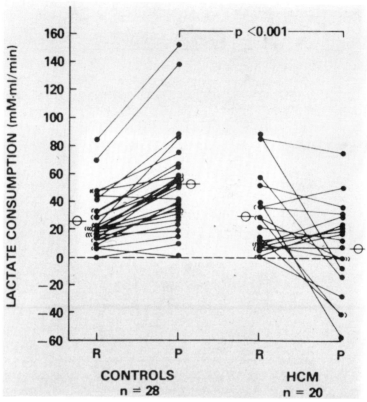

Figure 4. Individual values for lactate consumption in control subjects and in patients with hypertrophic cardiomyopathy measured at rest (R) and peak pacing (P). Patients below the dashed line have net lactate production. From Cannon et al. Circulation 1985;71:234-243.

Coronary sinus pH monitoring

In addition to the presence or absence of myocardial ischemia, coronary sinus lactate concentration is also determined by a number of factors such as substrate availability and adrenergic stimulation [33-34]. The timing of venous sampling is also critical as the maximal "washout" of acidic metabolites after a period of myocardial ischemia may occur immediately after the cessation of stress and last for only a few seconds [35-36]. A number of techniques theoretically overcome some of the short-comings of coronary sinus venous sampling; in particular the continuous monitoring of coronary sinus pH and oxygen saturation. Coronary sinus pH monitoring has been used in hypertrophic cardiomyopathy to demonstrate that chest pain following dipyridamole infusion is associated with a simultaneous fall in coronary sinus pH, confirming that pharmacological coronary vasodilatation can produce significant myocardial ischemia in patients with this disease [37] (figure 5). Although the clinical utility of this technique is currently limited by technical considerations, similar methods may provide the basis for future studies on myocardial ischemia in hypertrophic cardiomyopathy.

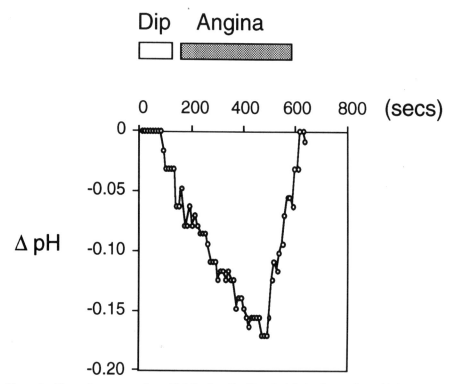

Figure 5. Change in coronary sinus pH following dipyridamole infusion in a patient with hypertrophic cardiomyopathy. From: Elliott et al. Heart 1996;75:179-183.

Significance of myocardial ischemia in hypertrophic cardiomyopathy

The evidence for myocardial ischemia in hypertrophic cardiomyopathy seems at first glance to be unequivocal, with pathological (small vessel disease, myocardial fibrosis), clinical (chest pain, ST segment change, perfusion defects), and metabolic (lactate extraction, coronary sinus pH), evidence for its existence. Unfortunately, as the preceding discussion has hopefully shown, the difficulties in detecting myocardial ischemia in individual patients have meant that its clinical significance remains uncertain. In a recent cross-sectional study of 23 young patients [38], reversible thallium-201 defects were detected in all patients with a history of cardiac arrest or syncope, supporting evidence from case reports that myocardial ischemia may be an important trigger for ventricular arrhythmia and sudden death in hypertrophic cardiomyopathy. However, a recent study from our own institution has failed to demonstrate any association between reversible perfusion defects and prognosis in young or old patients [25]. While differences in patient selection and imaging protocol may explain this disparity, it is more likely to be a reflection of the complexity of the mechanism underlying sudden death in this disease. It remains a source of constant personal fascination that the incredible mix of arrhythmogenic factors that make up the pathophysiology of hypertrophic cardiomyopathy is compatible with long periods of apparent clinical quiescence. While it is probable that myocardial ischemia is an important factor in precipitating sudden and often totally unexpected cardiac death, it is only one of several interdependent factors that ultimately result in fatal ventricular arrhythmia.

Conclusion

Although there are now sufficient clinical data indicating that myocardial ischemia occurs in patients of all ages with hypertrophic cardiomyopathy, the evidence that it plays a role in progressive left ventricular dysfunction and sudden death remains circumstantial. New imaging techniques combined with objective markers of myocardial ischemia will in the future determine the importance of myocardial ischemia in hypertrophic cardiomyopathy, and facilitate the development of more effective treatment algorithms.

References

1. Spirito P, Seidman CE, McKenna WJ, Maron BJ. The management of hypertrophic cardiomyopathy. N Engl J Med 1997;336:775-785.
2. Report of the 1995 World Health Organization/International Society and Federation of Cardiology task force on the definition and classification of cardiomyopathies. Circulation 1996;93:841-2.
3. Kimura A, Harada H, Park J-E et al. Mutations in the cardiac troponin I gene associated with hypertrophic cardiomyopathy. Nature Genetics 1997;16:379-382.
4. Watkins H, Thierfelder L, Hwang D, McKenna WJ, Seidman JG, Seidman CE. Sporadic hypertrophic cardiomyopathy due to de novo myosin mutations. J Clin Invest 1992;90:1666-71.
5. Frank S, Braunwald E. Idiopathic hypertrophic subaortic stenosis: clinical analysis of 126 patients with emphasis on the natural history, Circulation 1968;37:759-88.
6. McKenna WJ, Deanfield J, Faruqui A, England D, Oakley C and Goodwin J. Prognosis in hypertrophic cardiomyopathy. Role of age and clinical, electrocardiographic and hemodynamic features. Am J Cardiol 1981; 47: 532-8.
7. Wigle ED, Sasson Z, Henderson MA, Ruddy TD, Fulop J, Rakowski H, Williams WG. Hypertrophic cardiomyopathy: the importance of the site and extent of hypertrophy: a review. Prog Cardiovasc Dis 1985;28:1-83.
8. Gilligan DM, Chan WL, Ang EL, Oakley CM. Effects of a meal on hemodynamic function at rest and during exercise in patients with hypertrophic cardiomyopathy. J Am Coll Cardiol 1991;18:429-36.
9. O'Gorman DJ, Sheridan DJ Abnormalities of the coronary circulation associated with left ventricular hypertrophy. Clin Sci 1991;81:703-13.
10. Scheler S, Motz W, Strauer BE. Transient myocardial ischemia in hypertensives: the missing link with left ventricular hypertrophy. Eur Heart J 1992;13 (suppl D):62-65.
11. Tomanek RJ, Palmer RJ, Pfeiffer GL, Schreiber KL, Eastham CL, Marcus ML Morphometry of canine coronary arteries, arterioles and capillaries during hypertension and left ventricular hypertrophy. Circ Res 1986;58:38-46.
12. Davies MJ, McKenna WJ. Hypertrophic cardiomyopathy: pathology and pathogenesis. Histopathology 1995;26:493-500.
13. Maron BJ, Wolfson JK, Epstein SE, Roberts WC. Intramural ("small vessel") coronary artery disease in hypertrophic cardiomyopathy. J Am Coll Cardiol 1986; 8:545.
14. Tanaka M, Fujiwara H, Onodera T, Wu D, Matsuda M, Hamashima Y, Kawai C. Quantitative analysis of narrowings of intramyocardial small arteries in normal hearts, hypertensive hearts, and hearts with hypertrophic cardiomyopathy. Circulation 1987; 75: 1130-9.
15. Pichard AD, Mellor J, Teichholz LE, Lipnik S, Gorlin R, Herman MV. Septal perforation compression (narrowing) in idiopathic hypertrophic subaortic stenosis. Am J Cardiol 1977;40:310-4.

16. Brugada P, Bar FW, de Zwaan C, Green M, Wellens HJ. "Sawfish" systolic narrowing of the left anterior descending artery: an angiographic sign of hypertrophic cardiomyopathy. Circulation 1982;66:800-3.

17. Akasaka T, Yoshikawa J, Yoshida K, Maeda K, Takagi T, Miyake S. Phasic coronary flow characteristics in patients with hypertrophic cardiomyopathy: a study by coronary doppler catheter. J Am Soc of Echocardiography 1994;7:9-19.

18. Cannon RO, Dilsizian V, O'Gara P, Udelson JE, Schenke WH, Quyyumi A, Fananapazir L, Bonow RO. Myocardial metabolic, hemodynamic, and electrocardiographic significance of reversible thallium-201 abnormalities in hypertrophic cardiomyopathy. Circulation 1991;83:1660-67.

19. Elliott PM, Kaski JC, Prasad K, Seo H, Slade AK, Goldman JH, McKenna WJ. Chest pain during daily life in patients with hypertrophic cardiomyopathy: an ambulatory electrocardiographic study. Eur Heart J 1996;17:1056-1064.

20. Pasternac A, Noble J, Streulens Y, Elie R, Henschke C, Bourassa MG. Pathophysiology of chest pain in patients with cardiomyopathies and normal coronary arteriograms. Circulation 1982; 65:778.

21. Nicod P, Polikar R, Peterson KL. Hypertrophic cardiomyopathy and sudden death. N Engl J Med 1988; 318: 1255-7.

22. Camici P, Chiriatti G, Lorenzoni R, Bellina RC, Gistri R, Italiani G, Parodi O, Salvadori PA, Nista N, Papi L, L'Abbate A. Coronary vasodilatation is impaired in both hypertrophied and non hypertrophied myocardium of patients with hypertrophic cardiomyopathy: A study with Nitrogen-13 ammonia and positron emission tomography. J Am Coll Cardiol 1991;17:879-86.

23. Cannon RO, Rosing DR, Maron BJ, Leon MB, Bonow RO, Watson MD, Epstein SE. Myocardial ischemia in patients with hypertrophic cardiomyopathy: contribution of inadequate vasodilator reserve and elevated left ventricular filling pressures. Circulation 1985;71:234-437.

24. O'Gara PT, Bonow RO, Maron BJ, Damske BA, Van Lingen A, Bacharach SL, Larson SM, Epstein SE. Myocardial perfusion abnormalities in patients with hypertrophic cardiomyopathy: Assessment with thallium-201 emission computed tomography. Circulation 1987;76:1214-23.

25. Yamada M, Elliott PM, Gane J, Britten A, Kaski JC, McKenna WJ. Relation of thallium-201 perfusion abnormalities to clinical and prognostic markers in hypertrophic cardiomyopathy. Eur Heart J 1998;19: (in press).

26. Pitcher D, Wainwright R, Maisey M, Curry P, Sowton E. Assessment of chest pain in hypertrophic cardiomyopathy using exercise thallium-201 myocardial scintigraphy. Br Heart J 1980;44:650-6.

27. Rubin KA, Morrison J, Padnick MB, Binder AJ, Chiaramida S, Margouleff D, Padmanabhan VT, Gulotta SJ. Idiopathic Hypertrophic Subaortic Stenosis: Evaluation of anginal symptoms with Thallium-201 Myocardial imaging. Am J Cardiol 1979; 44: 1040-45.

28. Von Dohlen TW, Prisant LM, Frank MJ. Significance of positive or negative thallium-201 scintigraphy in hypertrophic cardiomyopathy. Am J Cardiol 1989;64:498-503.

29. Maddahi J, Abdulla A, Garia EV, Swan HJC, Berman DS. Noninvasive identification of left main and triple vessel coronary artery disease: Improved accuracy using quantitative analysis of regional myocardial stress distribution and washout of thallium-201. J Am Coll Cardiol 1986;7:53-56.

30. Camici P, Cecchi F, Gistri R, Montereggi A, Salvadori PA, Dolara A, L'Abbate A. Dipyridamole-induced subendocardial underperfusion in hypertrophic cardiomyopathy assessed by positron-emission tomography. Coronary Artery Disease 1991;2:837-41.

31. Nienaber CA, Gambhir SS, Mody FV et al. Regional myocardial blood flow and glucose utilization in symptomatic patients with hypertrophic cardiomyopathy. Circulation 1993;87:1580-90.

32. Grover-McKay M, Schwaiger M, Krivokapich J, Perloff JK, Phelps ME, Schelbert HR. Regional myocardial blood flow and metabolism at rest in mildly symptomatic patients with hypertrophic cardiomyopathy. J Am Coll Cardiol 1989;13:317-24.

33. Camici P, Marraccini P, Lorenzoni R et al. Metabolic markers of stress-induced myocardial ischemia. Circulation 1991; 83(5 Suppl):III8-13.

34. Gertz EW, Wisneski JA, Neese R, Houser A, Korte R, Bristow JD. Myocardial lactate extraction: multi-determined metabolic function. Circulation 1980;61:256-6.

35. Crake T, Crean PA, Shapiro LM, Rickards AF, Poole-Wilson PA. Coronary sinus pH during percutaneous transluminal angioplasty: early development of acidosis during myocardial ischemia in man. Br Heart J 1987;58:110-15.

36. Cobbe S. M., Poole-Wilson P.A. Continuous coronary sinus and arterial pH monitoring during pacing induced ischemia in coronary artery disease. Br Heart J 1982;47:369-74.

37. Elliott PM, Rosano GMC, Gill JS, Poole-Wilson PA, Kaski JC, McKenna WJ. Changes in coronary sinus pH during dipyridamole stress in patients with hypertrophic cardiomyopathy. Heart 1996;75:179-183.
38. Dilsizian V, Bonow RO, Epstein SE, Fananapazir L. Myocardial ischemia detected by thallium scintigraphy is frequently related to cardiac arrest and syncope in young patients with hypertrophic cardiomyopathy. J Am Coll Cardiol 1993;22:796-804.

Chapter 28

MICROVASCULAR ENDOTHELIAL DYSFUNCTION AFTER HEART TRANSPLANTATION

Giuseppe Vassalli and Augusto Gallino

The development of graft coronary artery disease is one of the most discouraging aspects in heart transplantation [1-4]. It is the third leading cause of death (after infection and allograft rejection) in the first year after transplantation, and the first leading cause of death in the subsequent years. Graft vasculopathy is manifested by a unique and unusually accelerated form of coronary artery disease which, in contrast to naturally occurring atherosclerosis, affects the whole length of the coronary vessels, including the small intramural branches [5,6]. Coronary lesions are detected angiographically in 50 percent of patients 5 years after transplantation [5], and intimal thickening can be detected by intravascular ultrasound imaging in a majority of patients with normal coronary angiograms [7,8]. Virtually all 5 year heart transplant survivors have histological evidence of coronary artery disease [6].

Coronary dysfunction as an early manifestation of graft vasculopathy has been observed in a significant proportion of cardiac transplant recipients even in the absence of coronary lesions. Together with a number of hemodynamic and structural factors, coronary dysfunction leads to a decrease in coronary flow reserve, which eventually results in myocardial ischemia during exercise. While myocardial ischemia can be manifested by exertional dyspnea or arrhythmia, anginal chest pain is rare because of the denervation of the cardiac allograft.

The present paper reviews recent advances in the understanding of the pathophysiological role of coronary dysfunction in cardiac transplant recipients. Recent reports on coronary flow reserve abnormalities after heart transplantation are discussed.

Epicardial coronary dysfunction in cardiac transplant recipients

Coronary artery dysfunction usually presents as a reduced vasodilator response or paradoxical constriction of epicardial coronary arteries in response to the administration of acetylcholine [9-14]. These abnormalities are potentially reversible even in vessels with intimal thickening [7], probably reflecting the episodic occurrence of endothelial injury. Coronary vasodilation in response to acetylcholine can be impaired as early as a few weeks after transplantation, even when flow-mediated vasodilation is normal [14]. Early coronary dysfunction resolves over the subsequent months in a majority of patients [15], suggesting that it might be due to an ischemic insult occurring around the time of transplantation. Although early coronary dysfunction is associated with an increased incidence of intimal thickening at 1 year posttransplantation [16], its predictive value for the subsequent development of graft vasculopathy is low [15,17].

The vasomotor response of epicardial coronary arteries to other vasodilator stimuli including substance P [18], cold pressor test [19], dynamic exercise [20] and increased blood flow [21] is also impaired in a substantial proportion of transplanted patients. However, flow-mediated vasodilation after intracoronary papaverine administration [21] or during tachycardic atrial pacing is maintained in patients with normal coronary angiograms [22].

The onset of coronary dysfunction after heart transplantation is related to the vasomotor stimulus used to detect it. Acetylcholine-induced vasodilation can be impaired very early after transplantation [15-17], whereas an abnormal response to substance P [18], cold [19] and dynamic exercise [20] is usually seen only one or more years after transplantation. A similar temporal pattern of coronary dysfunction in response to various stimuli has been described in nontransplanted patients with coronary arteriosclerosis [23], suggesting that the impairment of muscarinic acetylcholine-mediated vasorelaxation emerges early and selectively after endothelial injury.

Unlike acetylcholine, substance P, cold and dynamic exercise, which rely on a functionally intact endothelium to exert their vasodilator effect via the release of nitric oxide [24], the vasomotor effect of nitroglycerin, adenosine and dipyridamole, which is largely endothelium-independent, is intact in transplanted patients [13,20,21]. The selective impairment of endothelium-dependent vasodilation suggests that endothelial injury of epicardial coronary vessels occurs in cardiac transplant recipients.

Pathogenesis of graft endothelial dysfunction

The pathogenesis of graft endothelial dysfunction involves both transplantation-specific factors and generic vascular risk factors [1-4,25,26]. The simple observation that while transplanted vessels develop atherosclerotic changes, the host's native arteries are spared, suggested that immune-mediated mechanisms play a crucial role in the development of graft vasculopathy. This is supported by recent experimental data indicating that the induction of tolerance is able to prevent graft vasculopathy [27].

Coronary endothelium expresses both alloantigens that are recognized by circulating immune competent cells and, upon activation, adhesion molecules that facilitate cell binding to the endothelial surface [28]. Endothelial activation can be induced by a number of noxious factors including ischemia-reperfusion [29,30], the immune response to the allograft [31-36], cytomegalovirus infection [37,38], cyclosporine treatment [39,40], hyperlipidemia, insulin resistance, and hypertension [41,42].

The participation of specific inflammatory cell types in the genesis of graft vasculopathy was investigated in a mouse model in which carotid arteries were transplanted across multiple histocompatibility barriers into several mutant strains with selective immunological defects [34]. This approach revealed that an acquired immune response with the participation of CD4+ (helper) T cells, antibodies and macrophages is essential to the development of graft atherosclerosis. Donor-specific cytokine production by graft-infiltrating lymphocytes also induces and maintains graft vasculopathy in human cardiac allografts [35]. These findings are consistent with histopathological data from a retransplantation model showing that graft atherosclerosis begins in the early postoperative phase and progresses even in the absence of a continuous allogenic immunological drive [36].

Three factors determine the severity of coronary lumen narrowing in graft vasculopathy: immune-mediated intimal thickening, donor-transmitted lesions, and vascular remodeling. If donor disease is present at baseline, intimal thickening occurs in an eccentric manner with superimposition onto donor-transmitted lesions during the first year after transplantation, suggesting that these lesions may serve as a nidus for intimal thickening [43]. Although *de novo* lesions progress more rapidly than donor-transmitted arteriosclerosis, lesion severity is greater in patients with donor-transmitted disease 3 years after transplantation [44]. Moreover, vessels with donor arteriosclerosis do not undergo compensatory enlargement following intimal thickening [43]. Reports on vascular remodeling in graft vasculopathy are discordant, however. According to one study, one third of the increase in intimal area can be compensated by adventitial enlargement in the first year after transplantation [45]. In contrast, another study showed constrictive remodeling in vessels with intimal thickening in the first year after transplantation, with further constrictive remodeling with no increase in intimal lesions over the subsequent two years [46].

Graft microvascular dysfunction in response to physiologic stimuli

Coronary flow reserve is decreased in a substantial proportion of cardiac transplant recipients due to microvascular dysfunction and a number of hemodynamic and structural factors. These factors include tachycardia, hypertension, neurohumoral dysregulation, left ventricular hypertrophy, increased left ventricular end-diastolic pressure, epicardial coronary artery stenoses, obstructive microvascular changes, and allograft rejection. Acute rejection is associated with a marked decrease in coronary flow reserve presumably due to endothelial dysfunction, myocardial edema, and microthrombotic processes [47,48]. While coronary microvascular response to diltiazem is abolished during severe allograft rejection, nitroglycerin-induced vasodilation of epicardial coronary vessels is normal [49]. Flow reserve usually improves after successful treatment of the rejection [47].

Unlike changes in myocardial blood flow after pharmacologic vasodilation, coronary flow reserve measurements using physiologic vasodilator stimuli directly assess the ability of the coronary circulation to match an increase in myocardial oxygen demand with an increase in myocardial blood flow. Coronary flow reserve during bicycle exercise, determined by parametric imaging, is slightly decreased 3 months after transplantation, when exercise tolerance is markedly reduced, and is significantly decreased 2-6 years after transplantation, when exercise tolerance is almost normal (Figure 1) [20]. The decrease in flow reserve during exercise is significantly correlated with time after transplantation. In contrast, flow reserve measured with intracoronary papaverine as an endothelium-independent microvascular vasodilator is normal up to 6 years after transplantation. These data suggest that microvascular endothelial dysfunction is responsible, at least in part, for the decreased flow reserve during exercise. However, positron emission tomography studies with ^{13}N-ammonia [47,50-53] and ^{15}O-water [54,55] have shown an increase of myocardial blood flow at rest, which is linearly correlated to the rate-pressure product [51,56]. This appears to be a major determinant of the reduced flow reserve observed during exercise in transplanted patients [50]. Several other factors including left ventricular diastolic dysfunction [57-59], chronotropic incompetence [57], and neurohumoral dysregulation [60,61] potentially play a contributory role in the reduction of flow reserve during exercise. Left ventricular diastolic dysfunction and an abnormal volume status (resting pulmonary wedge pressure) and preload reserve (changes in left ventricular enddiastolic volume) may lead to an abnormal increase in left ventricular filling pressure during exercise. Neurohumoral dysregulation resulting from the loss of afferent neural information from cardiac mechanoreceptors leads to an exaggerated neuroendocrine response to exercise with an abnormal increase in plasma renin activity, atrial natriuretic peptide, norepinephrine and vasopressin [60,61].

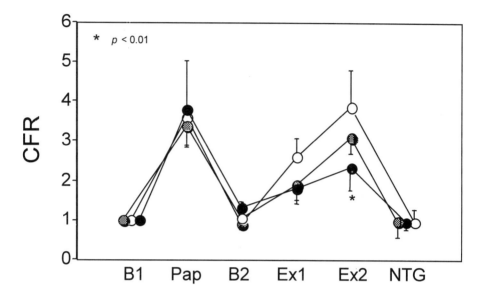

Figure 1. Decreased coronary flow reserve (CFR) during exercise in transplanted patients. CFR determined by parametric imaging after 10 mg intracoronary papaverine (Pap), at rest before the exercise (B2), during two levels of supine bicycle exercise (Ex1/2) and after 1.6 mg sublingual nitroglycerin (NTG; B1 = baseline) is shown for patients studied at 3 months (closed grey circles) and patients investigated 1-6 years after heart transplantation (closed black circles). Normal subjects are also shown (open circles). CFR during exercise is only slightly decreased (NS) early after transplantation but significantly reduced late after transplantation, whereas CFR measured with papaverine is normal at any time point (from: Vassalli G *et al. Circulation* 1997 [20]; reproduced with permission of the American Heart Association)

Both hyperemic blood flow and coronary flow reserve measured by positron emission tomography during a cold pressor test are decreased in transplanted patients [51]. In contrast, the increase in myocardial blood flow during maximal dobutamine stress is normal [52].

In summary, coronary flow reserve measured during dynamic exercise or a cold pressor test is decreased in transplanted patients due to multiple factors including an elevated blood flow at rest, microvascular endothelial dysfunction and diastolic left ventricular dysfunction.

Graft microvascular dysfunction in response to pharmacologic stimuli

Coronary flow reserve measured with acetylcholine [14,62,63] and substance P [21] is decreased in a significant proportion of transplanted patients. It is usually normal, however, when measured with endothelium-independent vasodilators such as adenosine [62,64,65] and papaverine [20,21,66]. Flow reserve determined with acetylcholine is normal 1 and 2 years after transplantation but is significantly decreased 3 years after transplantation, when flow reserve measured with adenosine is normal [62] (Figure 2). These data are consistent with graft microvascular dysfunction, which is supported by the fact that the impairment in acetylcholine-dependent flow reserve is partially normalized by L-arginine, a nitric oxide precursor [14] (Figure 3). This important observation indicates that graft endothelial dysfunction is potentially reversible, at least at an early stage. L-arginine administration has a similar effect on flow reserve in nontransplanted hypercholesterolemic patients [67].

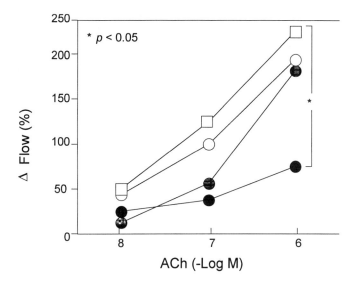

Figure 2. Abnormal coronary microvascular responses to acetylcholine in transplanted patients. Percent changes in coronary blood flow (Δ Flow) in response to serial administration of acetylcholine (ACh) in patients studied at 1 year (open circles), 2 years (closed grey circles) and 3 years after transplantation (closed black circles) and in normal subjects (open squares). Changes in coronary flow in response to acetylcholine are normal at 1 and 2 years after transplantation but reduced at 3 years. Flow responses to adenosine remain normal (modified from: Treasure CB *et al. Circulation* 1992 [62]; reproduced with permission of the American Heart Association)

Coronary flow reserve determined with dipyridamole is lower than with adenosine [65] and is slightly decreased in transplanted patients [65,68,69]. After correction for the increased myocardial blood flow at rest, however, flow reserve after dipyridamole administration is nearly normal in patients with normal coronary angiograms [47,54,55,69]. In contrast, it is decreased in vessels that exhibit a severe vasoconstriction in response to serotonin early after transplantation [68].

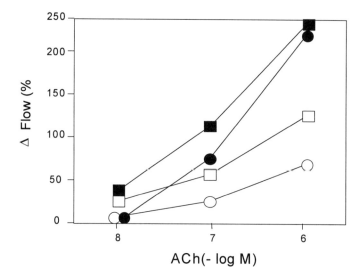

Figure 3. L-arginine administration improves coronary microvascular response to acetylcholine in transplanted patients. Percent changes in coronary blood flow (Δ Flow) in response to serial doses of acetylcholine (ACh) in transplanted patients with normal (closed symbols) or decreased coronary flow reserve (open symbols) before (circles) and after L-arginine infusion (squares). L-arginine improves the flow response to acetylcholine in patients with an impaired flow reserve (modified from: Drexler H *et al. Circulation* 1994 [14]; reproduced with permission of the American Heart Association)

Relationship between intimal thickening and coronary flow reserve

The relationship between structural changes in epicardial coronary arteries and flow reserve in transplanted patients is complex. Epicardial coronary vasodilation correlates with flow reserve after acetylcholine administration, suggesting that a common injury affects both large and small vessel endothelium [14]. An impaired coronary flow reserve is more likely to be improved by L-arginine in vessels with no intimal thickening [14]. Although the reversibility of endothelial dysfunction is related to the presence of intimal thickening, endothelial dysfunction (before L-arginine administration) is not always predicted by the degree of intimal thickening [14].

Flow reserve abnormalities during the cold pressor test are more marked in vessels with intimal thickening than in vessels with no structural changes [51]. Flow reserve as assessed by substance P [21] or dipyridamole [69] testing is normal in transplanted patients with normal coronary angiograms. When angiographic stenoses are present, regional flow reserve as assessed with dipyridamole is homogeneously reduced throughout the myocardium without a clear segmental relationship to coronary lesions. Similarly, abnormalities in left ventricular perfusion determined by Tl-201 myocardial SPECT do not correlate with the extent of intimal thickening early after transplantation, while a significant increase in the degree of scintigraphic abnormalities at 1-year post-transplantation is not accompanied by a parallel increase in coronary vessel wall alterations [70]. Flow reserve, assessed by adenosine or nitroglycerin administration, is normal in vessels with intimal thickening [71]. Histological abnormalities in small intramyocardial vessels are not correlated with intimal thickening or with endothelial dysfunction in epicardial vessels [72].

In summary, the microvascular response to acetylcholine is more often impaired in vessels with intimal thickening than in normal vessels, whereas the response to endothelium-independent vasodilators is maintained even in coronary arteries with intimal thickening.

Potential therapeutic approaches to endothelial dysfunction and graft vasculopathy

A number of strategies aiming at preventing the development of graft endothelial dysfunction and graft vasculopathy have been designed but, unfortunately, there is currently no established treatment for this disease. Potential therapeutic approaches include new immune modulatory drugs, corticosteroid-free or low-dose cyclosporine regimens, antibodies to vascular adhesion molecules, cytomegalovirus prophylaxis, vasodilators, and lipid-lowering drugs.

Rapamycin, an inhibitor of T-cell proliferation, reduced the degree of graft atherosclerosis in a clinical trial [73]. Tacrolimus (FK506) has a modulatory effect both on immune competent cells and on tissue factor expression in human monocytes/macrophages [74], which might be beneficial because coagulation is activated in graft vasculopathy [75]. The impact of a combination of FK506, mycophenolate mofetil, and prednisone on coronary flow reserve measured with acetylcholine is stronger than that of azathioprine, cyclosporine, and prednisone [76]. There are no histopathological or clinical differences between patients receiving FK506 and those on a cyclosporine-based regimen with lympholytic (ATG) induction [77]. In summary, none of the new immune modulatory agents has clearly improved on cyclosporine with regard to graft vasculopathy.

Monoclonal antibodies to vascular adhesion molecules inhibit the development of graft vasculopathy in experimental models [78,79] but their therapeutic role in the clinical setting is not yet established.

Cyclosporine-based, corticosteroid-free treatments avoid the atherogenicity of corticosteroids and are feasible in nearly 60% of transplanted patients [80-82]. Low-dose cyclosporine regimens [83] potentially attenuate the toxic effect of this drug on the endothelium [39,40]; however, a low-dose cyclosporine treatment started one year after transplantation does not appear to have any impact on coronary artery narrowing during the second and third year after transplantation [84].

Ganciclovir prophylaxis reduces the incidence of cytomegalovirus disease in transplanted patients and inhibits cytomegalovirus-enhanced atherosclerosis in an experimental model [85]. The best prophylactic effect might be achieved with a combination of ganciclovir and cytomegalovirus hyperimmune globulin [86], which seems to prevent allograft rejection through independent humoral mechanisms. However, a protective effect of gancyclovir treatment on graft vasculopathy in humans has not been demonstrated.

Oral L-arginine inhibits the development of primary atherosclerosis in experimental models [87,88] and L-arginine infusion improves the impaired graft microvascular response to acetylcholine in transplanted patients [14]. In an experimental model of severe alloimmune injury, however, oral L-arginine does not prevent intimal thickening despite a detectable enhancement of nitric oxide production [89]. Thus, there is currently no established role for L-arginine in the prophylaxis of graft vasculopathy.

Diltiazem, a calcium channel blocker, has attracted attention as a possible treatment for graft vasculopathy. A large randomized trial showed that diltiazem treatment started very early after transplantation reduces coronary artery narrowing, mortality from graft arteriosclerosis, and overall mortality in the first year after heart transplantation [90]. However, subsequent studies with smaller patient numbers have questioned the ability of a diltiazem treatment to prevent structural vascular changes, suggesting that its effect might be purely functional [91-93]. Angiotensin-converting enzyme inhibitors protect against graft vasculopathy in an experimental model [94] but their clinical value is unclear. Theoretically, vasodilator agents may have several beneficial effects including flow-mediated enhancement of nitric oxide production, vascular remodeling, and inhibition of smooth muscle cell proliferation [95].

The most significant advance in the prevention of graft vasculopathy is the use of 3-hydroxy-3-methylglutaryl coenzyme A inhibitors. These agents reduce both the incidence of coronary artery disease and overall mortality after heart transplantation [96,97]. Prospective studies have shown that pravastatin improves 1-year survival [96] and that simvastatin has a protective effect over a 4-year period [97]. Surprisingly, the effect of pravastatin on 1-year survival is independent from changes in lipid levels but is associated with a decreased incidence of severe allograft rejection, possibly reflecting a lower natural killer cell cytotoxicity [98].

In conclusion, prevention of graft coronary dysfunction and accelerated coronary artery disease in transplanted patients involves the optimal treatment of vascular risk factors, the use of corticosteroid-free regimens, the chronic administration of coenzyme A inhibitors and, possibly, of calcium channel blockers.

References

1. Billingham ME. Pathology and etiology of chronic rejection of the heart. Clin Transplant 1994;8:289-292
2. Valantine HA, Schroeder JS. Recent advances in cardiac transplantation. N Engl J Med 1995;333:660-661
3. Weis M, von Scheidt W. Cardiac allograft vasculopathy: a review. Circulation 1997;96:2069-2077
4. Vassalli G, Gallino A. Endothelial dysfunction and accelerated coronary artery disease in cardiac transplant recipients. Eur Heart J 1997;18:1712-1715
5. Gao SZ, Alderman EL, Schroeder JS, Silverman JF, Hunt SA. Accelerated coronary vascular disease in the heart transplant patient: coronary arteriographic findings. J Am Coll Cardiol 1988;12:334-340
6. Johnson DE, Gao SZ, Schroeder JS, DeCampli WM, Billingham ME. The spectrum of coronary artery pathologic findings in human cardiac allografts. J Heart Transplant 1989;8:349-359
7. Anderson TJ, Meredith IT, Uehata A, Mudge GH, Selwyn AP, Ganz P, Yeung AC. Functional significance of intimal thickening as detected by intravascular ultrasound early and late after cardiac transplantation. Circulation 1993;88:1093-1100
8. Popp RL. Intracoronary ultrasound in cardiac transplant recipients. In vivo evidence of "angiographically silent" intimal thickening. Circulation 1992;85:979-987
9. Nellessen U, Lee TC, Fischell TA, Ginsburg R, Masuyama T, Alderman EL, Schroeder JS. Effects of acetylcholine on epicardial coronary arteries after cardiac transplantation without angiographic evidence of fixed graft narrowing. Am J Cardiol 1988;62:1093-1097
10. Fish RD, Nabel EG, Selwyn AP, Ludmer PL, Mudge GH, Kirshenbaum JM, Schoen FJ, Alexander RW, Ganz P. Responses of coronary arteries of cardiac transplant patients to acetylcholine. J Clin Invest 1988;81:21-31
11. Yeung AC, Anderson T, Meredith I, Uehata A, Ryan TJ Jr, Selwyn AP, Mudge GH, Ganz P. Endothelial dysfunction in the development and detection of transplant coronary artery disease. J Heart Lung Transplant 1992;11:S69-S74
12. Nitenberg A, Benvenuti C, Aptecar E, Antony I, Deleuze P, Loisance D, Cachera JP. Acetylcholine-induced constriction of angiographically normal coronary arteries is not time dependent in transplant recipients. J Am Coll Cardiol 1993;22:151-158
13. Hartmann A, Weis M, Olbrich HG, Cieslinski G, Schacherer C, Burger W, Beyersdorf F, Schräder R. Endothelium-dependent and endothelium-independent vasomotion in large coronary arteries and in the microcirculation after cardiac transplantation. Eur Heart J 1994;15:1486-1493
14. Drexler H, Fischell TA, Pinto FJ, Chenzbraun A, Botas J, Cooke JP, Alderman EL. Effect of L-arginine on coronary endothelial function in cardiac transplant recipients: Relation to vessel wall morphology. Circulation 1994;89:1615-1623

15. Hollenberg SM, Burns DE, Klein LW, Costanzo MR, Parrillo JE, Johnson MR. Resolution of paradoxical coronary vasoconstriction at serial post-heart transplant studies. Circulation 1997;96(Suppl I):I-429 (abstr.)

16. Davis SF, Yeung AC, Meredith IT, Charbonneau F, Ganz P, Selwyn AP, Anderson TJ. Early endothelial dysfunction predicts the development of transplant coronary artery disease at 1 year posttransplant. Circulation 1996; 93:457-462

17. Aptecar E, Benvenuti C, Loisance D, Cachera JP, Nitenberg A. Early impairment of acetylcholine-induced endothelium-dependent coronary vasodilation is not predictive of secondary graft atherosclerosis. Chest 1995;107:1266-1274

18. Kushwaha SS, Bustami M, Lythall DA, Barbir M, Mitchell AG, Yacoub MH. Coronary endothelial function in cardiac transplant recipients with accelerated coronary disease. Cor Art Dis 1994;5:147-154

19. Benvenuti C, Aptecar E, Mazzucotelli JP, Loisance D, Nitenberg A. Coronary artery response to cold-pressure test is impaired early after operation in heart transplant recipients. J Am Coll Cardiol 1995;26:446-451

20. Vassalli G, Gallino A, Kiowski W, Jiang Z, Turina M, Hess OM. Reduced coronary flow reserve during exercise in heart transplant recipients. Circulation 1997;95:607-613

21. Mugge A, Heublein B, Kuhn M, Nolte C, Haverich A, Warnecke J, Forssmann WG, Lichtlen PR. Impaired coronary dilator responses to substance P and impaired flow-dependent dilator responses in heart transplant patients with graft vasculopathy. J Am Coll Cardiol 1993;21:163-170

22. Hanet C, Evrard P, Jacquet L, Goenen M, Robert A. Flow-mediated vasodilator response to tachycardia of epicardial coronary arteries is preserved in heart transplant recipients. Circulation 1993;88(Suppl II):II257-262

23. Zeiher AM, Drexler H, Wollschläger H, Just H. Modulation of coronary vasomotor tone in humans: progressive endothelial dysfunction with different early stages of coronary atherosclerosis. Circulation 1991;83:391-401

24. Berdeaux A, Ghaleh B, Dubois-Randé JL, Vigué B, Drieu La Rochelle C, Hittinger L, Giudicelli JF. Role of vascular endothelium in exercise-induced dilation of large epicardial coronary arteries in conscious dogs. Circulation 1994;89:2799-2808

25. Hosenpud JD, Shipley GD, Wagner CR. Cardiac allograft vasculopathy: Current concepts, recent developments, and future directions. J Heart Lung Transplant 1992;11:9-23

26. Libby P, Tanaka H. The pathogenesis of coronary arteriosclerosis ("chronic rejection") in transplanted hearts. Clin Transplant 1994;8:313-318

27. Orloff MS, DeMara EM, Coppage ML, Leong N, Fallon MA, Sickel J. Zuo XJ, Prehn J, Jordan SC. Prevention of chronic rejection and graft arteriosclerosis by tolerance induction. Transplantation 1995;59:282-288

28. Deng MC, Bell S, Huie P, Pinto F, Hunt SA, Stinson EB, Sibley R, Hall BM, Valantine HA. Cardiac allograft vascular disease. Relationship to microvascular cell surface markers and inflammatory cell phenotypes on endomyocardial biopsy. Circulation 1995;91:1647-1654

29. Murphy CO, Pan-Chih, Gott JP, Guyton RA. Coronary microvascular reactivity after ischemic cold storage and reperfusion. Ann Thor Surg 1997;63:20-26

30. Ibba Manneschi L, Formigli L, Tani A, Perna AM, Zecchi Orlandini S. Ultrastructural evidence of myocardial alterations in the course of heterotopic heart transplantation. J Submicrosc Cytol Pathol;1996:28:401-408

31. Salomon RN, Hughes CCW, Schoen FJ, Payne DD, Pober JS, Libby P. Human coronary transplantation-associated arteriosclerosis: evidence for a chronic immune reaction to activated graft endothelial cells. Am J Pathol 1991;138:791:798

32. Crisp SJ, Dunn MJ, Rose ML, Barbir M, Yacoub MH. Antiendothelial antibodies after heart transplantation: the accelerating factor in transplant-associated coronary artery disease? J Heart Lung Transplant 1994;13:81-91

33. Ferry BL, Welsh KI, Dunn MJ, Law D, Proctor J, Chapel H, Yacoub MH, Rose ML. Anti-cell surface endothelial antibodies in sera from cardiac and kidney transplant recipients: association with chronic rejection. Transpl Immunol 1997;5:17-24

34. Shi C, Lee W-S, He Q, Zhang D, Fletcher DL, Newell JB, Haber E. Immunologic basis of transplant-associated arteriosclerosis. Proc Natl Acad Sci USA 1996;93:4051-4056

35. van Besouw NM, Daane CR, Vaessen LM, Mochtar B, Balk AH, Weimar W. Donor specific cytokine production by graft-infiltrating lymphocytes induces and maintains graft vascular disease in human cardiac allografts. Transplantation 1997; 63:1313-1318

36. Izutani H, Miyagawa S, Shirakura R, Matsumiya G, Nakata S, Shimazaki Y, Matsuda H. Evidence that graft coronary arteriosclerosis begins in the early phase after transplantation and progresses without chronic immunoreaction. Histopathological analysis using a retransplantation model. Transplantation 1995;60:1073-1079

37. Grattan MT, Moreno-Cabral CE, Starnes VA, Oyer PE, Stinson EB, Shumway NE. Cytomegalovirus infection is associated with cardiac allograft rejection and atherosclerosis. JAMA 1989;261:3561-3566

302

38. Koskinen P, Lemstrom K, Bruning H, Daemen M, Bruggeman C, Hayry P. Cytomegalovirus infection induces vascular wall inflammation and doubles arteriosclerotic changes in rat cardiac allografts. Transplant Proc 1995;27:574-575

39. Bossaller C, Förstermann U, Hertel R, Olbricht C, Reschke V, Fleck E. Cyclosporin A inhibits endothelium-dependent vasodilatation and vascular prostacyclin production. Eur J Pharmacol 1989;165:165-169

40. Sudhir K, MacGregor JS, DeMarco T, Gupta M, Yock PG, Chatterjee K. Cyclosporin impairs release of endothelium-derived relaxing factors in epicardial and resistance coronary arteries. Circulation 1994;90:3018-3023

41. Vassalli G, Bracht C, Gallino A, Kiowski W, Turina M, Hess OM. Coronary vasomotion and flow reserve after heart transplantation. In: Annual Cardiac Surgery 1995, 8th Ed; ed.: Morton M, International Thomson Company, London 1995

42. Valantine HA. Role of lipids in allograft vascular disease: a multicenter study of intimal thickening detected by intravascular ultrasound. J Heart Lung Transplant 1995;14:S234-S237

43. Ziada KM, Kapadia SR, Crowe TD, Binak E, Motwani JG, Young JB, Nissen SE, Murat Tuzcu E. Three year ultrasound follow-up of donor transmitted coronary atherosclerosis in transplant recipients. Circulation 1997;96(Suppl I):I-65 (abstr.)

44. Wong C-K, Ganz P, Kobashigawa JA, Miller LW, Valantine-von Kaeppler HA, Ventura HO, Yeung HO, Yeung AC. Donor coronary disease serves as a nidus for intimal thickening and prevents adequate remodeling during the first year after transplant: a multicenter transplant intravascular ultrasound study. Circulation 1997,96(Suppl I):I-429 (abstr.)

45. Rieber J, Klauss V, Henneke KH, Kanig A, Spes CH, Sinzker H, Werner F, Meiser BM, Ackermann K, Angermann CE, Mudra H. Time dependent pattern of coronary artery remodeling in cardiac allograft vasculopathy: serial assessment by intravascular ultrasound. Circulation 1997;96(Suppl I):I-510 (abstr.)

46. Wener LS, Johnson JA, Tobis JM, Einhorn K, Inglish JA, Cassem JD, Currier JW, Koshigawa JA. Longitudinal remodeling in coronary arteries after heart transplantation. Circulation 1997;96(Suppl I):I-429 (abstr.)

47. Chan SY, Kobashigawa J, Stevenson LW, Brownfield E, Brunken RC, Schelbert HR. Myocardial blood flow at rest and during pharmacological vasodilation in cardiac transplants during and after successful treatment of rejection. Circulation 1994;90:204-212

48. Perrault LP, Bidouard JP, Janiak P, Villeneuve N, Bruneval P, Vilaine JP, Vanhoutte PM. Time course of coronary endothelial dysfunction in acute untreated rejection after heterotopic heart transplantation. J Heart Lung Transplant 1997;16:643-657

49. Dumont L. Experimental evidence that rejection, but not transplantation, modulates coronary reactivity to direct and indirect vasodilation. Can J Cardiol 1994;10:460-466

50. Krivokapich J, Stevenson L, Kobashigawa J, Huang S, Schelbert H. Quantification of absolute myocardial perfusion at rest and during exercise with positron emission tomography after human cardiac transplantation. J Am Coll Cardiol 1991;18:512-517

51. Kofoed KF, Czernin J, Johnson J, Kobashigawa J, Phelps ME, Laks H, Schelbert HR. Effects of cardiac allograft vasculopathy on myocardial blood flow, vasodilatory capacity, and coronary vasomotion. Circulation 1997;95:600-606

52. Rodney RA, Mancini DM, Lin J-W, Chou R-L, Bergmann SR, Cannon PJ. Myocardial blood flow response to maximal dobutamine stress in cardiac transplant patients. Circulation 1997;96(Suppl I):I-537 (abstr.)

53. Zhao XM, Delbeke D, Sandler MP, Yeoh TK, Votaw JR, Frist WH. Nitrogen-13-ammonia and PET to detect allograft coronary artery disease after heart transplantation: comparison with coronary angiography. J Nucl Med 1995;36:982-987

54. Rechavia E, Araujo L, De Silva E, Kushwaha S, Lammertsma A, Jones T, Mitchell A, Maseri A, Yacoub M. Dipyridamole vasodilator response after human orthotopic heart transplantation: quantification by oxygen-15-labeled water and positron emission tomography. J Am Coll Cardiol 1992;19:100-106

55. Senneff MJ, Hartman J, Sobel BE, Geltman EM, Bergmann SR. Persistence of coronary vasodilator responsivity after cardiac transplantation. Am J Cardiol 1993;71:333-338

56. Krivokapich J, Smith GT, Huang SC, Hoffman EJ, Ratib O, Phelps ME, Schelbert HR. ^{13}N-ammonia myocardial imaging at rest and with exercise in normal volunteers: quantification of absolute myocardial perfusion with dynamic positron emission tomography. Circulation 1989;80:1328-1337

57. Rudas L, Pflugfelder PW, Kostuk WJ. Comparison of hemodynamic responses during dynamic exercise in the upright and supine postures after orthotopic cardiac transplantation. J Am Coll Cardiol 1990;16:1367-1373

58. Paulus WJ, Bronzwaer JGF, Felice H, Kishan N, Wellens F. Deficient acceleration of left ventricular relaxation during exercise after heart transplantation. Circulation 1992;86:1175-1185

59. Kao AC, Van Trigt P 3rd, Shaeffer-McCall GS, Shaw JP, Kuzil BB, Page RD, Higginbotham MB. Allograft diastolic dysfunction and chronotropic incompetence limit cardiac output response to exercise two to six years after heart transplantation. J Heart Lung Transplant 1995;14:11-22

60. Braith RW, Wood CE, Limacher MC, Pollock ML, Lowenthal DT, Phillips MI, Staples ED. Abnormal neuroendocrine responses during exercise in heart transplant recipients. Circulation 1992;86:1453-1463

61. Masters RG, Davies RA, Keon WJ, Walley VM, Koshal A, de Bold AJ. Neuroendocrine response to cardiac transplantation. Can J Cardiol 1993;9:609-617

62. Treasure CB, Vita JA, Ganz P, Ryan TJ, Schoen FJ, Vekshtein VI, Yeung AC, Mudge GH, Alexander RW, Selwyn AP, Fish RD. Loss of coronary microvascular response to acetylcholine in cardiac transplant patients. Circulation 1992;86:1156-1164

63. Mills RM Jr., Billett JM, Nichols WW. Endothelial dysfunction early after heart transplantation: Assessment with intravascular ultrasound and Doppler. Circulation 1992;86:1171-1174

64. Kern MJ, Bach RG, Mechem CJ, Caracciolo EA, Aguirre FV, Miller LW, Donohue TJ. Variations in normal coronary vasodilatory reserve stratified by artery, gender, heart transplantation and coronary artery disease. J Am Coll Cardiol 1996;28:1154-1160

65. Chou TM, Sudhir K, Amidon TM, Klinski CS, DeMarco T, Chatterjee K, Botvinick EH. Comparison of adenosine to dipyridamole in degree of coronary hyperemic response in heart transplant recipients. Am J Cardiol 1996;78:908-913

66. McGinn AL, Wilson RF, Olivari MT, Homans DC, White CW. Coronary vasodilator reserve after human orthotopic cardiac transplantation. Circulation 1988;78:1200-1209

67. Drexler H, Zeiher AM, Meinzer K, Just H. Correction of endothelial dysfunction in coronary microcirculation of hypercholesterolemic patients by L-arginine. Lancet 1991;1546-1550

68. Preumont N, Lenaers A, Goldman S, Vachiery JL, Wikler D, Damhaut P, Degre S, Berkenboom G. Coronary vasomotility and myocardial blood flow early after heart transplantation. Am J Cardiol 1996;78:550-554

69. Wolpers HG, Koster C, Burchert W, van den Hoff J, Schafers HJ, Wahlers T, Meyer GJ. Koronarreserve nach orthotoper Herztransplantation: Quantifizierung mit N-13-Ammoniak und der Positronenemissionstomographie. Zeitschrift Kardiol 1995;84:112-120

70. Kerber S, Puschkas C, Jonas M, Janssen F, Heinemann-Vechtel O, Kosch M, Deng MC, Schober O, Scheld HH, Breithardt G. Can Tl-201 myocardial SPECT abnormalities in orthotopic heart recipients be explained by coronary vessel wall alterations assessed by intravascular ultrasound? Int J Cardiol 1996;57:91-96

71. Caracciolo EA, Wolford TL, Underwood RD, Donohue TJ, Bach RG, Miller LW, Kern MJ. Influence of intimal thickening on coronary blood flow responses in orthotopic heart transplant recipients. A combined intravascular Doppler and ultrasound imaging study. Circulation 1995;92:II182-II190

72. Clausell N, Butany J, Molossi S, Lonn E, Gladstone P, Rabinovitch M, Daly PA. Abnormalities in intramyocardial arteries detected in cardiac transplant biopsy specimens and lack of correlation with abnormal intracoronary ultrasound or endothelial dysfunction in large epicardial coronary arteries. J Am Coll Cardiol 1995;26:110-119

73. Goggins WC, Fisher RA, Cohen DS, Tawes JW, Grimes MM. Effect of single-dose rapamycin-based immunosuppression on the development of cardiac allograft vasculopathy. J Heart Lung Transplant 1996;15:790-795

74. Fuji S, Marutuka K, Sakamoto T. Tacrolimus hydrate FK-506 modulates expression of tissue factor in human monocyte/macrophage cell line: implication for cardiac transplant atherosclerosis. Circulation 1997;96(Suppl I):I-559 (abstr.)

75. Labarrere CA, Nelson DR, Pitts DD, Faulk WP. Endothelial activation, fibrin deposition and depletion of antithrombin and tissue plasminogen activator in arterioles with myocardial biopsies associated with development of transplant-induced coronary artery disease and graft failure. Circulation 1997;96(Suppl I):I-65 (abstr.)

76. Weis M, Wildhirt SM, Meiser BM, Schulze C, Uberfuhr P, von Scheidt W. Impact of immunosuppressive therapy on coronary endothelial function. Circulation 1997;96(Suppl I):I-510 (abstr.)

77. Tsamandas AC, Pham SM, Seaberg EC, Pappo O, Kormos RL, Kawai A, Griffith BP, Zeevi A, Duquesnoy R, Fung JJ, Starzl TE, Demetris AJ. Adult heart transplantation under tacrolimus (FK506) immunosuppression: histopathologic observations and comparison to a cyclosporine-based regimen with lympholytic (ATG) induction. J Heart Lung Transplant 1997;16:723-734

78. Akimoto H, Dalesandro J, McDonald TO, Thomas R, Rothnie CL, Allen MD. Antibody to VLA-4 reduces graft arteriopathy in rabbit carotid transplants. Circulation. 1995;92:Suppl I:I-497 (abstr.)

79. Brandt M, Steinmann J, Steinhoff G, Haverich A. Treatment with monoclonal antibodies to ICAM-1 and LFA-1 in rat heart allograft rejection. Transplant Internat 1997;10:141-144

80. Keogh A, Macdonald P, Harvison A, Richens D, Mundy J, Spratt P. Initial steroid-free versus steroid-based maintenance therapy and steroid withdrawal after heart transplantation: two views of the steroid question. J Heart Lung Transplant. 1992;11:421-427

81. Livi U, Luciani GB, Boffa GM, Faggian G, Bortolotti U, Thiene G, Mazzucco A. Clinical results of steroid-free induction immunosuppression after heart transplantation. Ann Thor Surg 1993; 55:1160-1165

82. Seydoux C, Berguer DG, Stumpe F, Hurni M, Ruchat P, Fischer A, Muller X, Sadeghi H, Goy JJ. Does early steroid withdrawal influence rejection and infection episodes during the first 2 years after heart transplantation? Transplant Proc 1997;29:620-624

83. Hausen B, Demertzis S, Rohde R, Albes JM, Schafers HJ, Borst HG. Low-dose cyclosporine therapy in triple-drug immunosuppression for heart transplant recipients. Ann Thor Surg 1994;58:999-1004

84. Vassalli G, Kaski JC, Tousoulis D, Kiowski W, Follath F, Turina M, Gallino A. Low-dose cyclosporine treatment fails to prevent coronary luminal narrowing after heart transplantation. J Heart Lung Transplant 1996;15:612-619

85. Lemstroem KB, Bruning JH, Bruggeman CA, Koskinen PK, Aho PT, Yilmaz S, Lautenschlager IT, Haeyry PJ. Cytomegalovirus infection-enhanced allograft arteriosclerosis is prevented by DHPG prophylaxis in the rat. Circulation. 1994;90:1969-1978

86. Valantine HA. Prevention treatment of cytomegalovirus (CMV) disease in thoracic organ transplant patients: evidence for a beneficial effect of hyperimmune globuline. Transplant Proc 1995;27(Suppl I):49-57

87. Taguchi J, Abe J, Okazaki H, Takuwa Y, Kurokawa K. L-Arginine inhibits neointimal formation following balloon injury. Life Sci 1993;53:PL387-392

88. Cooke JP, Singer AH, Tsao P, Zera P, Rowan RA, Billingham ME. Antiatherogenic effects of L-arginine in the hypercholesterolemic rabbit. J Clin Invest 1992;90:1168-117287

89. Gregory CR, Cooke JP, Patz JD, Berryman ER, Shorthouse R, Morris RE. Enhanced nitric oxide production induced by the administration of L-arginine does not inhibit arterial neointimal formation after overwhelming alloimmune injury. J Heart Lung Transplant 1996;15:58-66

90. Schroeder JS, Gao SZ, Alderman EL, Hunt SA, Johnstone I, Boothroyd DB, Wiederhold V, Stinson EB. A preliminary study of diltiazem in the prevention of coronary artery disease in heart-transplant recipients. New Engl J Med 1993; 328:164-170

91. Takami H, Backer CL, Crawford SE, Pahl E, Mavroudis C. Diltiazem preserves direct vasodilator response but fails to suppress intimal proliferation in rat allograft coronary artery disease. J Heart Lung Transplant 1996;15:67-77

92. Julius BK, Vassalli G, Sütsch G, Turina M, Kiowski W, Hess OM. Diltiazem in the prevention of graft atheromatosis. Circulation 1996;95(Suppl I):I-648 (abstr.)

93. Julius BK, Attenhofer CH, Sütsch G, Turina MI, Hess OM, Kiowski W. Diltiazem in the prevention of coronary graft atheromatosis: an intravascular ultrasound study. Circulation 1997;96(Suppl I):I-430 (abstr.)

94. Kobayashi J, Crawford SE, Backer CL, Zales VR, Takami H, Hsueh C, Huang L, Mavroudis C. Captopril reduces graft coronary artery disease in a rat heterotopic transplant model. Circulation 1993;88:286-290

95. Gibbons GH. Preventive treatment of graft coronary vascular disease: the potential role of vasodilator therapy. J Heart Lung Transplant 1992;11:S22-S27

96. Kobashigawa JA, Katznelson S, Laks H, Johnson JA, Yeatman L, Wang XM, Chia D, Terasaki PI, Sabad A, Cogert GA, Trosian K, Hamilton MA, Moriguchi JD, Kawata N, Hage A, Drinkwater DC, Stevenson LW. Effect of pravastatin on outcomes after cardiac transplantation. N Engl J Med 1995;333:621-627

97. Wenke K, Meiser B, Thiery J, Nagel D, von Scheidt W, Steinbeck G, Seidel D, Reichart B. Simvastatin reduces graft vessel disease and mortality after heart transplantation: a four-year randomized trial. Circulation 1997;96(Suppl I):I- (abstr.)

98. Valantine HA, Schroeder JS. HMG-CoA reductase inhibitors reduce transplant coronary artery disease and mortality: evidence for antigen-independent mechanisms? Circulation 1997;96:1370-1373

Index

a_2-receptors

abnormal adrenergic activity, 123

abnormal esophageal sensory perception, 33

abnormal pain perception, 61

abnormal redox state, 251

ACE gene, 232

ACE-inhibitors, 198

acid perfusion test, 37

adaptive LVH, 269

adenosine, 62, 119

afferent impulses, 65

algogenic substances, 63

ambulatory ECG monitoring, 6

aminophylline, 197

anaerobic glycolysis, 81

analgesic properties, 119

angina-like chest pain, 62

angiotensin II, 272

animal model, 96

anxiety disorders, 14

anxiety neurosis, 13

anxiety, 17

α-receptor blockade, 212

assessment of coronary blood flow, 161

ATP deficient states, 136

ATP, 135

autonomic nervous system, 211

autonomic overarousal, 17

barium radiology, 34

β-blockers, 195

benzodiazepines, 26

body cell mass, 146

brain evoked potentials, 64

calcium channel blockers, 196

capillary density, 244

cardiac chest pain, 2

cardiac metabolism, 84

cardiac syndrome X and microvascular angina, 1

cardiac work reserve, 159

cardio-esophageal reflex, 58

central nervous pathways, 78

chronic fatigue syndrome, 143

chronic pain, 65

chymase, 272

clinical features, 5

cognitive behavioral treatment, 24

cognitive factors, 20

concentric LVH, 270

contrast echocardiography, 163

coronary blood flow reserve, 159

coronary reserve in syndrome X, 167

coronary sinus pH, 287

coronary sinus thermodilution, 160

coronary sinus, 286

cortical activation, 61

critical closing pressure, 164

cytosolic citrate, 81

definition, 2

depression, 15

diagnostic approach, 154

diagnostic work out, 155

diffuse esophageal spasm, 37

dilated LVH, 270

diltiazem, 299

dobutamine stress, 177

Doppler catheter, 70

Doppler tip devices, 162

doxazosin, 74

dyslipidemia, 225

dysphagia, 34

echocardiography, 171

edrophonium test, 37

electrocardiographic changes, 5

electrocardiography, 283

306

endoscopy, 34
endothelial activation, 294
endothelial dysfunction, 92
endothelial function, 119
endothelins, 102, 106
esophageal balloon distension, 37
esophageal chest pain, 33
esophageal disease, 54
esophageal dysfunction, 53
esophageal manometry, 36
esophageal motility, 36
essential hypertension, 259
estradiol-17β, 115
estrogen deficiency, 115
estrogen replacement therapy, 115
estrogen replacement therapy, 200
estrogens, 115, 199
ET-1, 102
ETA, 104
ETB, 104
exercise-induced reflux, 39
extracardiac causes, 2

fatigue, 135
female prevalence, 6
fetal malnutrition, 244

ganciclovir, 299
glucose breakdown, 82
glucose uptake, 81
glycolysis, 81
glycolytic flux, 84
glycolytic metabolism, 230
graft microvascular dysfunction, 295
graft vasculopathy, 293

heart rate variability, 212
heart transplantation, 293
heterogeneity of flow, 73
hyperglycemia, 224
hyperinsulinemia, 221
hyperpolarizing factors, 91

hypertensive cardiomyopathy, 259
hypertensive hypertrophy, 273
hypertensive remodelling, 269
hypertrophic cardiomyopathy, 281
hyperuricemia, 229
hyperventilation, 17
hypochondriasis, 22
hysterectomy, 116

imipramine, 26, 198
increased cardiac sensitivity, 62
increased sympathetic activity, 211
increased sympathetic tone, 211
inert gas wash-out, 160
inflammatory disease, 251
insulin resistance, 221
ion leakage, 139
ionophores, 139
ischemia, 281
ischemic etiology, 76
ischemic myocardium, 82
isovolumic relaxation time, 178

lactate production, 84
lactate release, 69
lactate uptake, 84
lactate, 283
L-arginine, 92, 102
left ventricular function, 6
left ventricular hypertrophy (LVH), 259, 269
lifestyle, 188
linked-angina, 49, 54
lipid peroxidation, 124

management strategies, 203
menopause, 116
metabolic factors, 137
metabolic markers, 81
metabolic syndrome in women, 232
metabolic syndrome, 221
metabolism, 82
MIBG uptake, 153

MIBG, 126
microvascular dysfunction, 259
minimal coronary resistance, 165
misattribution, 20
multi-disciplinary approach, 209
myocardial blood flow, 69
myocardial glutamate uptake, 82
myocardial ischemia, 1

Na⁺-H⁺ exchange, 129
neuropeptide Y, 215
NIDDM, 221
nitrates, 196
nitric oxide, 91, 262
nociception, 61
nociceptive stimulation, 61
NPY, 215
nutcracker esophagus, 36

obesity, 223, 227
ophorectomy, 116
oral L-arginine, 299
ovarian insufficiency, 115
oxidative stress, 124
oxypurinol, 264

pain clinic, 209
panic disorder, 15
papaverine, 92
pathogenic hypotheses, 7
perception of pain, 119
perfusion defects, 136
pericardial effusion, 172
pericardial thickening, 172
perimenopausal symptoms, 116
PET neuroimaging, 77
pharmacological stress, 173
phosphofructokinase, 81
photon attenuation, 182
positron emission tomography, 69, 285
post-ischemic dysfunction, 174
potassium ion translocation, 136

potassium leakage, 124
prearteriolar dysfunction, 124
Prinzmetal's variant angina, 6
prostacyclin, 91
proto-oncogenes, 272
pseudo-angina, 1
psychiatric diagnoses, 15
psychiatric interventions, 24
psychiatric referral, 27
psychological abnormalities, 13
psychological consequences, 21
psychological factors, 19
psychological interventions, 24
psychological morbidity, 13
psychological treatment, 24

QT interval, 213
QT prolongation, 213
quality of life questionnaire, 189
quality of life, 187

radionuclide techniques, 181
rarefaction, 261
release of alanine, 82
reassurance, 20, 208
Reaven's syndrome X, 221
redox-sensitive genes, 251
regression of LVH, 276
relative wall thickness ratio, 172
remodeling, 261
replacement fibrosis, 272
resting energy expenditure, 145
risk factors, 251

silent ischemia, 77
single photon perfusion scintigraphy, 163
skeletal muscle biopsies, 137
slow flow, 182
small baby syndrome, 244
soldier's heart, 13
somatization, 22
steal, 124

strain gauge plethysmography, 262
subangiographic atheroma, 107
subspecialty referral, 208
substance P, 263
sudden death, 288
superoxide anions, 263
superoxide dismutase, 264
sympathetic denervation, 127
sympathetic drive, 211

Tc^{99} Tetrofosmin, 182
Technetium^{99}, 182
temporal summation, 64
thalamus, 61
thallium reverse redistribution, 71
thallium, 284
Thallium^{201} SPET, 182
total body potassium, 146
transesophageal echocardiography, 162
transmitral diastolic indices, 178
transmural "steal", 178
treatment of esophageal chest pain, 41

vascular endothelium, 91
vascular resistance, 260
vascular wall stress, 269

wall motion abnormalities, 174

Xenon-133, 182